Effective Risk Communication

The Role and Responsibility of Government and Nongovernment Organizations

CONTEMPORARY ISSUES IN RISK ANALYSIS

Sponsored by the Society for Risk Analysis

Volume 1 RISK EVALUATION AND MANAGEMENT
Edited by Vincent T. Covello, Joshua Menkes, and Jeryl Mumpower

Volume 2 DE MINIMIS RISK
Edited by Chris Whipple

Volume 3 CARCINOGEN RISK ASSESSMENT
Edited by Curtis C. Travis

Volume 4 EFFECTIVE RISK COMMUNICATION: The Role and Responsibility of Government and Nongovernment Organizations
Edited by Vincent T. Covello, David B. McCallum, and Maria T. Pavlova

Effective Risk Communication

The Role and Responsibility of Government and Nongovernment Organizations

Edited by

Vincent T. Covello

Center for Risk Communication
Division of Environmental Sciences
School of Public Health
Columbia University
New York, New York

David B. McCallum

The Institute for Health Policy Analysis
Georgetown University Medical Center
Washington, D.C.

and

Maria T. Pavlova

U.S. Environmental Protection Agency
New York, New York

Sponsored by
The Task Force on Environmental Cancer
and Heart and Lung Disease

Plenum Press • New York and London

Library of Congress Cataloging in Publication Data

Workshop on the Role of Government in Health Risk Communication and Public Education (1987: Washington, D.C.)

Effective risk communication: the role and responsibility of government and non-government organizations / edited by Vincent T. Covello, David B. McCallum, and Maria T. Pavlova; sponsored by the Task Force on Environmental Cancer and Heart and Lung Disease.

p. cm. —(Contemporary issues in risk analysis; v. 4)

"Proceedings of the Workshop on the Role of Government in Health Risk Communication and Public Education, held January 21-23, 1987, in Washington, D.C."—T.p. verso.

Includes bibliographies and index.

ISBN 0-306-48497-8

1. Health risk communication—Congresses. I. Covello, Vincent T. II. McCallum, David B., 1943- . III. Pavlova, Maria T. IV. Task Force on Environmental Cancer and Heart and Lung Disease (U.S.) V. Title. VI. Series.

RA423.2.W67 1987 89-30642

363.3'1—dc19 CIP

This limited facsimile edition has been issued for the purpose of keeping this title available to the scientific community.

10 9 8 7 6 5 4 3 2

Proceedings of the Workshop on the Role of Government in Health Risk Communication and Public Education, held January 21–23, 1987, in Washington, D.C.

Printed in the United States of America

Contributors

Frederick W. Allen Office of Policy Analysis, U.S. Environmental Protection Agency, Washington, D.C. 20460

Elaine Bratic Arkin The Institute for Health Policy Analysis, Georgetown University Medical Center, Washington, D.C. 20007

Michael Baram Center for Law and Technology, Boston University Law School, Boston, Massachusetts 02215

James D. Callaghan Consultant, New York, New York 10028

Caron Chess Environmental Communication Research Program, New Jersey Agricultural Experiment Station, Cook College, Rutgers University, New Brunswick, New Jersey 08903

Vincent T. Covello Center for Risk Communication, Division of Environmental Sciences, School of Public Health, Columbia University, New York, New York 10032

Christopher J. Daggett New Jersey Department of Environmental Protection, Trenton, New Jersey 08625

Baruch Fischhoff Department of Engineering and Public Policy, Carnegie-Mellon University, Pittsburgh, Pennsylvania 15213

Allan D. Franks State of Ohio Environmental Protection Agency, Columbus, Ohio 43266-1049

Peter D. Galbraith Connecticut Department of Health Services, Hartford, Connecticut 06106

Billie Jo Hance Environmental Communication Research Program, New Jersey Agricultural Experiment Station, Cook College, Rutgers University, New Brunswick, New Jersey 08903

Dale Hattis Center for Technology, Policy and Industrial Development, Massachusetts Institute of Technology, Cambridge, Massachusetts 02139

Barry L. Johnson Agency for Toxic Substances and Disease Registry, Public Health Service, Atlanta, Georgia 30333

Roger E. Kasperson Center for Technology, Environment, and Development, Clark University, Worcester, Massachusetts 01610

James R. Marshall Office of External Programs, U.S. Environmental Protection Agency, Region II, New York, New York 10278

James O. Mason Centers for Disease Control, Atlanta, Georgia 30333

David B. McCallum The Institute for Health Policy Analysis, Georgetown University Medical Center, Washington, D.C. 20007

Raymond R. Neutra California State Department of Health Services, Berkeley, California 94704

Ingar Palmlund Center for Technology, Environment, and Development, Clark University, Worcester, Massachusetts 01610

Maria Pavlova U.S. Environmental Protection Agency, Region II, New York, New York 10278

Peter M. Sandman Environmental Communication Research Program, New Jersey Agricultural Experiment Station, Cook College, Rutgers University, New Brunswick, New Jersey 08903

Robert J. Scheuplein Office of Toxicological Sciences, U.S. Food and Drug Administration, Washington, D.C. 20204

Paul A. Schulte National Institute for Occupational Safety and Health, Cincinnati, Ohio 45226

Paul Slovic Decision Research, Inc., Eugene, Oregon 97401

Arthur C. Upton New York University Medical Center, New York, New York 10016

Thomas Wilson Elkhart County Solid Waste Disposal, Elkhart, Indiana 46517

Alvin L. Young Office of Agricultural Biotechnology, U.S.D.A., Washington, D.C. 20250

Foreword

One of the greatest challenges facing those concerned with health and environmental risks is how to carry on a useful public dialogue on these subjects. In a democracy, it is the public that ultimately makes the key decisions on how these risks will be controlled. The stakes are too high for us not to do our very best.

The importance of this subject is what led the Task Force on Environmental Cancer and Heart and Lung Disease to establish an Interagency Group on Public Education and Communication. This volume captures the essence of the "Workshop on the Role of Government in Health Risk Communication and Public Education" held in January 1987. It also includes some valuable appendixes with practical guides to risk communication. As such, it is an important building block in the effort to improve our collective ability to carry on this critical public dialogue.

Lee M. Thomas
Administrator, U.S. Environmental Protection Agency,
and Chairman, The Task Force on Environmental
Cancer and Heart and Lung Disease

Preface

The Task Force on Environmental Cancer and Heart and Lung Disease is an interagency group established by the Clean Air Act Amendments of 1977 (P.L. 95-95). Congress mandated the Task Force to recommend research to determine the relationship between environmental pollutants and human disease and to recommend research aimed at reducing the incidence of environment-related disease. The Task Force's Project Group on Public Education and Communication focuses on education as a means of reducing or preventing disease.

The Project Group, chaired by Dr. Maria Pavlova of the U.S. Environmental Protection Agency, sponsored a workshop to explore existing federal risk communication activities, identify gaps in research and practice that need to be addressed, and develop effective strategies for interprogram and interagency cooperation in risk communication activities. The workshop, held in Alexandria, Virginia, on January 21–23, 1987, involved government policy-makers, program administrators, and public health professionals from federal, state, and local governments, as well as experts in risk communication from the academic community, citizen and environmental groups, media, business, and industry.

This report was compiled and edited by Dr. Vincent Covello of the Center for Risk Communication at Columbia University, Dr. David McCallum of the Institute for Health Policy Analysis at the Georgetown University Medical Center, and Dr. Pavlova. The views expressed are those of the individual authors and should not be construed as representing any official agency position.

The support of Dr. Scott Baker (U.S. Environmental Protection Agency and Chairperson of the Working Group of the Task Force on Environmental Cancer and Heart and Lung Disease) is recognized, and the expert assistance of Ms. Joanna Fringer, Ms. Kay Marshall, and Ms. Dori Steele (Technical Resources, Inc.) in the preparation of the manuscript is gratefully acknowledged.

Vincent T. Covello
David B. McCallum
Maria T. Pavlova

Contents

I

Overview

1

Principles and Guidelines for Improving Risk Communication

Vincent T. Covello, David B. McCallum, and Maria Pavlova

> If we think [the people] are not enlightened enough to exercise their control with a wholesome discretion, the remedy is not to take it from them, but to inform their discretion. (Thomas Jefferson, as quoted by William Ruckelshaus, 1983, p. 1027)

INTRODUCTION

In response to rising public concerns about health and environmental risks, government agencies have increasingly sought improved means for communicating risk information to individual citizens and public groups. Part of this increased interest in risk communication stems from current difficulties and frustrations (Ruckelshaus, 1983, 1987; Sandman, 1986; Thomas, 1987; Press, 1987; Covello and Allen, 1988; Slovic, 1987; Davies et al., 1987). Government officials are often frustrated by what they perceive to be inaccurate public perceptions of risk and unrealistic demands by the public for risk reduction. Citizens are often equally frustrated by the government's seeming disinterest in their concerns, unwillingness to take action, and reluctance or unwillingness to allow them to participate in decisions that intimately affect their lives.

Given the potential value of improved risk communication for addressing these problems, the Task Force on Environmental Cancer and Heart and Lung Disease (an inter-

The views expressed in this paper are solely those of the authors and do not necessarily represent the views of their agencies or organizations.

Vincent T. Covello • Center for Risk Communication, Division of Environmental Sciences, School of Public Health, Columbia University, New York, New York 10032. *David B. McCallum* • The Institute for Health Policy Analysis, Georgetown University Medical Center, Washington, D. C. 20007. *Maria Pavlova* • U. S. Environmental Protection Agency, Region II, New York, New York 10278.

agency group established by Congress in 1977 and chaired by the Environmental Protection Agency) sponsored a conference in January 1987 on the "Role of Government in Health Risk Communication and Public Education." The role of nongovernment organizations also was addressed. The conference had five major objectives: (1) to survey existing risk communication activities in the federal government; (2) to identify gaps in research and practice; (3) to examine organizational and institutional barriers to effective risk communication; (4) to foster greater understanding of risk communication objectives and approaches; and (5) to develop means for improving cooperation, collaboration, and coordination among federal agencies.

Conference participants included representatives from more than 14 federal agencies, as well as experts in risk communication from academia, citizen groups, the media, industry, and state and local government. Participants discussed a variety of risk communication issues, including methods to improve specific risk communication skills as well as fundamental issues of trust, credibility, and social responsibility. A basic point of discussion and debate was that improved risk communication can help agencies:

1. Reduce the likelihood that societal attention and resources will be diverted from important problems to less important problems.
2. Reduce the likelihood that individual and public attention will be diverted from significant risks to insignificant risks.
3. Reduce unnecessary human suffering due to high levels of anxiety, fear, outrage, and worry about risks.
4. Reduce levels of public outrage.
5. Reduce the likelihood of bitter and protracted debates and conflicts about risks.
6. Reduce unwarranted tension between communities and agencies.
7. Better understand public perceptions, needs, and concerns.
8. Better anticipate public responses to agency actions.
9. Better inform individuals and communities about important risks.
10. Better engage in dialogue with communities about risk issues.
11. Better inform individuals and communities about agency procedures, processes, and decisions.
12. Make more informed risk management decisions.

All of the participants agreed on the need for improved risk communication by government agencies; however, participants disagreed on the principal causes of risk communication problems. Some participants believed that risk communication problems arise primarily from the information sources (e.g., limitations of risk communicators and risk experts), while others believed that risk communication problems arise primarily from message design (e.g., limitations of scientific risk assessments), the delivery channel (e.g., limitations in the media or means by which risk information is transmitted), or the target audience (e.g., characteristics of the intended recipients of risk communications).

Despite disagreements on the origins of these problems, participants agreed that most risk communication programs lack clear objectives (i.e., informing people about risks, motivating individual action, stimulating emergency response, or contributing to the dispute resolution process). This shortcoming has contributed to a lack of clear guidelines for effective risk communication as well as a lack of clear standards and measures for evaluating risk communication programs.

After several days of analysis and discussion of issues, case studies, and commissioned papers, participants developed a broad and diverse set of risk communication principles and guidelines. Participants recognized, however, that many of these principles and guidelines are based on experience and observation, not on systematic research. Although research that bears on risk communication has been conducted, the number of studies specifically focused on risk communication is small. To date, little effort has been spent on developing or exploiting contributions from the relevant disciplines, on evaluating programs, or on examining the ethical and legal implications of government risk communication activities.

Because of the diverse goals and objectives of government risk communication programs, participants emphasized that only principles and guidelines—not rigid rules—could be developed at this time. Conference participants also recognized that some of the principles and guidelines may appear contradictory, such as the recommendations that government officials speak with one voice but also be open, frank, and honest. Many such tensions were noted during the conference but were partially resolved by agreement on three overriding principles.

First, citizens in a democracy have the right to participate in decisions that affect their lives, their property, and the things they value. Second, the goal of risk communication in a democracy should be to produce an informed public that is involved, solution-oriented, and collaborative; it should not be to diffuse public concerns or replace action. Third, risk communication is a two-way activity based on mutual respect, trust, and the open exchange of information. It is fundamentally these principles that distinguish risk communication efforts by government agencies from public relations efforts or attempts to manipulate public opinion.

Given the purposes of the conference, most of the discussion focused on principles and guidelines for use by government agencies. However, these principles and guidelines also apply to other organizations in the public and private sector. Although many of the principles and guidelines may seem obvious, they are continually and consistently violated in practice.

GUIDING RISK COMMUNICATION PHILOSOPHY AND ORIENTATION

Principles

1. Effective risk communication is an essential element in effective risk management.
2. Risk communication and risk management decisions are inextricably linked, but they require different expertise and resources.
3. Understanding how people perceive risks and how to communicate risk information effectively are keys to improving risk management.

4. What appears to be a simple risk management and communication problem actually may be an issue of enormous economic, social, and political complexity.
5. Interactive and participatory approaches to risk management and communication appear to offer the greatest promise of better, less controversial, and less divisive risk management decisions.
6. Critical elements in effective risk management and communication are the trust and credibility of the message source, the quality and clarity of the message design, the effectiveness and efficiency of the delivery channel, and the involvement and acceptance of the target audience.
7. Each of the participants in the risk communication process (e.g., government agencies, corporations, industry groups, unions, the media, scientists, professional organizations, public interest groups, and individual citizens) represents an important source of information about risks, risk assessment, risk management, and risk communication.
8. Government risk communication efforts often fail to address the distinctions that the public and the media consider important in judging and evaluating risks, including voluntariness, alternatives, controllability, familiarity, dread, origin (natural or manmade), benefits, fairness, catastrophic potential, and effects on economic welfare.
9. Government risk communication efforts often fail to address social, economic, and political issues and concerns that often accompany public debates about health risks, such as concerns about the effects of government actions on property values.
10. Individuals and communities have a right to know about the risks to which they are exposed and to participate in decisions that affect their lives, their property, and the things they value.
11. Risk communication is not a substitute for regulation or action.
12. Risk communicators are accountable to the public and should base their actions on principles of ethics.

Guidelines

1. Establish ongoing mechanisms and networks for sharing information among agencies about risks, risk assessment, risk management, and risk communication.
2. Coordinate government efforts aimed at increasing knowledge of risk communication processes and improving risk communication programs.
3. Establish a national agenda for risk assessment and risk communication research that identifies gaps and sets priorities.
4. Fund basic and applied risk communication research projects cooperatively.
5. Share in the planning and funding of research and demonstration programs.
6. Provide support for practical applications and social experiments in risk communication.
7. Hold regular workshops and seminars to discuss risk communication issues and experiences with representatives from industry, academia, labor unions, state

and local officials, citizen groups, and the media to (1) share information, (2) obtain a better understanding of each other's perspectives, (3) identify applied and research needs, and (4) solicit creative and innovative ideas.

8. Support the development of educational programs and materials on risk and risk assessment for children and young people.
9. Develop a government-wide code of ethics for risk communication.
10. Assign high priority to research aimed at understanding factors that enhance or diminish the effectiveness of risk communication, including basic and applied research on psychological processes (e.g., perceptions of risks and sources of risk information); sociological and political processes (e.g., community and group dynamics and processes); anthropological processes (e.g., symbolic meanings and cultural attitudes toward risks); economic processes (e.g., individual and group differences in the economic valuation of health and environmental consequences); risk comparisons (e.g., alternative formats for categorizing and comparing risks); mediation, negotiation, and public involvement processes (e.g., improved methods for identifying stakeholder values); legal issues (e.g., the legal basis for right-to-know legislation); and ethical issues (e.g., the meaning of informed consent and the societal and value implications of right-to-know legislation).

PLANNING AND EVALUATION

Planning and evaluation are generally given inadequate attention in government risk communication efforts. Only rarely are adequate resources and efforts devoted to identifying audiences, understanding problems, setting objectives, recruiting and training staff, pretesting messages, measuring success or failure, and learning from past mistakes. For a variety of internal and external reasons, rigorous and systematic evaluation activities are often neglected.

Principles

1. Risk communication efforts will be successful only if carefully planned and evaluated.
2. Planning and evaluation activities should be part of a continuous process aimed at assessing objectives and improving performance.
3. Rigorous evaluation is needed to measure success, identify program weaknesses, and improve current and future efforts.
4. Planning and evaluation activities require a substantial commitment of time, attention, and resources by top management.
5. The practical experience and knowledge of risk communication practitioners are an important yet underutilized source of information for developing and implementing risk communication programs and activities.
6. Public involvement and direct exchanges of information are another important yet

underutilized source of knowledge for identifying risk communication problems, understanding issues, and setting objectives.

7. Different risk communication goals and audiences require different risk communication strategies.
8. Training in risk communication skills can help avert or mitigate many risk communication problems.

Guidelines

1. Clearly identify and define the overall objectives of the risk communication effort, such as providing information to the public, motivating individuals to act, stimulating emergency response, or contributing to conflict resolution.
2. Clearly identify, define, and prioritize the specific interim and final objectives of the risk communication effort; without specific objectives, it is difficult to measure progress and make corrections.
3. Assign high priority to planning and evaluation efforts, including the establishment of special funding mechanisms for such activities.
4. Demonstrate your respect for the public and your sincerity by involving the public early, before important decisions are made about risk assessment activities, risk management strategies, and risk communication efforts.
5. Make it clear from the beginning how information derived from public participation activities will be used in policy decisionmaking.
6. Establish procedural safeguards to ensure that all parties with an interest or stake in the issue are involved and able to express their opinions.
7. Collate and synthesize existing knowledge on risk communication, including case studies, in a form that is readily usable by practitioners.
8. Classify and segment the different subgroups among the audience by sociodemographic characteristics (e. g., age, sex, income, occupation, education, family situation, places of residence, mobility, religion, and ethnicity), by psychological characteristics (e. g., attitudes, opinions, beliefs, values, and personality traits), and by behavioral characteristics (e. g., media exposure, membership or participation in organizations, and activity patterns).
9. Aim risk communications at specific subgroups.
10. Train staff—including technical staff—in communication skills.
11. Recruit spokespersons who are good at presentation and interaction.
12. Recognize that good risk communication is not just good communication.
13. Recognize and reward outstanding risk communication efforts by individuals and groups.
14. Pretest the risk communication messages for understandability, relevance, attention-getting ability, attractiveness, credibility, and acceptability to the target audience.
15. Carefully evaluate the interim and final results of risk communication efforts and programs.
16. Learn from past mistakes.

THE RISK COMMUNICATION PROCESS

The principles and guidelines that follow have been organized according to a model of the risk communication process that distinguishes between the message source, the message design, the delivery channel, and the target audience (Covello et al., 1986). Although conference participants found this model useful for structuring conference deliberations and for analyzing risk communication problems, participants also noted that the model could be misconstrued to imply that risk communication is a one-way activity, i.e., information flows from a source through a channel to an audience. The conference participants emphasized that effective risk communication must be understood as a two-way interactive process that is based on mutual respect and trust.

MESSAGE SOURCES

Government agencies are a major source of information on risks. In the last two decades, however, confidence and trust in government agencies as credible sources of risk information have declined. Contributing to this decline are the following perceptions: (1) regulatory agencies have been overly influenced by industry; (2) agencies are inappropriately biased in favor of promoting particular technologies; (3) agencies are not technically competent; (4) agencies have mismanaged health and environmental activities; (5) government agencies are bureaucratic, distant, cold, and uncaring; (6) government officials and experts have lied, presented half-truths, or seriously misrepresented facts in the past; and (7) government agencies, officials, and experts often disagree among themselves about important risk issues.

Principles

1. In communicating risk information, trust and credibility are a risk communicator's most precious assets.
2. The single most important problem undermining government risk communication efforts is the lack of trust and credibility.
3. Trust and credibility are difficult to obtain; once lost, they are almost impossible to regain.
4. Attention to details (e.g., dress, language used in risk communication materials, meeting location, and room arrangement) is often critical to effective risk communication.
5. Consistency within and among agencies at the federal, state, and local level is essential to effective risk communication.
6. Effective risk communication is often undermined by the failure of agencies to coordinate and consult in a timely manner; lack of coordination often results in conflicting messages and public confusion.
7. Collaborating and working with credible agencies and organizations can provide special access to target audiences, enhanced credibility for the risk communica-

tion effort, additional resources, and added expertise; it may also require large investments of time and resources, changes in the risk communication message or program, and loss of power and control.

8. Few things make risk communication more difficult than conflicts or public disagreements with other credible sources.

Guidelines

1. Devote substantial attention and resources to building trust and credibility.
2. Listen carefully to people and their concerns.
3. State your credentials; but do not ask or expect to be trusted by the public.
4. If you do not know an answer or are uncertain, say so.
5. Get back to people with answers.
6. Admit mistakes.
7. Disclose risk information as soon as possible (emphasizing any appropriate reservations about reliability), even when this means the release of uncertain or preliminary data; provide a realistic timetable for when better information will be available.
8. If in doubt, lean toward sharing more information, not less—or people may think you are hiding something.
9. Identify and candidly discuss data uncertainties, strengths, and weaknesses, including those identified by other credible sources.
10. Recognize and address the "hidden agendas," symbolic meanings, and broader social, economic, and political considerations that often accompany and complicate the task of risk communication.
11. Identify worst-case estimates as such, and cite ranges of risk estimates when appropriate.
12. Identify with the audience and avoid violations of community norms (e.g., attire and language).
13. Always try to include a discussion of risk management actions that are under way or can be taken.
14. Whenever possible, present options that give people a sense of personal control over the risk situation.
15. Tell people what you cannot do and why.
16. Promise only what you can do, and be sure that you do what you promise.
17. Closely coordinate all inter- and intraorganizational communications.
18. Transmit official communications through a single credible spokesperson or through persons specifically designated by that spokesperson.
19. Use credible intermediaries and involve them in the risk communication program.
20. Devote effort and resources to building bridges with other organizations.
21. Try to issue communications jointly with other trustworthy sources, such as credible university scientists, physicians, trusted local officials, and opinion leaders.

MESSAGE DESIGN

It is impossible to develop an effective message without detailed, in-depth knowledge and understanding of (1) characteristics of the target audience, including information about their knowledge, attitudes, perceptions, behavior, beliefs, values, needs, and concerns; and (2) characteristics of the community in which the target audience resides, including information about social networks, opinion leaders, and community dynamics. The most effective risk messages are those designed for a specific audience.

Principles

1. The design of effective risk messages is often complicated by multiple, competing objectives, including the individual's and community's "right to know," the duty and obligation to protect public health, the costs of unnecessarily alarming people, and the possible consequences of either premature or delayed action.
2. Technical language and jargon are useful as professional shorthand but can pose substantial barriers to successful risk communication with the public.
3. Risk messages should always be pretested for content, clarity, and effect.
4. The most effective risk messages are those that clarify, not simplify, complex risk information.
5. Graphs and other visual materials represent an important but underutilized means for communicating risk information.
6. Risk comparisons are a useful tool for informing and educating people about risks; however, the simplicity and intuitive appeal of risk comparisons may be deceptive.

Guidelines

1. Recognize the power of subtle changes in the way risk information is communicated; use such power and knowledge ethically and responsibly.
2. Recognize, respect, identify, and address people's values, preferences, and concerns.
3. Use simple, nontechnical language.
4. Use vivid, concrete images, examples, and anecdotes that communicate on a personal level and make technical risk data come alive.
5. Avoid distant, abstract, and unfeeling language about death, injuries, and illnesses.
6. Use innovative ways—including graphics and other visual aids—to attract the attention of the target audience.
7. Reinforce messages by presenting them several times through multiple formats.
8. Avoid messages intended to arouse fear and anxiety.
9. Whenever possible, include concrete information about specific actions that people can take, even it if is only to tell them where to go to get further information or assistance.

10. Make it easy for people to obtain further information.
11. Present a fair and balanced message that accurately describes the strengths and weaknesses of both sides of a risk issue or a risk debate.
12. Develop messages that recognize, respect, and address the fears, emotions, and concerns of people.
13. Use risk comparisons carefully and intelligently to help put risks in perspective; use risk comparisons only if (1) they are targeted to a specific audience; (2) they take into account target audience needs, concerns, and level of knowledge; (3) they are specific in their intent; (4) they acknowledge and discuss all assumptions and uncertainties in the calculation of comparative data and caution against drawing unwarranted conclusions; (5) they present different measures of risk (e.g., annual mortality rates and lost life expectancy) to illustrate the effects of alternative ways of expressing comparative risk data; (6) they are targeted to substances, products, or activities that are similar or related; (7) they respect distinctions that people consider important in evaluating risks; and (8) they do not attempt to preempt or prejudge decisions by individuals and communities about the acceptability of the risk being compared.

DELIVERY CHANNELS

The news media are prime transmitters of information on risks. They play a critical role in transmitting risk information to the public, in setting agendas, and in determining outcomes. However, the news media represent only one message delivery channel. Other channels include interpersonal networks (e.g., peers and fellow employees), social networks (e.g., voluntary, community-based, and professional organizations), direct advertising, public service announcements, entertainment media, libraries, health fairs, local government agencies, public meetings, one-on-one contacts and counseling, health professionals, community networks, posters, videotapes, pamphlets, and brochures. Despite their potential effectiveness, these and other alternative communication channels are often underutilized by government agencies. The most effective communication efforts are those that exploit the strengths of specific communication channels.

Principles

1. All message delivery channels for communicating risk information have counterbalancing strengths and weaknesses.
2. Three factors are critical in choosing the most effective mix of communication channels: the content of the message, the characteristics of the media,and the characteristics of the specific target audience.
3. Some channels are more appropriate than others for specific issues and messages.
4. Some channels are more likely than others to reach specific target audiences.
5. Some channels are more feasible than others given program resources.
6. The mass media are not a single, monolithic entity; there are many types of mass media organizations, each with its own interests, information needs, concerns, priorities, and audiences.

7. The news media are generally more interested in politics and conflict than in risk; more interested in simplicity than in complexity; and more interested in danger than in safety.
8. News organizations represent only one among many mass media channels for communicating risk information; other mass media (e.g., entertainment and advertising) play an equal if not larger role in communicating risk information.

Guidelines

1. Select channels that are appropriate for the message, that are likely to reach the target audience, and that are feasible given program resources.
2. Communicate through channels that are perceived to be credible by the target audience.
3. Use multiple media strategies for communicating and reinforcing risk information, including public service announcements on television and radio, instructional television and radio programs, news coverage, and information brochures mailed directly to people's homes.
4. Use interpersonal and social networks (e.g., peer and social relationships, fellow workers and fellow students, teachers, religious and community leaders, doctors, and employers) to support and reinforce messages.
5. Establish telephone hot lines, toll-free numbers, and other mechanisms to control the spread of rumors and other misinformation.
6. Meet the needs of the media: be open with and accessible to reporters; respect their deadlines; provide information tailored to the needs of different news media, such as graphics and other visual materials for television; anticipate questions and provide relevant background materials; follow up on stories with praise or criticism as warranted; try to establish longstanding relationships with specific editors and reporters.

TARGET AUDIENCES

Government agencies often fail to target their risk communications to specific audiences. Only rarely are attempts made to characterize target audiences by their sociodemographic characteristics, knowledge of the subject, primary sources of information, attitudes, perceptions, concerns, and preferences. Although a variety of techniques exist for obtaining such information (e.g., techniques for segmenting audiences, for testing message penetration, and for measuring response), they are seldom used by government agencies.

Principles

1. If you do not listen to people, you cannot expect them to listen to you.
2. The public is not a single, monolithic entity; there are many publics, each with its own interests, information needs, concerns, and priorities.

3. If people are sufficiently motivated, they are quite capable of understanding complex risk information.
4. Information about audience characteristics can be obtained through a variety of techniques, including surveys, exploratory group sessions (focus groups), checklists, demographic profiles, and in-depth personal interviews.
5. People consider many factors in evaluating and judging the acceptability of risks, including catastrophic potential, reversibility, persistence, immediacy of consequences, impact on future generations, impact on children and other sensitive or vulnerable populations, victim identity, familiarity, understanding, scientific uncertainty, dread, voluntariness, controllability, clarity of benefits, equity, institutional trust, attributability, type of evidence, and personal stake (see Table 1); for

Table 1. Factors Involved in Public Risk Perception[a]

Factor	Conditions associated with increased public concern	Conditions associated with decreased public concern
Catastrophic potential	Fatalities and injuries grouped in time and space	Fatalities and injuries scattered and random
Familiarity	Unfamiliar	Familiar
Understanding	Mechanisms or process not understood	Mechanisms or process understood
Uncertainty	Risks scientifically unknown or uncertain	Risks known to science
Controllability (personal)	Uncontrollable	Controllable
Voluntariness of exposure	Involuntary	Voluntary
Effects on children	Children specifically at risk	Children not specifically at risk
Effects on future generations	Risk to future generations	No risk to future generations
Victim identity	Identifiable victims	Statistical victims
Dread	Effects dreaded	Effects not dreaded
Trust in institutions	Lack of trust in responsible institutions	Trust in responsible institutions
Media attention	Much media attention	Little media attention
Accident history	Major and sometimes minor accidents	No major or minor accidents
Equity	Inequitable distribution of risks and benefits	Equitable distribution of risks and benefits
Benefits	Unclear benefits	Clear benefits
Reversibility	Effects irreversible	Effects reversible
Personal stake	Individual personally at risk	Individual not personally at risk
Scientific evidence	Risk estimates based on human evidence	Risk estimates based on animal evidence
Origin	Caused by human actions or failures	Caused by acts of nature or God

[a]Adapted from Covello, von Winterfeldt, and Slovic, 1986.

example, risks that are perceived to be voluntary are accepted more readily than those that are perceived to be imposed; risks that are perceived to be under individual control are accepted more readily than those perceived to be under government control; risks that are perceived to be fair are accepted more readily than those perceived to be unfair.

6. Public concerns about risks are a function of the perceived level of risk; the level of outrage (a combination of several factors including fairness, benefits, alternatives, control, and voluntariness); and the perceived effects of the issue on individual and social welfare (e.g., adverse effects of negative publicity on community property values and tourism).
7. People in the community are often more concerned about issues such as trust, credibility, competence, control, voluntariness, fairness, caring, and compassion than mortality statistics and the details of quantitative risk assessment.
8. Regardless of how well you communicate risk information, some members of the audience will never be satisfied.

Guidelines

1. Do not make assumptions about what people know, think, or want done about risks.
2. Devote time and allocate sufficient resources to find out how people are thinking and behaving, including their knowledge, attitudes, activity patterns, beliefs, and values. Use techniques such as interviews, surveys, and focus groups.
3. Devote time and allocate sufficient resources to understand those factors in the environment or community that facilitate or present obstacles to effective risk communication.
4. Acknowledge and respond (both in words and with actions) to the emotions and feelings that people express e.g., anxiety, fear, anger, outrage, and helplessness.
5. Acknowledge and respond to the distinctions that people view as important in evaluating risks.
6. Let people know that you understand what they said, and address their concerns as well as your own.
7. Use data about target audience characteristics to develop alternative risk communication strategies, to plan communication efforts, and to evaluate program effectiveness.
8. Develop and support programs that are aimed at improving general scientific literacy and knowledge of risk assessment principles.
9. Never let your efforts to inform people about risks prevent you from acknowledging—and saying—that any illness, injury, or death is a tragedy.

SUMMARY AND CONCLUSIONS

As attested to by recent events (see, for example, the case studies in this volume), the consequences of ignoring or violating risk communication principles and guidelines can be substantial. These include (1) bitter and protracted risk debates and conflicts; (2) high levels of public outrage; (3) the diversion of societal attention and resources from important problems to less important problems; (4) the diversion of individual attention from significant risks to insignificant risks; and (5) unnecessary human suffering due to high levels of anxiety, fear, outrage, and worry.

One cause for optimism is that risk communication is no longer a neglected topic within government (see, for example, Ruckelshaus, 1987; Press, 1987; Thomas, 1987; Covello and Allen, 1988; and Chapters 2 and 7 of this volume). It is now widely recognized that risk communication is a field worthy of government recognition, attention, and resources in its own right. It is also widely recognized that past mistakes may have exacerbated risk communication problems and conflicts. In many cases, government agencies have simply not been effective in communicating risk information to the public.

The principles and guidelines presented here represent an attempt to address these problems. They also represent an attempt to stimulate discussion, dialogue, and debate in a field that is still in its infancy. While federal agencies have learned from their mistakes, the current challenge is to master and apply these lessons in order to improve risk communication and risk management activities.

ACKNOWLEDGMENTS. We are indebted to Frederick Allen, Ann Fisher, Detlof von Winterfeldt, Peter Sandman, Caron Chess, Billie Jo Hance, and Paul Slovic for allowing us to draw on their insights in preparing this paper.

REFERENCES

Covello, V. T. and F. W. Allen. 1988. Seven cardinal rules of risk communication. Washington, D.C.: Environmental Protection Agency, Office of Policy Analysis.

Covello, V. T., D. von Winterfeldt, and P. Slovic. 1986. Communicating scientific information about health and environmental risks: problems and opportunities from a social and behavioral perspective. In *Uncertainties in Risk Assessment and Management*. Ed. V. Covello, L. Lave, A. Moghissi, and V. R. R. Uppuluri. New York: Plenum.

Davies, J. C., V. T. Covello, and F. W. Allen (eds.). 1987. *Risk Communication*. Washington, D.C.: The Conservation Foundation.

Press, F. 1987. Science and risk communication. In *Risk Communication*. Ed. J. C. Davies, V. T. Covello, and F. W. Allen. Washington, D.C.: The Conservation Foundation, pp. 11–17.

Ruckelshaus, W. D. 1983. Science, risk, and public policy. *Science* 221(4615): 1026–1028.

Ruckelshaus, W. D. 1987. Communicating about risk. In *Risk Communication*. Ed. J. C. Davies, V. T. Covello, and F. W. Allen. Washington, D.C.: The Conservation Foundation, pp. 3–9.

Sandman, P. M. 1986. *Explaining Environmental Risk*. Washington, D.C.: U.S. Environmental Protection Agency, Office of Toxic Substances.

Slovic, P. 1987. Perception of risk. *Science* 236(4799): 280–285.

Thomas, L. M. 1987. Why we must talk about risk. In *Risk Communication*. Ed. J. C. Davies, V. T. Covello, and F. W. Allen. Washington, D.C.: The Conservation Foundation, pp. 19–25.

II

Perspectives on Government Risk Communication

2

The Federal Role in Risk Communication and Public Education

James O. Mason

The interpretation and communication of risk factors are now recognized as essential parts of the process of risk assessment and risk management. In our society, it cannot be otherwise. Collectively, the public must decide which risks are acceptable. Individually, each person makes risk management decisions every day in the context of his or her life.

The government's responsibility in risk communication is to help ensure that decisions of public policy and personal practice are based on the best available information. We probably will never achieve this ideal in risk communication, but we are doing better than in the past. As federal agencies, we are working more effectively together. For example, recently the Environmental Protection Agency (EPA) and the Centers for Disease Control (CDC) released a joint report to the public on the health risk of radon. Communication among federal agencies is absolutely essential for effective communication with the public. Federal agencies are collaborating more closely with state and local counterparts and cultivating a less adversarial and more collegial relationship with the media. We also are beginning to involve the concerned public in the risk communication process by sharing information at the earliest feasible stage. These are procedures we must continue to follow.

One thing is certain: the public is eager to learn about risks. The journal of the American Academy for the Advancement of Science (AAAS), *Science*, entitled its October 1985 issue on risks, "Playing the Odds: A Worrier's Guide to the 20th Century." Indeed, we sometimes appear to be a nation of perpetual worriers.

How did we get this way, especially at a time when we are living longer and healthier lives than ever before? It might be useful to consider briefly the backdrop against which our risk communications are projected and interpreted. As we seek to create an en-

James O. Mason • Centers for Disease Control, Atlanta, Georgia 30333.

lightened awareness of relative risk, we need to take into account risk perceptions that are already in the public eye.

In the second half of the twentieth century, mankind has had to cope, as never before in our long and perilous history, with the potential for self-destruction—the mushroom cloud that shadows us all. This reality imperceptibly conditions our response to other risks. Exhortations to control the controllable or prevent the preventable must contend with a pervasive sense of impotence in the face of nuclear destruction. We need not surrender to this sense of impotence, but we cannot afford to forget it.

The public's profound uneasiness about the presence of ionizing radiation also is related to the fear of nuclear destruction. Real or illusory, concern about radiation damage haunts the public, especially in the light of evidence that it can affect future generations. Three Mile Island dramatized this perceived threat a few years ago, and Chernobyl burned it into our consciousness in 1986. The nature of radiation—silent, invisible, and undetected by the five senses on which we depend—enhances its menace.

The fear of toxic chemicals in the environment fits into the same category; reports of the tragedy in Bhopal, India, crystallized this concern. Residents in our nation's cities and towns began eyeing "the factory" with suspicion and asking the following questions: What is it really producing? Might it leak? Might it explode? What substances may be oozing into our soil, washing into our river, or contaminating our wells? These same concerns apply to toxic dumps; Love Canal and Times Beach have been added to the public's vocabulary.

Our task of risk interpretation in these areas can be seen as an uphill struggle against preexisting perceptions. In many cases our studies may show that these fears are baseless or exaggerated, but simply stating this will not dispel them.

At CDC, which is the operating agency of the Public Health Service primarily concerned with the prevention of disease and promotion of health, we deal with three sets of risks. These risks differ significantly in a number of ways but all require careful interpretation to a variety of publics. The three sets are the risk of infectious disease; the risks associated with personal health-related behaviors; and the risks associated with environmental hazards both in the workplace and in the community.

INFECTIOUS DISEASE

The risk of infectious disease represents mankind's oldest and most familiar health hazard. Throughout past centuries, even though the level of knowledge was low, savants and healers sought to explain diseases as best they could to a frightened populace that was eager to seize on any clue that might enhance their chances of survival. Smallpox was attributed to disturbances in the ambient air, to "animalcules" that overheated the blood, to perverse actions of various deities, and to retribution for sin. Each explanation suggested a possible line of remedial action, and these were assiduously pursued. Most of them, of course, proved notably ineffectual.

In the late eighteenth century when Edward Jenner discovered that smallpox could be prevented by immunization, he attracted the attention of scientists in many parts of the world. Thomas Jefferson wrote the following to him from America in 1806: "Future nations will know by history only that the loathsome smallpox has existed and by you has been extirpated."

Today smallpox is gone—eradicated by a worldwide program that is among man's great achievements. However, it took nearly two centuries after Jenner's initial discovery of a true preventive measure. A substantial part of the task of smallpox eradication involved communicating risk interpretation to a great variety of publics, including health professionals and policy-makers.

In our own lifetime, we have witnessed dramatic reductions in the toll of many other communicable diseases, especially the infectious diseases of childhood that are amenable to prevention through immunization. Polio, a scourge much feared in my own childhood and early adulthood, is almost gone from most developed countries. But even these types of diseases are subject to continuing challenges of communication concerning relative risk. Pertussis is another case in point. Before the development of an effective and generally safe vaccine, whooping cough was a widespread and serious illness of childhood, which was sometimes fatal and could lead to serious and lasting neurological and respiratory consequences.

It has been 50 years since the public read the news stories heralding a vaccine, and most of today's parents have never seen a case of pertussis. Recently, however, many of them have seen dramatic presentations about the risk of the vaccine on television. It is instant news when a judge awards hundreds of thousands of dollars to the parents of one child whose brain damage is possibly attributable to immunization for this disease, but it is not considered news when thousands of cases of pertussis do not occur thanks to the vaccine. In these circumstances, it is not easy to communicate the concept of relative risk in such a way as to convince parents that it is important for their children to receive vaccines. There is a risk from the vaccine; however, the risk from the disease is far greater.

In a different context, we have similar difficulties in convincing budget makers about the importance of funding proven prevention programs in the face of a declining incidence of infectious diseases and their consequences. Each year the battle for funding for prevention programs is fought as if for the first time. Meanwhile, highly visible and dramatic treatment interventions, such as organ transplants, receive the attention of the public and budget makers alike. This pattern represents a major distortion in the perception of relative risk and public health.

One dimension that affects the public perception of risk is newness. We learn to live with the presence of familiar risks and diseases, with varying degrees of discomfort. However, public interest and anxiety are greatly heightened when a new risk appears. The most recent and dramatic example of this phenomenon is AIDS. People devour every scrap of information they can find about AIDS, and the media sources search for items to appease this hunger.

AIDS poses a formidable set of challenges for risk communication and interpretation. Its recent dramatic appearance and its high fatality rate would in themselves command instant and continuing interest. In addition, the specific characteristics of this particular disease carry the potential for sensationalism and controversy. Taken together, these factors require a very high degree of sensitivity in the face of a seemingly insatiable thirst for information on the part of the general public, the groups at high risk, and the various media that serve them.

The responsibility of a government agency in dealing with a problem of this nature is easy enough to state. We need to communicate both what we know and what we do not know through channels that will reach the audiences that need the information, in ways that will be meaningful to them. If there is an action message or something that people can do to protect themselves, we need to be especially clear and persuasive about that component.

SELF-IMPOSED RISKS

I would like to touch briefly on the other types of health risks mentioned earlier. In terms of clear and present danger, the risks we impose on ourselves through daily lifestyle choices are by far the most significant risks. Cigarette smoking alone accounts for more than 300,000 excess deaths in the United States every year. By any rational measure, it is by a large margin our greatest cause of preventable mortality. Alcohol abuse also is directly implicated in many thousands of excess deaths per year, a disproportionate share of them in the younger age groups. Finally, simple failure to use seat belts probably accounts for 20,000 unnecessary accident fatalities each year.

Yet, perhaps because they are self-imposed and apparently controllable, these risks seem less frightening than the intangible, insidious threats that are perceived in the environment. A person who smokes two packs of cigarettes a day, has three drinks after work, and then drives home with his seat belt unbuckled may be deeply and actively concerned about the health risks of Three Mile Island or a chemical plant in his part of town.

These behavioral choices, which rank at the top of any hierarchy of relative risks, present a different kind of communications problem. Over the years, the public has become almost universally aware of the self-imposed perils of cigarette smoking. The release of the first *Surgeon General's Report on Smoking and Health* in January 1964 commanded the front pages of newspapers for days. It continued to stay in the news while claims and counterclaims were advanced by health officials and industrial spokespersons, and it reemerged as a major news item in the early 1970s in connection with cigarette advertising.

Today, local campaigns to legislate restrictions about where and when smoking will be permitted make the local news. The annual issuance of a new *Surgeon General's Report* on a specific aspect of smoking creates an occasion for press attention, as in the case of this year's report that stresses the hazards of passive smoking. However, since these findings only reinforce earlier disclosures, they are short-lived.

Nevertheless, information about smoking has become a part of a broader network of people-to-people communication. Nonsmoking areas, once furiously resisted, are now commonplace, and the heroes and heroines of films and TV dramas almost never smoke anymore. Children are so well briefed on smoking hazards that they often become the educators of their parents. It is clear that we have won a number of significant victories in the Public Health Service's goal of a smoke-free society by the year 2000. The goals of a government agency in this situation are to keep reinforcing, to capitalize on trends, and to furnish accurate and supportive information to its growing number of allies.

The public perception of the risks related to alcohol abuse has had a different history. Although most of the essential facts have been well established and widely disseminated for years, they are getting more attention now than ever before. This is not happening because of any new scientific knowledge, but because the association between drinking and traffic deaths has generated a powerful wave of public agitation for legislative action to raise the legal drinking age, enforce existing laws more stringently, and impose heavier penalties. As a political issue, this problem is getting the attention it deserves.

RISKS FROM ENVIRONMENTAL HAZARDS

When we examine the risks from environmental hazards, a somewhat different set of concerns is introduced. A 1985 report to the Secretary of Health and Human Services entitled "Risk Assessment and Risk Management of Toxic Substances" identifies three categories of public concern: (1) concerns of individuals about the health effects of toxic chemicals; (2) concerns of individuals, communities, and organizations about the activities of industry and local, state, and federal governments in the control of hazardous materials and the management of the health risk posed by these substances; and (3) scientific concerns about the appropriateness and correctness of the methods used in assessing the risk of toxic substances.

The first two concerns cited above are directly relevant to the topic of risk communication, as there is widespread anxiety in relation to environmental hazards. Some of these anxieties may be exaggerated, but they have a basis in reality. The enormous increase in production of new goods and services, with their resultant benefits, also has brought potential hazards. Virtually everyone accepts the concept that some risk is inevitable, but the public has some legitimate questions and expectations. They feel entitled to know what toxic substances are present, how exposures occur, and what levels are safe. Most importantly, they feel that someone must be responsible for managing these risks, since they as individuals are powerless to do so. This "someone" who must be responsible is usually expected to be a government agency. Government agencies are expected to explain the situation and to fix it if necessary.

PRINCIPLES OF RISK COMMUNICATION

Four principles are critical to carrying out the government's role in risk communication. These principles are derived from CDC's experience in infectious diseases, life-style choices, and environmental hazards and are as follows: credibility of the source; quality of the message; use of intermediaries; and involvement of the concerned public.

Credibility is difficult to establish, easy to lose, and almost impossible to regain once lost. In risk communication, credibility must be based on a willingness to share good science and an apolitical approach to knowledge. Risk communicators have suffered from credibility gaps in the past. What we say, as well as what we do not say, is often greeted with skepticism. This skepticism frequently occurs when we are trying to put risks in perspective. It almost seems as if the public wants its worst fears to be confirmed. For example, if we report that a perceived risk is indeed real, we tend to be believed. However, if we report that the perceived risk has been exaggerated, we often face suspicion.

The most effective way to deal with the credibility problem is to tell "the truth, the whole truth, and nothing but the truth" every time; however, this is easier said than done. Unfortunately, we almost never know the whole truth, and one of the most difficult three-word sentences to pronounce is "I don't know." It is doubly difficult if the interrogator thinks that you do know but are not talking, or if you are unclear about what you really know and what you believe to be true. Almost every scientist or health official occasionally strays across the frontier between fact and opinion. Unfortunately, the opinions frequently appear in the headline or in the resulting story.

Another problem related to telling the truth has to do with self-protection. In what has been described as a litigious society, acknowledging error may have very serious consequences. However, in many circumstances, evasion merely delays the inevitable, and candor pays dividends in future credibility. A good example occurred recently, when officials of the National Institutes of Health were confronted with a tragic situation in which an error in treatment caused the death of a child. They immediately and unequivocally accepted full responsibility for the error, which enhanced their credibility and reflected well on health officials.

Credibility is closely linked with the quality of the message, which is based on good science that is clearly and accurately presented. However, risk communication often forces us to translate good science into information that is easily understood by the lay public. In some cases that is not a desirable situation.

In the environmental field, we place heavy emphasis on quantitative data. As scientists, we tend to be acutely uncomfortable with data that cannot be solidly quantified, but as public health officials we do not always have the luxury of waiting. Nearly 30 years ago, during the First National Conference on Air Pollution, the Surgeon General, Leroy Burney, said: "In law, the suspect is innocent until his guilt has been proved beyond reasonable doubt. In the protection of human health, such absolute proof often comes late." Sometimes, risk communication consists of the best available data, candid acknowledgment of the data's limitations, and reasonable inference about the outcome.

Our success in risk communication usually depends on the use of intermediaries, especially the news media. Over the years, with only a few exceptions, we at CDC have found that this can be a productive partnership. Conscientious scientists, health professionals, and journalists share common ground in the conviction that the public has the right to know about risks that may affect them. We sometimes differ on questions such as how much and how soon, but there is little disagreement with the premise. We believe that a well-informed public is better equipped to make both individual and collective decisions that will reduce health risks and enhance survival.

Both scientists and risk communicators share the desire to be the first to get into print. "Publish or perish" seems to be inherent in both lines of work, and this mutual imperative results in more information being rapidly disseminated to the public. However, the different responses evoked by the pressure to publish highlight the differences between the two groups. The health professional who is reporting on a single study in the scientific literature has the luxury of explaining the limitations of the data and the qualifications of the results. By contrast, the science writer usually faces a tighter deadline and a more diffuse audience. Science writers may ask questions that scientists find naive or discomforting, but these are the questions their readers will want answered. They communicate with both the scientific world, in which gray is commonplace, and the public, which is accustomed to black and white. These journalists are valuable allies and should be viewed and treated with respect.

Experience has taught us one important lesson: if we put out information by our own initiative and on our own terms, the results are usually good. In contrast, bad stories almost always result from leaks or from sources with special axes to grind. We need to follow what our experience has taught us and get messages out as early as possible.

Risk communication is most effective if the people concerned are involved from the earliest possible stage. When the public knows our plans and is included in the process, our goals can become their goals and the outcomes are more likely to be comprehended and accepted.

This volume will make a vital contribution to environmental health and safety by highlighting the importance of risk communication and interpretation. As health professionals, we have much to learn from each other, so that the public can benefit from our information. Ultimately, it is their decisions that will shape our environment.

REFERENCES

Hopkins, D. R. 1983. *Princes and Peasants: Smallpox in History*. Chicago: University of Chicago Press, p. 310.

Smoking and Health Report of the Advisory Committee to the Surgeon General of the Public Health Service. Public Health Service publication 1964;1103.

Proceedings: National Conference on Air Pollution. Public Health Service publication 1959;654:5.

3

Communicating with the Public on Health Risks

Arthur C. Upton

Communication with the public on health risks dates from ancient times. Early examples can be found in the Bible. For centuries, warning signs and labels have been in general use to inform the public about various risks to health.

In recent years, communication about health risks has been complicated by new and unfamiliar types of hazards and by public confusion and apprehension about the magnitudes of the threats. One has only to recall Agent Orange, asbestos, dioxin, ethylene dibromide (EDB), Love Canal, Three Mile Island, Bhopal, Chernobyl, and AIDS to appreciate how intensely the public has reacted to different health "crises" during the past decade. The psychological, economic, and sociopolitical impacts of such crises have been staggering and often out of proportion to the actual or potential health impacts. To this extent, the crises have brought to light inadequacies in communication that demand the serious attention of all concerned (Covello et al., 1983).

ROOTS OF THE PROBLEM

A major source of present difficulty is the complexity of the cause–effect relationship for many of today's risks to health. In contrast to drowning, for example, where the cause of death is obvious and occurs promptly, the effects of a toxic agent may not appear until months, years, or decades after exposure. The effects of a toxic agent may appear in the form of a small increase in the risk of a disorder that can also arise through other causes. Moreover, in any given affected individual, there are usually no distinguishing features by which the disorder (e.g., leukemia or birth defect) can be attributed conclusively to the

---

Arthur C. Upton • New York University Medical Center, New York, New York 10016. Preparation of this report was supported in part by grant ES 00260 from the National Institute of Environmental Health Sciences, grant CA 13443 from the National Cancer Institute, and Special Institutional Grant 009 from the American Cancer Society.

toxicant, as opposed to some other cause. In addition, the magnitude of the risk for a given level of exposure is almost always a subject of scientific debate, especially at low doses where estimates may vary by orders of magnitude and where the existence of a threshold cannot be excluded. Because of these complexities, estimates of the risks associated with low-level exposure to toxic agents are difficult to convey accurately and in proper perspective to members of the public.

Another difficulty stems from the confusion that is caused by disagreements among experts over the magnitude of a given risk. Although, in the face of uncertainty, scientific controversy is to some extent inevitable if not desirable, the public is not able to judge the merits of opposing views. Furthermore, it is the extreme views that capture attention, particularly those that magnify projected risks. When such views, irrespective of their scientific soundness, challenge those of responsible authorities, the credibility of the latter suffers.

Another factor affecting the reception of a communication on health risk is the context in which it is presented. In principle, no risk is acceptable if it is readily avoidable or if no benefit is to be gained by taking the risk. To interpret and judge a risk properly, therefore, the risk must be considered in the context of relevant risk-benefit relationships, taking into account not only the risk itself and the presumed benefits to be gained by taking the risk, but the risks and benefits of alternative courses of action. This, of course, is complicated by social, philosophical, ethical, and economic questions, since the risks and benefits may not be distributed equitably and since individuals often differ in their attitudes toward both risks and benefits.

Also affecting the acceptability of a given risk is the extent to which it is perceived to be involuntary, unfamiliar, catastrophic, uncontrollable, and scientifically uncertain. Hence, these questions need to be addressed in a risk communication if the issue is to be treated adequately.

REMEDIAL APPROACHES

Although there is general agreement on the need for improving communication with the public on health risks, the overall strategy for doing so has yet to be determined. Only recently has there been a general awareness of the need, as reflected in conferences, workshops, and study groups devoted to the subject. Clearly, the time has come for a systematic and concerted attack on the problem. In recognition of this fact, the Third Task Force for Research Planning in Environmental Health Science included a Subtask Force on Information Exchange in the Environmental Health Sciences (National Institute of Environmental Health Sciences, 1986). The recommendations of this Subtask Force, summarized briefly in the following, are timely and pertinent.

The Subtask Force identified the following six general principles to be observed in communicating with the public on risks to health: (1) the uncertainty in the information that is conveyed must be specified, along with the reasons for the uncertainty; (2) the information must be conveyed in perspective and in proper context; (3) new as well as traditional means of communication (e.g., computers, videotapes, and so on) should be exploited to help people "find out how to find out"; (4) a communication can be most effective when it reflects an understanding of what the public wants to know; (5) accurate dissemination to and among disparate groups (workers, teachers, students, physicians, consumer advocates, and the like), requires appropriately specialized communication programs; and (6) when information is released to the public, the potential regulatory and scientific uses of the information, as well as any policy implications it may have, should be indicated.

Among more than 20 specific measures to improve risk communication that were recommended by the Subtask Force, the following are especially noteworthy:

1. A comprehensive public survey should be carried out and repeated periodically to assess the environmental health awareness of groups varying in age, occupation, and locale and to assist in creating better public information exchange and outreach programs.
2. An interagency advisory committee should be created to strengthen communication on environmental health matters in and out of government.
3. Educational programs emphasizing issues in environmental health, reading lists, slide shows, computer software, videocassettes, and other information materials should be made available to schools, school administrators, and librarians, including educational materials aimed at elementary students through the twelfth grade.
4. An independent clearinghouse for environmental health information, with a computerized data base and information readily accessible to the media and other users, should be established.
5. Seminars on risk assessment and risk management should be conducted for science writers, congressional aides, decision makers, and opinion leaders.
6. A series of forums for professionals should be held to promote the exchange of opposing views about environmental health information and its policy implications.
7. Pilot education programs for the public and for special groups, including television broadcasts and a national telephone hotline with a toll-free number, should be established to provide information on specific environmental health problems.
8. An independent body in a staff relationship with Congress (similar to the Office of Technology Assessment) should be created to provide ongoing assessment of the impact of health research on public policy decisions and to help guide legislative action.
9. Provision should be made for the periodic review and evaluation of environmental health information exchange programs.

While the above recommendations would undoubtedly be helpful, what will ultimately be needed is the development of a stronger epidemiological and toxicological science base, as well as a new body of knowledge on risk communication, with appropriate institutional mechanisms and educational programs for informing the public. Our experience with alcohol abuse, cigarette smoking, and use of seat belts testifies dramatically to the limitations of present day risk communication techniques in combatting entrenched habits and powerful psychological drives. The demands of technology and the laws that have been enacted in response to them (e.g., the "right-to-know" law) require that we move swiftly to improve our effectiveness in risk communication.

REFERENCES

Covello, V. T., W. G. Flamm, J. V. Rodricks, and R. G. Tardiff, eds. 1983. *The Analysis of Actual Versus Perceived Risks*. New York: Plenum Press.

National Institute of Environmental Health Sciences. 1986. *Human Health and the Environment: Some Research Needs*. Report of the Third Task Force for Research Planning in Environmental Health Science. NIH Publication No. 86-1277. Washington, D.C.: U.S. Government Printing Office, pp. 335–43.

4

The Role of Risk Communication in Environmental Gridlock

Christopher J. Daggett

This is a particularly timely volume, given the growing difficulties that health and science experts, government officials, business representatives, and public interest groups are having with the communication of risk factors to the press and to the general public. Analysis of the risk communication process also is imperative in light of the increasing awareness that risk communication problems, along with several other factors, contribute to the general difficulty that we have in this country in forging coherent, lasting solutions to our most intractable environmental problems. Let us examine risk communication today in the context of this larger phenomenon and address how improvements in risk communication can help us out of the bind environmental policy-makers at all levels of government are experiencing. We face imposing obstacles in moving toward more effective risk communication strategies.

First of all, risk assessment is a far-from-perfect art, and scientific consensus on dose-response is a rare commodity. For example, a National Academy of Sciences report on saccharin concluded that over 70 years the expected number of cases of human bladder cancer resulting from daily exposure to 120 milligrams of saccharin could be anywhere from 0. 22 to 1,144,000. Given the imperfections of risk assessment, it is obvious that communicating the results of these assessments is, and will continue to be, an inherently difficult task.

Compounding this fact, however, is the peculiar and often irrational way that the general public perceives environmental and health risks; for example, many people are not comfortable with mathematical probability as a guide for living. If you inform people that their risk of developing cancer from a 70-year exposure to a certain carcinogen at ambient level ranges between 10^{-5} and 10^{-7}, their response may be, "Okay, but can I drink the water?"

Christopher J. Daggett • New Jersey Department of Environmental Protection, Trenton, New Jersey 08625.

We also know that people tend to overestimate the probability of unfamiliar, catastrophic, or well-publicized events but tend to underestimate the probability of unspectacular or familiar events, which claim only one victim at a time. For example, many people are afraid to fly with commercial airlines, but very few people are afraid to drive in cars. These kinds of attitudes defy all of the known statistics.

Generally, people appear to respond most negatively when the degree of risk is unknown and the consequences are particularly dreadful. This is a constant problem in the complex world of toxic waste, and even expert advice does not seem to help in this area. People will throw themselves in front of bulldozers to keep a hazardous waste facility out of their community, even with experts' assurances of its safety. Yet people living under a high dam on an earthquake fault will ignore the experts' warnings.

The way in which risk is described also can influence perceptions. Workers probably would be worried to know that their occupational exposure would double their risk of cancer, but they might not worry as much if they knew that it would increase their risk from 1 in a million to 2 in a million.

In addition, public perception of risk varies with the degree that the risk is viewed as either voluntary or involuntary. People tend to accept a far greater risk from the voluntary decision to drive an automobile than they will from the involuntary breathing of exhaust from someone else's car. The classic example of this is cigarette smoking; most of EPA's field engineers have found themselves at one time or another being accused of child poisoning by a chain-smoking parent.

CURRENT EXAMPLES

A recent complicated case that illustrates public thinking about potential risks involves the State of New Jersey's attempts to store and ultimately dispose of 7200 tons of slightly radioactive soil. The soil had originally been recovered from excavation around homes in Montclair and Glen Ridge, near where a radium-processing facility once operated.

The State's first option, albeit a temporary one, was to store the soil in a safe facility at a West Orange armory. When the plan was presented at a town meeting, hundreds of angry residents shouted it down. Since that avenue was blocked, New Jersey looked outside its borders for a permanent storage site. Only three commercial sites nationwide can accept low-level radioactive waste—in South Carolina, Washington, and Nevada.

The South Carolina site did not have the storage capacity for the waste. Of the two remaining sites, the Nevada site was the least costly for New Jersey's purposes, so a contract was signed with the owners and a permit secured from the State of Nevada. However, when word spread regarding the shipment of the soil into Las Vegas, it became a politically hot issue, even though the soil is less radioactive than materials that are routinely deposited at the site. The City of Las Vegas and Clark County, backed by the Governor of Nevada, sued to stop the shipment. New Jersey, in turn, sued Nevada for violating interstate commerce laws.

Currently, the case is before a special master of the U. S. Supreme Court, but the final outcome is probably years away. Meanwhile, a plan to send the soil to the Washington site also ran into difficulty after the site's operators decided that it was not radioactive enough for their limited storage space.

Recently, New Jersey's Department of Environmental Protection (DEP) proposed to secure an appropriate site within the State, where the soil would be blended with "clean" soil to lower its radioactivity level and then used to restore an old quarry. After a thorough search, DEP settled on a site in Vernon Township, a selection that was approved by the DEP's Science Advisory Board. The DEP also obtained EPA approval of the soil-blending concept. When the State went public with this proposal, however, it encountered intense public opposition as well as a lawsuit. The State prevailed in the court battles that followed, all the way up to and including the New Jersey State Supreme Court. The decision of the State's highest court did not sway the thousands of angry protesters in Vernon who demonstrated in opposition to the DEP's plan. Faced with the threat of violence, the State abandoned the Vernon plan. A criteria board was then established to locate a site, and the entire process started again. Finally, DEP was able to dispose of this material by having it blended with material of a higher level of radiation and then disposed of in a licensed facility that could accept the resulting mix.

This case is extremely complicated, but it is interesting in terms of risk communication and how public reaction to it compares with the reaction to the recently discovered, naturally occurring radon in our region and throughout the country. An example of this is a case in Clinton, New Jersey, where naturally occurring uranium in the earth was producing radon levels in homes that were more of a health threat than the blended soil in the Vernon case. Yet there was little public alarm or outcry about this radon in Clinton. Instead, the local authorities, the State, and EPA were able to work together to produce a well-conceived and well-executed approach to the problem.

ENVIRONMENTAL GRIDLOCK

It appears that it is not always the objective health dangers that determine public reaction as much as the circumstances that surround the issue and how they shape public perception of risk. However, a larger issue is also at stake. Cases like the Vernon Township situation illustrate not only risk communication problems, but a fundamental breakdown in the environmental decisionmaking process that poor risk communication can help create. One of our most pressing environmental issues at the national, regional, and even local level is called environmental gridlock, for lack of a better description. There is a broad consensus that we face numerous environmental threats but that consensus is not working toward practical, lasting solutions. One feels frustration when looking at the worsening problems around us and our inability to find solutions to them.

The most obvious manifestation of this issue is in the debate over what to do about hazardous waste. Clearly, this is a problem that requires some long-term, comprehensive solutions. This country churns out approximately 250 million tons of hazardous waste every year. This is in addition to all the waste generated in previous years that sits in leaking landfills or other inadequate facilities, as well as the waste that has been coming out of the Superfund cleanup program over the last few years.

State and national polls indicate that the public is fully aware of the need to do something about hazardous waste and to do it quickly. Yet that awareness seems to pale in comparison to the ire inspired under the "not-in-my backyard" (NIMBY) banner in the selection of sites for hazardous waste disposal facilities. Everyone wants something done with the waste, as long as their community is not involved in the solution.

This NIMBY syndrome is compounded by public opposition to innovative technological approaches to disposal problems. For example, incineration of hazardous waste at sea has been practiced in Europe for several years, but the application of ocean incineration in this country has been met with vehement opposition. Some of this opposition has been generated in the coastal states that are nearest to the proposed off-shore incineration site, which is simply another version of NIMBY. However, widespread resistance has come from public activists who question the idea of ocean incineration itself. They argue that a method that removes 99.9999% of the waste incinerated is less than ideal. They may be right, but the question is whether we can afford to wait for ideal solutions. At any rate, the debate over ocean incineration has dragged on for so long that one of the two companies in the United States able to provide this service went out of business waiting for final approval, and the other firm sued EPA in order to force the issuance of regulations to govern the process, and later announced its intention to abandon its quest.

Environmental gridlock is not confined to the hazardous waste issue; in Region II and elsewhere, it also characterizes the debate over commercial development of some of our most vital wetlands and waterfront resources. The development project for the western shoreline of Manhattan, commonly known as the Westway Project, caused protracted legal battles that spanned more than 14 years before resulting in a deadlock in 1985.

Unfortunately, cases like the Westway Project, ocean incineration, and sites for hazardous waste facilities are no longer the exceptions; in fact, they are becoming the norm. This gridlock situation is the result of several converging circumstances and historical factors. The kinds of pollutants we are currently dealing with are less understood and less visible than the more obvious, conventional pollutants that we successfully battled in the early 1970s. Consequently, solutions today are inevitably more difficult than they were before. We also have seen a growing mistrust of the government (some of it well founded), which undermines effective compromises. In addition, press coverage of these issues is colored by a natural tendency to highlight unusual, startling news at the expense of mundane information, however pertinent it may be.

THE FAILURE OF RISK COMMUNICATION

One of the most significant factors contributing to environmental gridlock is the problem of risk communication. In fact, poor communication of risk is at the heart of each of the previous gridlock examples. Improving risk communication procedures can help to loosen gridlock situations and find solutions to this dilemma. Steps can be taken to improve risk communication to create a more informed public and, in turn, a more informed public debate.

First, it is obvious that we, as risk communication professionals, have to do a better job of organizing our scientific risk information before we attempt to disseminate it. If we are careless with our own data, it will have a ripple effect throughout the risk communication process. In addition, we should determine the audience to whom we are targeting our information, which means being more aggressive in assessing the demographics of a community and its information needs. Once this is accomplished, we can tailor risk communication messages to the targeted audience. We also should consider in this process the particular media sources that we use to promote our messages. Regardless of popular perceptions, media sources are no more uniform than the various publics they serve. The specific needs, capabilities, understanding, and biases vary for television, radio, newspapers, and special-interest publications, as well as for science reporters and general-assignment reporters. Each risk communication effort should be followed up to determine what perception the message has created and what, if any, behavior changes have resulted. This is a crucial strategy for guiding future risk communication strategies.

Beyond these procedural improvements, the overall context of risk communication strategies should be assessed. The risk communication efforts of the EPA and the state agencies have been hindered in the past by the failure to open up our decisionmaking process to public scrutiny. Although we have made tremendous strides in this regard in recent years, additional efforts are necessary. We have to be honest with the public about the information we have and, perhaps more importantly in the uncertain world of risk, we also need to be frank with the public about the information we lack.

Finally, we need to be aware of the fact that communication, by definition, is a two-way process. We should actively solicit information from the affected public and, where appropriate, include it in our deliberations. It may be difficult to build the necessary trust and give-and-take relationship between risk communicators and the public, but it seems to be the only way to solve situations like the one that occurred in Vernon Township, New Jersey.

In Region II, EPA recently undertook a pilot communication project that incorporates these ideas. An environmental public education initiative was developed in Toms River, New Jersey. Toms River was selected because the community faces a wide variety of environmental problems, largely due to the presence of a local chemical facility of the Ciba-Geigy Corporation. The facility is quite complex because it is a Superfund site and it has a unit that is permitted under the Resource Conservation and Recovery Act, a sewage treatment plant, and an ocean outfall pipe.

The goals of the Toms River project have been to identify the concerns of citizens, to develop responses to those concerns, and to communicate the responses through a variety of mechanisms, including one-on-one sessions, public meetings, library exhibits, and pamphlets and flyers. We will use whatever means of communication we deem most effective for this project.

This is a project with long-term payoffs, and we do not know yet how effective it will be in facilitating future risk communication in the area. However, we have received some positive feedback from the community, and we are going to continue with efforts of this kind.

As we work toward improved risk communication, we need to remember that the goal is not to change people's opinions about controversial environmental issues. The goal is to change the way we discuss these issues, make the discussions accurately reflect the risks we face and the available options, and enable us to make effective decisions.

Thomas Jefferson anticipated many of the policymaking problems we are facing today when he said, "If we think [the people] not enlightened enough to exercise their control with a wholesome discretion, the remedy is not to take it from them, but to inform their discretion." This concept is what effective risk communication is all about. There is no way to succeed in this task overnight, and some of our most problematic issues are ahead. However, the increased awareness that something has gone awry in the way that we make and communicate environmental decisions in this country is encouraging. We can look forward to the new research and ideas that this awareness will no doubt generate.

5

Risk Communication: Moving from Theory to Law to Practice

Michael Baram

Risk communication has become a central feature of public policy for dealing with health, safety, and environmental hazards in the United States and the European Community (EC). New laws in both industrial societies now establish an extensive set of risk communication duties for government and industry, and provide the public with various rights of access to risk information held by private firms and public agencies.

These recent developments are based on a diverse set of policy considerations. For example, risk communication is viewed by many as a moral imperative, since essential fairness and social justice require that a person has a responsibility not to permit his activities to create an undue risk of harm to the health and well-being of others, and should thereby inform and warn persons at risk.

In industrial democracies, risk communication can also be held forth as a political imperative, since democracy is premised on the exercise of choice by an informed citizenry in governmental processes. Thus, the responsibility to inform and warn persons concerned about risk from technological initiatives is imposed on government, and rights to such information vested in the public.

Risk communication is also seen as a suitable response to people's fears of technology and its uncertain impacts on their interests. People fear most what they cannot see, understand, or control, and risk communication enables people to better cope with technology. Risk communication is also now needed to enable the public to choose wisely among competing products in the marketplace, since private firms now use risk publicity to compete successfully, offering products advertised as less risky than those of their

---

Michael Baram • Center for Law and Technology, Boston University Law School, Boston, Massachusetts 02215. This paper is based on research supported by the European Community Research Center and the U.S. Environmental Protection Agency.

competitors, such as low-salt and low-fat foods, safer cigarettes, safer automobiles, and safer energy systems.

Finally, risk communication is seen as a means of supplementing traditional methods for dealing with risky technologies and their health, safety, and environmental hazards. The traditional methods of regulation and tort liability rules to prevent, punish, and deter risky activities have obvious limitations to their effectiveness and involve what many now feel are excessive growth and costs for governance, and excessive losses for industry and its insurers. Attention is now returning to first principles, that risk communication can be used to provide protections without excessive government growth or industrial liability.

Thus, several policy considerations and social goals support the recent enactment of laws requiring various risk communication systems. Legal measures enacted in the United States and the European Community now require various forms of risk communication and provide duties for government and industry and rights for the public, in three risk contexts: consumer risk from hazardous products, worker risk from hazardous workplaces, and community risk from industrial hazards, which include sudden accidents and gradual releases of harmful substances.

CONSUMER RISK

Various federal laws and regulatory programs in the United States require the manufacturers of certain products (e. g., drugs and pesticides) to provide labels and other information for informing consumers about product risks and safe use practices. In addition, any person may invoke his or her rights under the Freedom of Information (FOI) law to gain access to information on product risks (e. g., auto crash test data) held by federal agencies, subject to trade secret and other limitations, although much of this information may be of ambiguous significance as to risk. In the 12 member nations comprising the EC, the "Sixth Amendment" requires this form of risk communication for a broad range of products, and recent amendments proposed in the EC would even impose tactile labeling to communicate risk to the visually impaired consumer.

In both legal systems, however, a more pervasive and potent force for risk communication by product manufacturers has long been at work, namely, product liability law. In our 50 states and in the 12 EC nations, tort and contract theories govern commerce in products. These doctrines establish the communication duties and rights that apply to the manufacturers, purchasers, consumers, and users of products. In general, they afford compensation and other remedies to persons injured by products if they can provide evidence of harm, causation, a product defect or unduly dangerous feature, and fault on the part of the manufacturer.

However, many states, and the newly promulgated EC Directive on Product Liability, have eliminated the need to establish fault or negligence on the part of the manufacturer, thereby creating a "strict products liability" doctrine. Under strict products liability, the injured user or purchaser faces only two evidentiary hurdles: proof of causation and product defect. In numerous state court decisions, a product defect (making it unreasonably hazardous) has been found to arise from the manufacturer's failure to adequately warn and provide safe use instructions to purchasers and users. Because workers may also be injured by products in their employment, they may also rely on strict products liability law to secure compensation from the manufacturer, and many now do so, as this decade of asbestos litigation indicates so vividly.

The result has been a surge in products liability litigation against manufacturers by consumers, users, and workers, with failure to warn and provide adequate safe-use instructions as the main liability argument. This has led to large compensatory damage awards for failure to adequately warn, and even larger awards of punitive damages when the failure to warn was intentional or reckless.

Certain criteria favorable to persons at risk are used in the courts to determine if company communication practices were adequate in such cases. For example, one criterion deals with the foreseeable probability and magnitude of harm by requiring that the greater the incidence and seriousness of harm that is foreseeable on the basis of manufacturer expertise, the more precise, clear, and obvious the warning must be to be found adequate. Another criterion deals with the utility of the warning, by requiring that the greater the benefit (risk reduction) it would produce, the more likely it is to be needed. Other criteria deal with excessive product promotion, which may negate the effect of the warning provided.

Some courts have also responded to manufacturer defenses of scientific uncertainty about risk or remoteness of harm as reasons for not warning, by holding that the seriousness of the risk alone, irrespective of incidence, should govern the warning decision; a warning should provide "what a reasonable person would want to know," and manufacturers must not wait for scientific certainty.

These successful private actions for personal injury not only compensate the injured, they also deter or prevent risks over time. The rational corporation must now seek to avoid such liability and other losses by use of improved risk analysis of products and risk communication. Thus, duty to warn has become a potent force for industrial risk analysis and communication.

WORKER RISK

With regard to worker risk, as noted above, products liability law promotes risk communication by manufacturers to workers in "downstream companies" that purchase the manufacturer's products for employee use.

But, in addition, government regulations now assure that minimal forms of risk communication be used by the manufacturers and importers of hazardous chemicals, and by the downstream firms that purchase and use these chemicals in manufacturing processes. In the United States, the Hazard Communication Rule enacted by the Occupational Safety and Health Administration (OSHA) requires that a manufacturer or importer of any of some 2000 designated chemicals provide labels and Material Safety Data Sheets (MSDSs) for such chemicals to their own workers who may be subject to exposure to such chemicals, and to downstream firms that purchase and use such chemicals. The downstream firms must make the labels and MSDSs available to their own workers and conduct programs to educate workers about safe use. Similar requirements have been established for the 12 member nations of the EC by the EC's Sixth Amendment.

The OSHA rule on hazard communication, therefore, establishes a worker's "right to know" in many sectors of industry, but conflicts in certain respects with laws enacted for similar purposes by over 25 states. Industry has turned to the courts to resolve these conflicts and, in opposition, state officials and unions have argued to preserve the state laws and to expand the scope of the OSHA rule.

Both parties have had some success. The courts have held that OSHA's rule preempts state law, insofar as the state law also deals with the manufacturing sector of industry regulated by OSHA, a position favorable to industry seeking a uniform set of risk communication requirements across the nation. But the courts have also ordered OSHA to expand the scope of its rule to cover transportation, construction, and other industrial sectors if warranted by sufficient evidence of worker illness due to their lack of information. The courts have also ordered OSHA to narrow the protection of trade secret information that the original OSHA rule generously provided. OSHA is now revising its rule, and the states are now conforming their laws to the OSHA rule.

Thus, an extensive set of federal and state laws governing risk communication in the worker risk sector is in place, empowering workers with a right to know that has considerable potential for preventing job-related illnesses. This right will become ever more expansive as new workplace hazards are identified.

COMMUNITY RISK

As for the community risk sector, legal developments have been rapidly emerging in response to the Seveso accident at a Hoffmann-La Roche plant, the Bhopal accident and the Institute, West Virginia release of chemicals (both at Union Carbide plants), and other industrial accidents involving hazardous materials. Thus, the EC has enacted its "Seveso Directive" and, in the United States, EPA, roughly 25 states, trade associations, municipalities, and Congress have enacted various programs for accident risk communication and emergency response planning.*

These diverse legal measures have some common features. Several require industry self-evaluation of accident hazards at facilities that handle particularly volatile and toxic chemicals (178 named chemicals in the EC, 402 in the United States) and development of improved methods for accident prevention and emergency response on a facility-specific basis. All require that this information be provided to designated national, state, and local officials, who will evaluate the information, use their authority to impose additional safety measures at particular facilities, and develop community emergency response programs using state, local, and regional officials and industry managers as key actors with site-specific expertise.

The EC and U.S. systems will be implemented over the next few years, and numerous problems are foreseeable. Since each facility is unique and requires special attention, it will not be possible to rely on generic criteria in evaluating safety and accident potential. Use of risk analysis will raise the question, "how safe is safe enough?" Many state and local officials are inadequately trained or have inadequate resources, and in many instances no such officials have even been designated. The emergency plans to be

*Congress enacted a federal Community Right-to-Know law in October 1986.

drawn up will be of variable quality, and few will be tested by costly and disruptive public evacuation exercises, raising the issue of their adequacy and reliability. Confusion and conflicts arising from multiple levels of government involvement will have to be resolved.

Special problems for industry will also arise regarding the protection of confidential or trade secret information about chemical processes and management systems, despite provisions in all these laws affording some protections for trade secrets. Management will face government intrusion on a new and particularly threatening level, as government officials and their consultants will now be evaluating and forcing changes in internal company practices and risk management systems. Indeed, some see these new laws as providing, in essence, for government licensing of chemical facilities. This diffusion of responsibility for plant safety between industry and government will raise, in turn, the issue of how to allocate liability when a plant accident occurs despite the joint efforts of industry and public officials.

Community members seeking access to accident risk information will be presented with several new opportunities and obstacles, since most of these laws in the United States provide for citizen access to much, but not all, of the information to be provided by industry to government. Thus, community right-to-know doctrines will be tested and, to the extent they are affirmed, may chill industrial safety analyses and disclosures of the results to government.

The EC's Seveso Directive, in contrast, provides for some information disclosure to citizens by government but only on a narrow, need-to-know basis (e.g., information on how to respond to an accident). By insulating industry from citizen intrusion under a community right-to-know banner, the EC may actually promote better industrial self-evaluation, disclosure, and cooperation with government, and more effective accident control and emergency plans. However, trust in such a government-industry partnership is lacking in the United States.

THE LARGER ISSUES

Beyond the legal issues that arise in the process of implementing duty to warn, right to know, and other doctrines lie several larger issues that deal with the quality and utility of risk communication.

First, there is the issue of reluctance to disclose uncertain information about risk. Persons responsible for risky activities are reluctant to disclose risk information that may confuse or distress the public, or arouse it to take legal, political, or economic actions against the activity. Reluctance to disclose was most apparent at Chernobyl, where it led to anxieties, confusion, harms, economic dislocations, and produced public furor at a level perhaps greater than what would have occurred had disclosures been made.

Health and environmental scientists in government agencies are also reluctant to disclose uncertain or inconclusive risk information because of their concern about possible controversy and their sense of professional responsibility. Thus, in Massachusetts, the Department of Public Health was attacked by many because it withheld the findings of incomplete cancer risk studies it had done on several communities. These studies indicated certain above-average cancer rates but were scientifically inconclusive, and agency officials felt it would be professionally irresponsible to generate anxieties and controversies unless more conclusive findings were reached, a response that did not satisfy critics.

Perhaps such reluctance to disclose should be addressed by recalling the judicial rule in products liability law concerning the duty to warn. As discussed earlier, some courts have held that the duty to warn or disclose should be based on what a reasonable person would want to know, and not on scientific certainty.

A second issue pertains to the distinction between risk information and hazard information. Virtually all the legal requirements discussed have been mislabeled as "risk communication" requirements, when in reality consumers, workers, and community residents are given abstract hazard information in most cases, without the exposure and health response information that would enable them to make a careful personal assessment of their risk. What happens next is unclear, but it seems that persons given hazard information develop mental models of "worst case scenarios" that then stimulate anxiety and conflict.

For example, the MSDS required by OSHA is a succinct form of communication replete with hazard information for workers. It should be reconsidered so that it provides more than abstract data about molecular weight, flash point, and toxicity, and becomes a true risk communication with information that a worker should know in order to make a personal evaluation of risk and a personal choice about work habits and exposure conditions on the job. However, it is obvious that translating hazard information into risk information is an extremely difficult task.

Coping with this problem raises a third issue: should "learned intermediaries" be positioned between the disclosers and receptors of risk information to help translate hazard attributes into more personal risk evaluations? The concept of the learned intermediary for risk communication is found in the law dealing with the prescribing of drugs for patient use in medical care. Hazard attributes disclosed by drug companies in package inserts are usually inadequate for properly informing a patient seeking to make a personal decision about drug use and risk. Hence, products liability law applicable to drugs has developed the concept that the company must disclose hazards to the physician and the consumer, but that the prescribing physician is the learned intermediary and is legally responsible for understanding the hazard attributes and properly communicating them in the form of personal risk information to the patient, so that the patient may make a properly informed personal choice.

Although flawed in practice in many respects, perhaps the learned intermediary concept could be adapted to fit the new workplace and community contexts for risk communication, with medical and public health professionals as learned intermediaries for workers and citizens.

Finally, we need to look at an important policy issue. To what extent should risk problems be dealt with by risk communication instead of by government regulation? For many types of hazards, risk communication seems to be equitable, efficient, and effective and therefore a justified substitute for government regulation. For other types of hazards, it may be unsuitable as a regulatory substitute. Instinctively, one feels that a serious risk such as radon in homes is a prime candidate for a risk communication approach, whereas nuclear reactor safety requires strong and enforceable regulation with ancillary communication measures. Perhaps such feelings hinge on whether the receptor of a risk communication can then act on the new information to voluntarily and effectively reduce the risks of concern, on either a personal or collective basis, and in a timely fashion. Therefore, new policy initiatives calling for risk communication instead of risk regulation should be carefully assessed in terms of their risk-reducing merits.

Thus, we stand on the threshold of the risk communication era, replete with promises, performance problems, and opportunities to resolve many of the technological risk issues that afflict industrial society.

6

Hazard versus Outrage in the Public Perception of Risk

Peter M. Sandman

One goal of risk communication is to produce in the audience the appropriate level of concern and action. That is, risk communicators sometimes want to tell people to take a risk seriously—wear a seat belt, quit smoking, cut down on fats, check their homes for radon or their water for lead and take action if the level is high. On the other hand, risk communicators sometimes want to tell people not to worry so much about a risk. One would expect that at least one of these tasks would be a simple one, but it turns out that they both can be very difficult.

HAZARD VERSUS OUTRAGE

Scientists and managers who study risk for a living are consistently irritated that the public seems to worry about the "wrong" risks, which is often true when mortality statistics are used as the standard. But rather than see this as a perceptual distortion on the part of the public, it is more useful and accurate to see it as an oversimplification on the part of the scientists and managers.

In other words, the concept of risk means a lot more than mortality statistics. Let us take the classic definition of risk—how many people are how likely to incur how much damage if we do X—and call that "hazard." Hazard is what risk assessments are designed to estimate. Now, let us call everything else that goes into lay people's risk perceptions "outrage." Outrage is everything that is relevant about a risk except how likely it is to be harmful.

Is anything else relevant? Consider this example: virtually everyone would rather drive home from a party on the highway than walk home on deserted streets. We feel safer

Peter M. Sandman • Environmental Communication Research Program, New Jersey Agricultural Experiment Station, Cook College, Rutgers University, New Brunswick, New Jersey 08903.

in our cars, not because we miscalculate the relative likelihood of a fatal mugging versus a fatal car crash, but because the possibility of getting mugged strikes us as an outrage, while we accept the possibility of an auto accident as voluntary and largely controllable through good driving. (Approximately 85% of Americans consider themselves better than average drivers; optimistic bias is one reason why serious hazards tend to be underestimated.) Similarly, a household cleanser, however carcinogenic, seems a lot less risky than a high-tech hazardous waste treatment facility because the former is familiar and under one's own control, whereas the latter is exotic and controlled by others.

Here, then, is the fundamental premise of my argument: Expert risk assessments ignore outrage and focus on hazard, but citizen risk assessments are more a product of outrage than of hazard. That is, we consistently underestimate the hazard of risks that are low-outrage and overestimate the hazard of risks that are high-outrage. We do this because we care about outrage.

COMPONENTS OF OUTRAGE

Much research has been conducted on what is being defined here as outrage. Some of the key variables that determine the level of our outrage follow.

Voluntary versus Involuntary

Most environmental risks, like muggings, are involuntary and therefore enormously objectionable; on the other hand, people who voluntarily assume risks naturally tend to consider them acceptable and thus underestimate the hazard as a result. Voluntariness is correlated with acceptability. Natural risks, such as geological radon, fall into the middle position on this issue. They are more outrageous than a voluntary risk but much less outrageous than a risk imposed by somebody else.

Familiar versus Exotic

A carcinogenic household cleanser is not going to evoke as much of an outraged reaction as a new, strange-looking, high-tech industrial facility. Familiar surroundings lead to underestimation of risk, as does familiarity with the risk itself.

Dreaded versus Not Dreaded

It is not fully understood why some outcomes are so much more dreaded than others, but it is a fact that they are. For instance, there is a case where an environmental manager has let stand a false, or at least questionable, impression that certain industrial effluents are carcinogenic because the effluents are in fact associated with other health problems like asthma and emphysema. People don't worry much about asthma and emphysema; it is only the incorrect association with cancer that causes them to be regulated.

Diffuse in Time and Space versus Focused in Time and Space

This is one of the main reasons why airline safety arouses so much more public concern than auto safety, the statistics notwithstanding. Airline passengers die in larger bunches. Consider cigarettes as an example. If all smokers died on October 13 in Chicago, we would long ago have outlawed smoking.

Controlled by the Individual versus Controlled by the "System"

This is connected to voluntariness, but it also has to do with who protects against the risk. Most people believe they are better than average drivers, so as long as they control the car they feel fairly safe. In fact, people who feel the solution is in their own hands are often so reassured by this that they feel little need to actually carry it out. Putting oneself in the hands of a corporation or the government provokes a very different level of concern.

Fair versus Unfair

This is also connected to voluntariness, since a coerced risk is bound to feel unfair. But it also has to do with whether the risks and the benefits are going to the same people. Hazardous waste facilities, for example, typically accept imported waste and often export the profits to nonlocal owners. The unfairness of a community stuck with all the risk and little of the benefit exacerbates the community's assessment of the risk.

Morally Irrelevant versus Morally Relevant

Some risks are just risks; others are wrongs or evils as well. The distinguishing characteristic of moral imperatives, of course, is that they are to be obeyed without counting the cost. This has happened with many kinds of environmental risk. To many ears it now sounds callous, if not immoral, to assert that cleaning up a river or catching a midnight dumper is not worth the expense, that the cost outweighs the risk, that there are less expensive ways to save lives. Consider an analogy—the police do not always catch child molesters, but they know not to argue that an occasional molested child is an "acceptable risk."

It is best to think of health risk (i. e., hazard) and outrage as two completely independent variables. The greater the outrage, the more public concern there will be about risk—regardless of whether the situation is or is not a serious health hazard. The less the outrage, the harder it will be to generate public concern—again, regardless of whether or not the hazard is serious.

THE POLITICS OF HAZARD, OUTRAGE, AND RISK COMMUNICATION

Below is a 2 × 2 matrix that illustrates the four main possible combinations of hazard and outrage. It is an oversimplification, of course, but a useful way to think about risk communication.

	High outrage	Low outrage
High hazard	1	2
Low hazard	3	4

The cases in box 4 obviously create no problem. Box 1 should contain the consensus issues, where everybody unites against the "bad guys." The interesting boxes, of course, are 2 and 3. In box 2 are all the serious risks that are nearly impossible to get people excited about—smoking, not wearing a seat belt, geological radon, etc. They kill people, but they do not interest people very much. In box 3 fall the interesting, politically "sexy" issues that are relatively less important in terms of health. They are genuine outrages, but small threats to health.

This matrix poses a very serious problem for environmental groups. In days past, there were plenty of environmental issues in box 1. Environmental groups could—and did—harness and shape public outrage in order to focus attention on serious hazards, and the results included a lot of critical environmental legislation.

There are still some issues in box 1, but increasingly environmentalists are stuck with difficult choices between box 2 and box 3. Low-outrage hazards do not increase membership or contributions. An environmental group that focuses on low-outrage hazards has left politics and gone into the education business—a much less exciting business. On the other hand, focusing on low-hazard outrages involves less environmentalism and more community organizing. Mobilizing against outrage is an important public service even when the hazard is low—but environmentalists are truest to their heritage when they are saving lives and preserving ecosystems as well as fighting for fairness and community control. The dilemma for environmental groups can be seen in their failure (with some exceptions) to respond strongly to geological radon and in their strained effort to stake out a livable position on the siting of new hazardous waste facilities.

While environmental groups are at least aware of the dilemma, it is apparently invisible to most of government and industry. Government, in particular, often assumes that hazard is the only component in risk issues. It systematically ignores the factors that contribute to outrage—and in the process, all too often, it triggers more outrage. Government insists on ignoring the psychological and political dimensions of risk, everything from failing to give the community some control over the decision, to refusing to acknowledge the legitimacy of emotions, to insisting on telling people they have no business worrying about toxic waste if they smoke or ski or drive. A good example of self-defeating government behavior involved community people who were very nervous about barrels of low-level radioactive waste. Some local bus drivers asked for dosimeters to check their exposure as they drove past the storage site. The agency involved hotly refused on the grounds that there was no measurable exposure and it would be "bad science" to "take their foolish objections seriously" by giving the citizens a chance to find out for themselves.

In summary, advocacy groups build citizen outrage intentionally because that is what they do best. Government agencies too often build citizen outrage unintentionally because they feel it would be bad science to pay attention to psychological reality. Therefore, the general public continues to get more and more outraged about certain risks at the expense of certain other risks, and all too often these are (in hazard terms) the wrong risks.

The solutions are obvious, although not easy. First, we need to teach people about hazard, to help them understand which are the serious risks. Despite what some believe, people are able to understand risk data. Consider the correlation between what a weather forecaster predicts about the probability of rain and the number of people who carry umbrellas the next morning. Teaching people about hazard is the long-term solution.

Second, we have to do everything we can to make serious hazards outrageous. The furor over second-hand smoke, for example, is the best thing that has happened to the campaign against smoking and has probably saved thousands of smokers' lives.

Third, we have to stop contributing to the outrage of insignificant hazards. As long as government and industry manage low-hazard risks in genuinely outrageous ways—without consulting the community, for example—citizens will continue to overestimate these risks and activists will continue to mobilize against them.

Reducing the issue of public risk perception to hazard versus outrage is not to suggest that this summarizes all that is known about the issue. But it is a way of beginning to understand the regularity in public perception and public response to risk. Any risk communication we undertake will be more successful if we realize that we are talking about outrage, not just about hazard.

III

Government Risk Communication Programs

7

The Government as Lighthouse

A Summary of Federal Risk Communication Programs

Frederick W. Allen

Since early times, certain activities have been undisputed as important functions of governments, such as conducting foreign relations and warfare and managing a monetary system. Another classic function of government has been to operate lighthouses, which can be considered one of the first and archetypical kinds of risk communication. A light or a foghorn indicates that danger is present. The lighthouse provides an interesting analogy for the various risk communication programs that the federal government has developed since the founding of the Republic.

The primary source of information for this paper is the Inventory of Government Risk Communication Programs (Appendix A). The inventory is a first attempt to summarize federal risk communication efforts. It is not comprehensive and should not be used to derive statistically significant conclusions. Rather, the inventory is intended to highlight the innovative, unique, or particularly interesting aspects of the wide variety of government risk communication programs. For each agency, the inventory includes background information; an overview of the agency's risk communication messages, target audiences, and communication channels and selected programs; a brief summary of research, planning, and evaluation activities; and identification of information resources.

In reviewing the inventory, several observations become apparent regarding the role of the federal government in risk communication (these also apply to state and local government). The first and most significant point is the number and variety of risk communication programs. Most of the programs have certain unique aspects, which indicates that much can be learned from their diversity. This diversity underscores the fact that a program that works for one agency may not necessarily work for another. The conditions under which agencies and programs within an agency operate help to explain why these

---

Frederick W. Allen • Office of Policy Analysis, U. S. Environmental Protection Agency, Washington, D. C. 20460. The opinions expressed here are the author's and not necessarily those of the agency.

programs are so different. In that respect, our government has come a long way from the simple operation of lighthouses.

The second observation is that risk communication is perhaps one of the least understood functions of government. While foreign relations, national defense, and economics are intensively researched and studied, risk communication is an area of government activity that has not been adequately studied or understood. This is especially significant in light of the third observation, which is that risk communication is potentially one of the most powerful domestic functions of government. Therefore, risk communication deserves much more attention.

OBJECTIVES AND FOCUS OF RISK COMMUNICATION

Much of the diversity in federal risk communication programs can be attributed to the differences in the missions and mandates of the 14 agencies* that are described in the inventory. Their risk communication activities range from single advisories on specific chemicals to comprehensive multimedia programs that address broad issues. The amounts of resources that are devoted to these different programs also vary widely.

In examining the reasons for these different efforts, it is useful to think of a continuum where at one end government is requiring people to do something and at the other government is exhorting people to do something. Risk communication usually falls on the exhortation end, but requiring and exhorting are not mutually exclusive activities and often operate together. In addition, risk communication can serve to correct a lack of information or enhance available information, so that individuals can make appropriate decisions.

At CPSC, for example, information and education activities may accompany a mandatory or voluntary standard or be completely separate. Information and education efforts also may be in response to an imminent hazard where it is difficult to identify the people affected (e.g., people who possess a product) and thus may require a general information campaign to inform the public.

At EPA, the decision to develop an advisory or risk communication program may stem from jurisdictional responsibilities or limitations. For example, an office may develop an advisory (1) if the risk is outside EPA's area of regulation, as in the case of certain occupational risks; (2) as an interim measure while regulatory action is pursued; (3) if the nature of the risk makes standards infeasible; or (4) in response to requests from regional, state, and local constituencies.

The federal risk communication programs also have a variety of focuses. In general,

*Agencies surveyed were the Agency for Toxic Substances and Disease Registry (ATSDR), Centers for Disease Control (CDC), Consumer Product Safety Commission (CPSC), Environmental Protection Agency (EPA), Food and Drug Administration (FDA), National Center for Health Statistics (NCHS), National Cancer Institute (NCI), National Heart, Lung, and Blood Institute (NHLBI), National Institute for Occupational Safety and Health (NIOSH), Nuclear Regulatory Commission (NRC), Office on Smoking and Health (OSH), Occupational Safety and Health Administration (OSHA), the United States Air Force (USAF), and the U.S. Department of Agriculture (USDA).

Specific information regarding foci, program types, audiences, information dissemination, and materials is presented on a program-by-program basis in Tables 1 to 5.

Table 1. Focus of Risk Communications

Agency	Focus of risk communications
ATSDR	Health effects of exposure to toxic chemicals at Superfund sites
CDC	Public health: disease and injury prevention and health promotion
CPSC	Consumer protection and product safety
DoD	Exposure to toxic chemicals around military installations
EPA	Exposure to toxic chemicals
FDA	Exposure to chemicals in food, pharmaceuticals, and cosmetics, and risks from medical equipment
NCHS	Morbidity and mortality data
NCI	Cancer prevention and control
NHLBI	Prevention and control of heart, lung, and blood diseases
NIOSH	Occupational safety and health
NRC	Safety issues associated with nuclear materials
OSH	Health consequences of tobacco use
OSHA	Occupational safety and health
USDA	Food production and protection and nutrition

most of the programs focus on exposure to toxic chemicals in the workplace or environment; disease prevention related to life-style factors such as smoking and diet; or product safety and consumer protection (see Table 1). The primary objective or intended effect of most programs fall into the following general categories enumerated by Vincent Covello (see Table 2):

1. Information and education.
2. Behavior change and protective action.
3. Disaster warning/emergency information.
4. Joint problem solving/conflict resolution.

Table 2. Typology of Program(s)

Agency	Education and information	Behavior change and protective action	Disaster warning and emergency information	Conflict resolution and problem solving
ATSDR	X		X	
CDC	X	X	X	X
CPSC	X	X		
DoD	X		X	X
EPA	X	X	X	X
FDA	X	X		
NCHS	X			
NCI	X	X		
NHLBI	X	X		
NIOSH	X	X	X	
NRC	X		X	
OSH	X	X		
OSHA	X	X	X	
USDA	X	X		

All of the agencies described in the inventory have information and education programs. Most of the agencies also are involved in action or behavior change activities; therefore, they are confronted with the difficulties of changing behavior even when people are knowledgeable about a risk. (According to OSH, nearly everyone who smokes believes that smoking is hazardous to their health.) Additionally, many of the agencies have programs to warn people about disasters and provide emergency information. However, very few of these federal agencies have joint problem-solving or conflict resolution activities, which suggests that this an area deserving of attention. Clearly, risk communicators must recognize the appropriate category for their programs, if the programs are to be effective.

Target Audiences

Federal risk communication programs also vary in terms of their target audiences. It is evident that there are many publics—local publics, patients, workers, health professionals, the media, industry, and many others—and each public has its own unique characteristics. The different agencies use various means to understand and reach these various audiences (see Table 3).

The National Cancer Institute (NCI), for example, routinely conducts market research focusing on citizens' risk concerns. In the 1970s, people were concerned about chemicals in the environment as a cause of cancer. In the 1980s, the concerns have shifted to life-style factors (e.g., smoking and diet), and NCI's education programs have changed accordingly. The National Heart, Lung, and Blood Institute employs focus groups, interviews, questionnaires, and surveys to track the public's attitudes and behaviors, particularly among high-risk groups.

Communication Channels

It also is apparent from the inventory that different agencies rely on varied channels and vehicles for information dissemination, including direct mail, the mass media, trade associations and labor unions, manufacturers and retailers, intermediaries, local and state government agencies, clearinghouses, and hotlines (see Table 4). Many of the agencies surveyed emphasized the importance of identifying their audiences' regular sources of information before planning a communication program and selecting appropriate channels.

The agencies also are paying particular attention to the groups they work with and the intermediaries they select. Several are focusing on increasing the involvement of health professionals in the risk communication process, and, indeed, the medical community, public health groups, and voluntary health agencies often are willing to distribute materials developed by the agencies. Other agencies have involved industry, labor organizations, and trade associations in their risk communication programs as a means of fostering cooperation and using available resources. For example, NIOSH, through its New Directions Grants Program, is involving labor and trade organizations in the delivery of safety and health services to target populations with special needs. In addition, there are a number of instances in which agencies with common interests have formed networks to de-

Table 3. Target Audiences

Agency	General public: National	General public: Local	Workers	Health professsionals	Health educators	Community leaders	International state and local health agencies	Industry	Media	Other government agencies	Special target groups
ATSDR		X		X	X		X			X	Persons living near Superfund sites
CDC	X	X	X	X	X	X	X	X		X	
CPSC	X			X	X		X	X		X	Elderly, infants, children
Dod		X	X			X					Communities near military bases
EPA	X	X	X	X	X	X	X	X	X	X	
FDA	X	X		X				X			
NCHS	X			X			X			X	
NCI	X			X	X		X		X		High-risk populations
NHLBI	X			X	X		X		X		High-risk populations
NIOSH			X	X	X		X	X		X	
NRC	X	X	X	X					X		
OSH	X			X	X				X		Adolescents, pregnant women, children, smokers
OSHA			X	X	X			X			
USDA	X	X		X	X		X				

Table 4. Channel/Vehicle of Information Dissemination

Agency	Media: Print	Media: Radio	Intermediaries: Voluntary health agencies	Health professionals and educators	State, regulatory and local agencies	Industry: Trade association manufacturers	Clearinghouse/ data base	Other
ATSDR			X	X			X	Public meetings, registries
CDC	X		X	X	X			
CPSC	X	X	X	X		X		
DoD	X				X			Community public meetings
EPA	X	X	X	X	X	X	X	Community public meetings
FDA	X		X	X		X		
NCHS	X						X	Other government agencies
NCI	X	X	X	X	X		X	
NHLBI	X	X	X	X	X			
NIOSH	X					X	X	
NRC	X							
OSH	X	X	X	X		X	X	
OSHA	X		X	X	X	X		
USDA	X				X			

velop a shared risk communication program with broad messages; EPA, NIOSH, and OSHA, for instance, have collaborated in an effort to inform brake-and-clutch auto mechanics about the risks of asbestos exposure. Indeed, one of the results of the January 1987 Workshop on the Role of Government in Health Risk Communication and Public Education was the formation of the Interagency Group on Public Education and Communication, which includes 15 federal agencies and is under the auspices of the Task Force on Environmental Cancer and Heart and Lung Disease.

Message Development

Federal agencies develop their messages in several ways, depending on the specific risk situation and the target audience. One of the lessons that has been learned by federal agencies, often the hard way, is that it is important to set realistic, achievable aims and goals, instead of attempting to cure all cancer or eliminate all pollution.

Another lesson in message development that has been learned by NIOSH and a number of other agencies, including EPA, is how difficult it is to make the risk seem real when the risk is chronic and the basic evidence is derived from animal studies. It is much easier to develop a message to which the audience will listen if there is a clear, acute risk to humans.

It is also interesting to observe that while all of the agencies surveyed are trying to communicate with the public about different kinds of risks, fewer than half pretest their messages before they are executed. Generally, agencies develop messages on the basis of their experience and how they think the audience will react, without first pretesting them. This practice should be changed.

Materials and Products

Many agencies rely on printed materials, including news releases, to distribute their messsages, primarily because of costs. Some agencies also develop broadcast materials, which are much more expensive but are useful in certain cases. Some of the agencies also have been creating user-friendly data bases, which can be useful to specialized audiences (see Table 5).

Evaluation

The whole area of risk communication is probably one of the least understood functions of government. A major reason for this is that, as the inventory indicates, federal agencies do little evaluation of their risk communication programs. This mirrors the fact that they do little pretesting.

Many reasons exist for this lack of program evaluation. Evaluation requires assessing the goals of risk communication activities, which is difficult if the programs lack clearly stated objectives. In addition, risk communication programs may be eliminated if they are shown to be ineffective, rather than reorganized and improved. Evaluation also is difficult because many confounding factors are involved in such an analysis. Surveys can provide

Table 5. Products and Materials

Agency	Labels	PSAs	Press releases	Articles	Hotline	Brochures/ publications	Advisories	Audiovisual	Data base	Fact sheets	Miscellaneous
ATSR						×	×		×		
CDC			×	×		×					
CPSC	×	×	×	×	×	×	×			×	Newsletter
DoD		×		×			×			×	
EPA	×	×	×	×	×	×	×	×	×	×	Workshops, public meetings
FDA	×		×	×		×	×				
NCHS						×				×	Public reports
NCI		×	×	×	×	×		×	×	×	Press kits
NHLBI		×	×	×	×	×		×		×	Press kits
NIOSH						×	×	×	×		
NRC			×								Media seminars
OSH		×		×		×	×	×	×	×	
OSHA	×					×	×	×			
USDA				×		×				×	

information on change, but it is difficult to attribute that change to one specific campaign or another. In addition, many people working in risk communication programs have not been trained to perform evaluations.

The costs involved in doing evaluations also can be high, and the attitude of many agencies is that, given their limited budgets, they should focus on simply getting the message out and hope that it is effective. However, the costs do not always have to be high, and the activity itself should not be considered optional. The CPSC actually has been required by its congressional oversight committees to perform program evaluations; evaluation activities should be required more often. In some current EPA projects, we are trying to build into the planning stages some provision for evaluating the effectiveness of risk communication activities. Federal, state, and local agencies should include an evaluation component in their risk communication programs. Finally, as more programs incorporate evaluation components, there will be a need to study the results in order to develop guidelines for improving risk communication and choosing the most appropriate types of activities for a particular campaign.

Let Us Be Lighthouses

Evaluation is important because risk communication is potentially one of the most powerful domestic functions of government. It could be argued that it can actually outrank regulation as a powerful tool because, ultimately, regulation and many government programs are based on what the public wants. The government has a strong opportunity, through its risk communication programs, to play a role in helping the public determine what it wants.

It is clear, therefore, that we all need to give risk communication a good deal more attention. Let us be lighthouses pointing out not only danger but also the best channels for our organizations to take into the harbors.

8

Qualitative Risk Assessment

Experiences and Lessons

Barry L. Johnson

The purposes for presenting this chapter are twofold. The first is to discuss the Agency for Toxic Substances and Disease Registry (ATSDR) programs that bear on the subject of health risk communication and public education. The second is to share some of ATSDR's experiences and lessons gained from our health assessment program.

The central thesis of this chapter is that risk communication and public education must begin by appreciating that we, as agents of the government, are dealing with people—not abstract entities, not "demographic groups," not political constituents, but people in the mainstream of our nation's society. If we fail to understand their concerns, feelings, mistrust, and uncertainties, and do not factor these into our actions, we will surely fail to communicate with them, or help them to achieve any level of education about health risk. Please note that I said communicate with, not communicate to, the public. There is a vast difference between the two.

ATSDR'S PROGRAMS RELEVANT TO RISK COMMUNICATION

The ATSDR was created in 1980 with the passage of the Comprehensive Environmental Response, Compensation, and Liability Act (also known as Superfund). The intent of Congress was to create a federal public health agency that would specialize in the health effects of hazardous substances in the environment. In this regard, the agency was to work as an independent agency with the Environmental Protection Agency (EPA) and the states to assess and communicate the effects on public health of uncontrolled releases of haz-

Barry L. Johnson • Agency for Toxic Substances and Disease Registry, Public Health Service, Atlanta, Georgia 30333.

ardous substances into the environment. The ATSDR provides public health services to other government agencies, the private sector, and the general public on issues related to hazardous substances, and supports research that enlarges the base of knowledge about the effects of hazardous substances on human health. The ATSDR does not perform risk management, nor is it a regulatory agency.

The Superfund law of 1980 specified five areas of principal responsibility for ATSDR. These five areas, and their relevance to risk communication and public education, are as follows:

Health assessments—The ATSDR health assessment is the evaluation of data and information on the release of hazardous substances into the environment in order to assess any current or future impact on public health, develop health advisories or other health recommendations, and identify studies or actions needed to evaluate and prevent human health effects.

Medical consultation—The ATSDR provides medical and public health consultation and advice to EPA, the Coast Guard, the states, and local health officials in instances of emergency releases of hazardous substances. An example would be a transportation mishap in which an organic chemical is released into the environment. A 24-hour service is staffed by physicians, toxicologists, environmental health scientists, and public health advisors to respond to such incidents. When contacted, ATSDR advises on the public health implications presented by the release. Risk communication involves primarily emergency response officials and local medical care providers, although on occasion the agency is also contacted by local news media.

Information development—The agency is charged under Superfund to develop, maintain, and distribute information on hazardous substances. The ATSDR provides funds, advice, and assistance to the National Library of Medicine (NLM) and others in their development of computerized data bases on hazardous substances. Our vision is to further enhance the NLM toxicological data base and to make it more widely available to the states and the general public.

Exposure registries—The Superfund Act mandates ATSDR to establish and maintain a national registry of all persons exposed to hazardous substances. Communicating to the public the purposes of these registries, establishing criteria, and assessing benefits to individuals for participating in a national registry are procedures that must be carefully considered. Such registries will be essential if relationships between exposure to environmental toxicants and resulting health effects are to be better understood. The information gained from the registries will need to be communicated back to the registrants. This is another important way to educate the public about hazardous substances.

Research—The agency is authorized by Superfund to develop information on associations between exposure to hazardous substances and effects on human health. This is interpreted to be a research directive, since much remains to be learned about the human health effects of uncontrolled environmental toxicants, especially the long-term effects of low-level exposure to toxicants known to be toxic at higher exposure levels. The ATSDR therefore supports or conducts epidemiological and toxicological research intended to clarify associations between exposure and health effects. The outcome of this research becomes very important in the conduct of risk assessment and, ultimately, risk communication.

In addition to these five responsibilities given to ATSDR under Superfund, the Superfund Amendments and Reauthorization Act of 1986 (SARA) added, or revised, these three responsibilities:

Health assessments—ATSDR is required to conduct, by December 10, 1988, a health assessment of each site on the National Priorities List (NPL). Moreover, any site added to the NPL must obtain a health assessment within one year. The act also permits an individual citizen to petition for a health assessment of a site. Obviously, communication about health assessment findings to the public becomes an exercise in risk communication.

Toxicological profiles—The ATSDR and EPA are required under SARA to rank the most hazardous substances at Superfund sites, after which ATSDR, in cooperation with EPA, will develop a toxicological profile for each ranked chemical. The profiles will be useful in communicating health risk and in public education.

Medical education—Medical education materials are to be developed that can be used by health care providers in attending to persons exposed to hazardous substances and by medical educators for their use in medical school curriculae.

ATSDR HEALTH ASSESSMENTS

The agency's health assessments are our principal statements on health risk. The ATSDR conducts health assessments of releases of hazardous substances, most often from waste sites. These health assessments are qualitative risk assessments, performed by a multidisciplinary team of physicians, toxicologists, environmental health scientists, and public health advisors. The agency renders an opinion on the health implications of the release of a hazardous substance, based on environmental sampling data, toxicity data, plume migration estimates, pathways of human exposure, and human populations at risk of exposure. These data are normally furnished by EPA but are sometimes supplemented by data from state or local agencies.

The product of the health assessment is a report to EPA, copied to the applicable state agency, that states ATSDR's opinion of the health implications of the evaluated site and provides recommendations as to health actions to take in order to reduce exposure to hazardous substances. The ATSDR often accompanies EPA and state officials into meetings with the public to discuss health risks associated with individual sites. These contacts with the public are sometimes preceded by visits from our staff to the site of concern. The purpose is to obtain information (e.g., human exposure information) not otherwise available.

EXPERIENCES AND LESSONS

From these site visits and appearances at public meetings have come experiences and lessons that are worth sharing. The ATSDR's experience suggests that the public has little understanding of numerical estimates of risk. That is not to say that ATSDR does not accept such estimates; indeed, ATSDR accepts the value of any useful, credible process to set priorities for risk management. However, those using quantitative estimates of risk are obligated to inform the affected public of any limitations or uncertainties of their methods and estimates. Further, the use of estimates of comparative (i.e., relative) risk is not always persuasive to the public. A public that is anxious about a waste disposal site is not going to be impressed when that perceived risk is compared to the risk of not using a seat belt.

What the public does accept is a candid, honest expression of risk when expressed by a source they trust. Trust is central to successful risk communication. Other principles of communication that ATSDR has observed are as follows:

First, the communication must be credible to those receiving the message, or the message, regardless of its accuracy or urgency, will not be heard. One sometimes unappreciated contributor to credibility is constancy of appearance by government agents. To be more specific, the public can relate to persons they get to know. One example is that of a small mining community in a western state. The town was built on top of a former mine tailing site, and the soil is contaminated with lead, arsenic, and zinc. Several meetings were held with the residents over a two-year span, but only one of three government agencies had its same representative at all meetings. It should be obvious which agency was perceived as credible by the town's residents.

Second, the message must be accurate and honest, one based on contemporary knowledge and accepted scientific methods. If the message is wrong, that fact will soon become known, as there are usually persons waiting to critically evaluate it.

Third, the message must be presented in language that can be understood by those receiving it. Risk messages couched in technical or government jargon will not be effective. In this regard, the news media can be of great assistance in helping to communicate health risk in terms understandable to the public.

Fourth, the message must be developed by using input from those affected by it. This means listening to members of the public who express concern about their exposure to hazardous substances, keeping them apprised of, and involved in, study designs and progress, and presenting and discussing study outcomes with them.

Finally, the effectiveness of any communication from a health assessment should be evaluated after its release. The ATSDR evaluates its communications by asking regional staff to conduct follow-up interviews with persons involved with, and affected by, the risk communication.

These simple principles, when applied with an appreciation for the importance of the public's concern and rights, will enhance risk communication but will not always guarantee success. Success comes from gaining experience in communication, evaluating its effectiveness, and attempting to do better in the future based on what has been learned.

9

De Minimis *Risk from Chemicals in Food*

Robert J. Scheuplein

The concept of *de minimis* risk is based on the idea that certain risks involving exposures to carcinogens are too small to cause concern. If this idea has merit, it will require a real effort in risk communication to gain public acceptance. It will involve asking the public to unlearn certain fears concerning carcinogens that federal agencies are in part responsible for creating.

Before discussing *de minimis* risk, communicating food-borne risk should be placed in the context of the Food and Drug Administration's (FDA's) special history of dealing with chemicals in foods. Potential risk from food has been a matter of public concern since 1879 when the first bill "For Preventing the Adulteration of Articles of Food and Drink" was introduced in Congress. In contrast to this long history, the statutes that govern newer agencies such as the Environmental Protection Agency (EPA), Occupational Safety and Health Administration (OSHA), National Institute of Occupational Safety and Health (NIOSH), and Consumer Protection and Safety Commission (CPSC) have been in existence for 25 years or less. If one looks at the capability of the public to develop strong attitudes and perceptions of chemical risk over a longer time span, it is quite impressive. The 82-year history of the Food, Drug and Cosmetic Act shows quite clearly that the public, through the media, is capable of understanding risk, responding to perceived outrages, and effectively lobbying Congress to force appropriate legislative changes.

During the period from 1879 when the first congressional bill was introduced until 1906 when the Federal Food and Drug Act was enacted into law, Americans were becoming increasingly concerned over the safety of their food supply for several reasons, all relating to the fact that much of the food was no longer produced in the home or in the neighborhood and that incidents of adulteration had increased. Unwholesome imports

Robert J. Scheuplein • Office of Toxicological Sciences, U.S. Food and Drug Administration, Washington, D. C. 20204.

were being "dumped" into the United States, and domestic food was being debased by intentional substitution of inferior substances. Damage was concealed and some food was simply filthy. Proponents of the 1906 act were also alarmed by the accumulating number of unfamiliar chemicals that were added to preserve food and improve its appearance and texture, a problem created by the necessity to store food longer and transport it further.

The notion of adulteration, originally intended to apply more to intentional debasement of food for profit, came to embrace the addition of "unsafe chemical additives" that seemed to be provided more for the producer's convenience than the consumer's. The 1906 statute's central idea was the prevention of acts by food producers, motivated either by greed, carelessness, or ignorance, that caused ordinarily wholesome food to become unsafe or that resulted in its misrepresentation. There was no expressed intent to improve the safety of natural food as selected and prepared by individuals. If improved health or less risk could be had through better nutrition or a better selection of foodstuffs, this was not perceived in 1906 as a matter for federal intervention. Even now, despite the probably significant risks associated with traditional dietary practices, there is still no great public clamor for federal intervention in the use or the preparation of common foods. As an example of the accepted reality of such risk, consider the following statement from the 1982 National Academy of Sciences (NAS) Report, "Diet, Nutrition, and Cancer":

> . . . although the formula is still not known, we do have some estimate of the benefits it . . . [a precise formula for modifying the diet to minimize the incidence of cancer] . . . would bestow. Judging from the observed differences in cancer rates among populations with different diets, it is highly likely that the United States will eventually have the option of adopting a diet that reduces its incidence of cancer by approximately one-third, and it is absolutely certain that another third could be prevented by abolishing smoking. . . .

The risks the NAS are talking about are many orders of magnitude—thousands of times larger—than the carcinogenic risks quoted for some food additives and contaminants, e.g., saccharin and polychlorinated biphenyls (PCBs). Are people unaware of these facts? Is it really because of poor government efforts at communication? Or is it that we tend to respond negatively to information that implies that we should change the comfortable habits of a lifetime? On these matters, is it federal intervention that is less likely to be welcomed and the risk that is more likely to be accepted?

REVISION OF THE FOOD AND DRUG ACT

Inadequacies in the 1906 act were recognized from the start and from time to time bills were presented to rectify this or that omission. But particularly during the golden glow of the 1920s, the political climate was not conducive to reform. The depression aggravated the continuing evils. Sharpened competition led to more outrageous advertising claims, which were immune from policing under the 1906 act. Radio, hardly having time to develop an advertising code, filled the airwaves with false therapeutic promises. Inflated promotion and product cheapening affected other industries as well, especially cosmetics, on which the 1906 law was silent.

A few days after he was inaugurated in 1933, President Franklin D. Roosevelt authorized a revision of the Food and Drug Act. It took five years for the revised act to become law. In the case of both the 1906 and the 1938 acts, the regulated industries lobbied with greater effectiveness than did consumers. Women's organizations in both decades were the most important and steadfast of consumers' champions. In the end, the passage of legislation depended on public pressure felt in Congress, generated in each case by a dramatic threat to public health. In 1906, it was the fear of impure meat dramatized by Upton Sinclair's exposé, *The Jungle*, a book that horrified consumers with its portrayal of conditions in the meat-packing industry. In 1937, the "Elixir of Sulfanilamide" disaster resulted from a misguided effort to provide a liquid dosage form for one of the first "wonder drugs," sulfanilamide. The company chemist had tested the solvent, diethylene glycol, for appearance, fragrance, and flavor, but not for safety. Over 100 people died and many hundreds were made seriously ill.

The 1938 act and its interpretation by FDA substantially broadened FDA's authority in the direction of protecting the consumer from unsafe food per se, rather than acting solely in response to an act of food adulteration by a food manufacturer or distributor. For the first time, the law contained a provision that prohibited the marketing of even a traditional food if it were shown to be "ordinarily injurious," i.e., harmful to typically healthy individuals under ordinary conditions of use. No intervening act of adulteration was required and no foreign substance need be added, but the ordinarily injurious standard of safety was lower than that for added constituents. Natural toxic constituents in food, such as oxalic acid in rhubarb or solanine in potatoes, could be deemed adulterants only if the food contained them in sufficient quantity to be considered ordinarily injurious. Added constituents, on the other hand, were made subject to the far stiffer "may render injurious" standard. Under this provision, FDA need show only the existence of some significant possibility that the food could be injurious to the health of a consumer.

The 1938 act also authorized FDA, for the first time, to permit the presence of safe levels of poisonous and deleterious added substances if such substances were necessary in the production of food or if they were unavoidable even under good manufacturing processes. The FDA has taken the position that it may, under this section of the act, establish tolerances or action levels for environmental contaminants. Examples are aflatoxin in corn and peanuts, DDT in fish, and PCBs in fish and shellfish. The tolerance is established by considering the contaminant's toxicity, the extent to which its occurrence can be controlled, and the capability of analytical methods to measure the contaminant and enable enforcement of the tolerance. The practical significance of this provision is that a contaminant, such as aflatoxin, is permitted in food at a risk that is probably significantly higher than it would be if it were a direct food additive and regulated as such.

This original triad of provisions for the three categories of food substances, which are traditional foods, additives, and unavoidable additives or contaminants, has been amended several times since 1938, usually to separate out a particular class of added substances for special regulatory attention. For example, Congress required the registration and licensing of pesticides under the Pesticide and Chemical Act of 1954. In 1958, the Food Additives Amendment established a similar preclearance scheme for direct and indirect additives (processing or packaging migrants). The same preclearance scheme was extended to color additives in 1960 and to animal drugs in 1962. These amendments reversed the legal burden of proof demanded under the law and fundamentally changed the regulation of intentional additives in the United States. The FDA was no longer required to show that a marketed additive might be injurious to consumers; instead the sponsor had to provide experimental evidence to FDA demonstrating that the additive would be safe for its intended use prior to receiving approval for marketing.

THE DELANEY CLAUSE AND DE MINIMIS *RISK*

The safety standard for additives [sec. 402(a)(1) and sec. 409] was a demonstration of a "reasonable certainty of no harm" under anticipated and foreseeable levels of exposure. In addition, carcinogenic additives were banned under the Delaney Clause, which states that no additive shall be deemed safe if it is found to induce cancer when ingested by humans or animals. This applied to food additives, color additives, and animal drug residues.

The purpose in presenting this discussion of FDA's food safety standards is to illustrate a few facts: the statutory provisions permit greater risk or less assurance of safety for substances of greater perceived value (traditional food); they permit less risk for inherently unnecessary substances, no matter how useful (additives); and they tolerate intermediate risk for necessary or unavoidable substances (contaminants). These statutory provisions enacted over a period of almost 80 years represent a series of risk-benefit judgments by Congress. There are many reasons to suppose that the public currently is more aware and more actively interested in such matters, but these provisions, enacted in every case only after extensive public hearings and extensive media attention, show that historically public opinion is capable of influencing such decisions and from time to time modifying the way the risks are controlled.

The FDA now faces the question of how to interpret the Delaney Clause under circumstances radically different from those at the time of its enactment. We now realize that many foods and some food additives contain carcinogens at extremely low levels, levels that are far below threatening levels and possibly below any toxicologically significant level at all. The FDA's response has been to adopt a risk assessment approach to the interpretation of the general safety standards and a *de minimis* approach to the application of the Delaney Clause. In essence, the FDA has judged that it can determine whether the potential human risk from exposure to an animal carcinogen is so trivial as to be the functional equivalent of no risk at all.

A lively debate is now under way concerning the legality of the *de minimis* interpretation, and that issue is pending in the U.S. Court of Appeals. The issue involves important scientific, policy, and legal questions, including the following:

1. Are methods scientifically adequate to assess carcinogenic risks with sufficient accuracy?
2. What constitutes a "safe" or trivial level of human exposure to such substances?
3. Is it appropriate as a matter of policy for FDA to change prior interpretations of its statute if necessary to achieve that law's basic policy goals?
4. Is the *de minimis* doctrine correctly applied in the face of the absolute language of the Delaney Clause?

These questions are not easy to resolve and FDA is anxiously awaiting the court's decision. The FDA's basic premise is that *de minimis* situations are being exempted from a statutory command in order to implement, not to escape, the legislative design. All food additives at some level will inevitably contain carcinogenic impurities. Our analytical methods are now capable of detecting substances at the parts per trillion level. A literal interpretation of the statute could force FDA to ban hundreds of useful additives because they contain trace levels of carcinogens. Many of these occur at levels that are orders of magnitude lower than naturally occurring carcinogens found in traditional foods that are routinely permitted. The *de minimis* approach may be regarded as a controversial attempt to try to make scientific sense of the law in the face of these findings and in the absence of any recent explicit instructions from Congress. The *de minimis* approach is an exercise of an agency's discretion in the face of a law that many believe has become unworkable in accurately communicating the risk from chemicals in food. Only time will tell whether the courts and the public decide that it is still workable.

10

Interactions between State and Federal Programs

Peter D. Galbraith

Milton Russell, Assistant Administrator of the Environmental Protection Agency (EPA), said, "Real people are suffering and dying because they don't know when to worry and when to calm down. They don't know when to demand action to reduce risk, and when to relax because the health risks are trivial or simply not there." He went on to note that failure in risk communication can have several negative effects, including (1) diversion of societal attention and resources from important health or environmental problems; (2) diversion of personal attention from real risks that can be reduced to insignificant risks; (3) unnecessary human suffering due to high levels of anxiety and worry; and (4) defensive indifference or the attitude that if everything causes cancer, why do anything?

HISTORY

As the controversy over ethylene dibromide (EDB) and the "killer muffins" began to unfold, William Ruckelshaus, Administrator of the EPA, approached the Association of State and Territorial Health Officers (ASTHO) indicating the need for collaboration between EPA and the state health officers. While much was accomplished to enhance collaboration, there is a long way to go. The Environmental Protection Agency and state health officers now communicate much more effectively and health officers continue to work well with the Public Health Service and the Centers for Disease Control. However, the loop involving the three entities has not been closed, leaving considerable gaps in environmental public health and thus increased opportunity for lack of harmony in risk communication. The application of better science would also be a meaningful outcome of closing the loop.

Peter D. Galbraith • Connecticut Department of Health Services, Hartford, Connecticut 06106.

The State/EPA relationship has benefited tremendously from the creation of a permanent ASTHO Environment Committee, the inclusion of a health officer on EPA's State/EPA Committee, which meets quarterly, and the addition of health officials on a variety of EPA task forces and advisory groups.

If significant progress in risk communication is to be made, a great deal more attention needs to be paid to the issue of acceptable risk and relative risk. The traditional wisdom is that voluntary risks, such as smoking and use of alcohol, are acceptable, and nonvoluntary risks, such as EDB in grain products or alar in apples, are not. How then does one explain minimal public reaction to one of the most significant environmental risks over the past decade—radon?

A balanced perspective on relative risk needs to be addressed in elementary school. Children need to understand at an early age that life years lost before age 65 are 1.6 million per year from smoking, 1.5 million from alcohol, and 1.3 million from injuries. These, plus unintended pregnancy, obesity, improper nutrition, and handguns, would be high on the list of most public health officials when enumerating significant risks. The public would probably come up with a different list. The computerized health risk assessment developed in Rhode Island and used throughout Connecticut and numerous school districts in the country provides an exciting model for bringing this issue into the classroom.

Other research needs include perception of risks and benefits, comparative risk, sources of risk communication that are perceived to be most credible, the best communicator in a crisis, and the most effective means of presenting disagreements among experts. The latter is a problem health experts create for themselves day in and day out, EDB being an excellent example.

RISK ASSESSMENT/RISK MANAGEMENT

A tremendous amount of attention has been paid to the rudimentary science of risk assessment, which is the source of many risk communication problems. At the state level, most of the problems are created as risk management decisions are made. Some believe that one molecule of a chemical is too much, while others see more significant risks in other areas. Thus, the public gets confused and develops an attitude of defensive indifference.

Another area that should be examined as we seek to improve risk communication is the language of risk assessment and risk management. The presumption is that a risk exists and the process merely involves quantifying the risk. Also, as scientists, we do not feel comfortable saying that it is acceptable to eat the muffins or that there is no risk in letting your child go to school with a child who has AIDS. We choose to use a language that will satisfy our colleagues versus the public that we are trying to reassure.

STATE/FEDERAL COLLABORATION

Both the federal and state governments learned a great deal as to how they can benefit from improved collaboration during the EDB situation. As the issue of the pesticide alar was addressed in August 1985, we benefited from what had been learned, yet there were significant gaps and mistakes on both sides that complicated the risk communication tasks involved. The recent issue of lead in drinking water is an example of a risk communication problem that was created by the manner in which it was announced. The announcement came from the federal government with no warning to the states. It was perceived as an acute risk by many members of the public, who believed that they had been poisoning their children for many years as a result of the pipes in their homes. Instead, the federal and state governments could have developed a message and a strategy that together would have resulted in a more accurate and balanced communication. Radon is a case in which this kind of collaboration has worked well.

Just about every State Health Department has at least one and usually two electronic communication devices that could be used to facilitate risk communication efforts.

As agencies work together on joint releases of information regarding risks, they have an opportunity both from the federal and the state perspectives to recognize that sometimes the presentation and the resulting public perceptions may be as important as the findings themselves. This gives the opportunity to anticipate difficult questions and be better prepared to deal with them.

ESTIMATING RISK WITH NUMBERS

The use and abuse of numbers is something that both the federal and state governments should pay attention to. Frequently, when estimating the number of cancers that a substance may cause, the upper bound limit will be used, with no indication that the lower limit may indeed be zero. The use of these numbers also suggests a degree of precision in risk assessment that usually does not exist.

When talking about environmental contaminants, one rarely knows the whole truth, yet rarely does one simply say the answer to a question is not known. All too often, one gets into the area of personal opinion, which is what makes the headline, versus good science. Admitting error is often even more difficult.

The press often lets health risk experts get away with bad science, as do other health experts. The scientific experts are eager to dismiss a position based on bad science as simply a difference of opinion between two experts. The press should ask the follow-through questions such as: Is it safe to eat the apples? Should citizens move away from a chemical plant? What can a person do to reduce the risk?

In conclusion, it should be noted that although many of the recommendations for improved risk communication seem obvious, nonetheless they are continually and consistently violated. A simple commitment to joint federal/state press releases on sensitive issues would be a significant step forward in improving risk communication.

11

Interactions between Community/Local Government and Federal Programs

Thomas Wilson

The purpose of this chapter is to illustrate both the risk assessment needs of local officials and the ways in which we can help other levels of government with the risk communication process.

The health department of Elkhart County is a medium-sized health department in a medium-sized county. The population of Elkhart County is about 143,000 people. Our perspective may be more rural than that of risk communicators at the state and federal levels.

Our first experience with risk assessment occurred in 1979. At that time, some residents noticed a bad taste and funny smell in their water and had the water analyzed at a private laboratory. It was determined that benzene and several petroleum-related materials were in their drinking water.

Once we started investigating and determined that there was in fact a problem, people began to ask us questions about what all this meant to them in terms of health effects. What were the risks in drinking this water. We immediately looked for somebody to help us with the problem because, being a local agency, we did not have the funds or the capabilities to do the type of work that we knew would be necessary in that situation. As a result, we received health effects information from the Environmental Protection Agency (EPA) Region V. At that time, we were using Suggested No Adverse Response Levels* as a means of communicating potential risk.

Since that first case in 1979, the local health department has been involved in 39

*Suggested No Adverse Response Levels, now called Health Advisories, describe concentrations of contaminants in drinking water at which adverse effects would not be anticipated to occur. They are developed from data describing noncarcinogenic endpoints of toxicity and do not incorporate quantitatively any potential carcinogenic risk from such exposure. They are not legally enforceable federal standards.

Thomas Wilson • Elkhart County Solid Waste Disposal, Elkhart, Indiana 46517.

separate groundwater contamination cases within Elkhart County. We have also been involved in a variety of acute exposure cases related to the accidental release of hazardous materials. All these cases required some type of risk communication, i.e., an attempt to communicate to people what the potential health effects could be. Most of the information that we have used came from federal agencies.

Before describing the assistance we received from federal agencies, it will be useful to describe the background of local agency personnel and their very definite need for education in risk communication and risk assessment.

Local agency personnel bring a variety of backgrounds to their jobs. Our academic training comes from a wide variety of science and health programs. In my particular division, we carried out 12 different programs that ranged from traditional food protection to groundwater protection. We functioned as generalists and did not have a lot of specialized knowledge. We spent our time performing a variety of tasks in many different areas. Therefore, local agency personnel must rely on others for special cases. In our area, we relied on the State Departments of Health and Environmental Management and the EPA for specialized knowledge, training, and action.

We are readily accessible to the public because we live within the communities we serve. We meet our constituents in the grocery stores, at cocktail parties, wherever we go. When people have a problem and recognize us, they come up and talk to us about it. We also have contacts with local information systems. In our area, the various media have designated reporters to work directly with local government agencies.

We can be a mirror of the attitudes and concerns of our communities. We may even be a part of the exposed population. Our office is located in Elkhart, Indiana, where the municipal water supply has been contaminated with trichlorethylene for a number of years. The city is just now bringing that matter to resolution by developing treatment facilities for the water supply.

The interaction that occurred between our agency and the federal government happened in two ways. We were provided with technical and financial assistance. Technical assistance came in the form of laboratory services, a variety of field work and investigative procedures, and education. Again, there is a definite need for the education of local officials. All these activities have been vital to the resolution of our environmental contamination cases.

We solicited technical help in almost every groundwater contamination case that was identified. Our initial contact, generally because of protocol, was with a state agency. They would either then contact a federal agency on our behalf or ask us to make the contact directly. As time went on and we were able to develop relationships with various personnel at EPA's Region V, we began to ask for help directly. Because most of the federal agency offices are in Chicago or Indianapolis, our approach was to try to develop as much information as we could prior to the initial contact.

The risk communication process is intertwined with investigative work. As our investigations developed, the levels of contamination changed, the involved area expanded, or new contaminants were identified. Rarely did we progress through an investigation without developing data that required reinterpretation or new interpretation of the potential health effects. As soon as a change occurred, we would again ask for help from the EPA. Once we communicated to the people that they were exposed to different contaminants or that the levels had increased, their questions about potential health effects surfaced again.

We received a variety of tools from federal agencies to help us. One of the most useful to us was what we called exposure interpretation sheets. These were developed by the health effects specialists at EPA (see Table 1). They gave us this information as background material. They were one- to three-page letters that consolidated information developed by the National Academy of Sciences, the National Institute for Occupational Safety and Health, and the National Cancer Institute. The sheets also included a discussion section that gave various time-related exposure limits. Exposure limits, no matter how reliable, are something the public demands. They have to have some benchmark through which to gauge their exposures if they are going to be able to understand what all this information means to them.

Environmental Protection Agency representatives were also involved in conducting investigative procedures. Personalizing the activities is extremely important. Most of these required contact with the exposed population on an individual basis. It was impossible to go into a home and take a water sample without spending some time talking about the contamination case, and the potential health effects.

We usually tried to send one of our representatives along with the federal agency personnel during this process. This served two purposes: it helped educate us, and it also promoted a feeling of confidence among the concerned citizens. People like to be able to meet and talk to agency personnel. All agencies are under close scrutiny by the public. Individuals were quick to crtiticize if the investigation appeared to lack coordination.

We received periodic briefings by EPA representatives. These discussions were informal and often involved well-publicized problems outside our area. The staff developed into a good community resource. They were able to provide accurate answers or referrals for questions from the media or concerned citizens.

We also participated in different types of meetings. These ranged from strategy meetings of representatives from a variety of government agencies to publicly announced informational meetings where we would meet with people from the community and try to explain a problem to them.

Local agency personnel can be an important part of the risk communication process, but they need to have training in order to do this effectively. Our department got into the process out of necessity. We did a good job of investigating and determining that we had problems. Once we started talking to people about the fact that contaminants were in their drinking water, they wanted to know what the health effects were. It was important for us to be able to give them that information. We never really established a formalized communication process; it simply evolved over the course of time.

Local agency personnel can also serve as a buffer. People who need to talk to someone generally will call their local agency representative first. In addition, we can reduce the workload. In our area, we had multiple contamination cases that involved the same type of materials. After having worked through one particular case, be it benzene or trichlorethylene, we were then able to communicate directly with people without having to involve federal agencies first.

We also received financial assistance to communicate with the public about health risks, which was very important to us. In 1980, the Michigan Area Council of Govern-

Table 1. EPA Exposure Interpretation Sheet for 1,2-Dichloroethane: Recommended Limits in Drinking Water

1,2-Dichloroethane (DCE) has been evaluated in *Drinking Water & Public Health,* (National Academy of Sciences, 1977). The following includes reevaluation of that material, based on current evaluation concepts and the 1977 National Cancer Institute biosassy.

DCE is used in the manufacture of vinyl chloride and tetraethyl lead; as an insecticide, tobacco flavoring, and ingredient in paint and varnish removers; and in metal degreasing, chemical synthesis, and ore flotation.

DCE is slightly soluble in water ($^1/_{120}$). An EPA survey of 80 water samples analyzed showed DCE concentrations ranging from 0.02 to 6.0 micrograms (μg) per liter (U.S. EPA, 1975–560 4-75-5PB. 260961). Finished water in New Orleans showed the presence of 8.0 μg/liter (8 ppb).

DCE is rapidly absorbed from oral or pulmonary exposure and in mice. DCE is metabolized through liver dehalogenation and oxidation to the chloroacetic acid excretory product. In relation to other, similar compounds, DCE is slowly exhaled, due to greater lipid solubility, and has a greater tendency toward accumulation. The principal target organs in the mouse are liver, kidney, and adrenals.

Exposure in Man

The National Institute for Occupational Safety and Health has estimated that some 2 million workers may be exposed to DCE. Exposure in man to high concentrations of DCE results in irritation of the eyes, nose, and throat, with prolonged exposure affecting the central nervous system, liver, kidney, and adrenals. Accidental human ingestion of a single dose of 0.5–1.0 g/kg body weight (20–50 ml) has resulted in fatality. The autopsy showed liver necrosis as well as focal degeneration of the adrenal tissue and general necrosis.

Investigators have reported hemorrhagic lesions of most organs, and a depletion of clotting factors and thrombocytopenia in a DCE-poisoned patient. Hypocoagulability of blood may be a sensitive index of DCE exposure: chronic low-level exposures may produce these same symptoms. The recommended U.S. standard for occupational exposure to DCE is 5.0 ppm, since abnormalities have been described from exposure of as low as 10 ppm, and ranging up to 200 ppm.

Exposure in Animals

Carcinogenicity. In 1977, the National Cancer Institute (NCI) released data resulting from bioassays on rats and mice. Technical grade DCE was given postorally in corn oil at two dosage levels to male and female animals of each species. Untreated and vehicle controls were also evaluated. The animals received the following doses: 95 and 47 mg per day for rats of both sexes. The mice received 95 and 47 mg/kg per day (low dose) and 299 and 149 mg/kg per day (high dose). The dosage schedule was once a day, 5 times per week, for 78 weeks. Mammary and stomach tumors were diagnosed in DCE-fed rats, while mice showed a dose-dependent increase over the controls of hepatocellular carcinomas. Both species exhibited an increase in lung tumors.

Mutagenicity. DCE is considered to be a weak mutagen based on changes occurring in *Salmonella typhimurium* (TA 1530, TA 1535, and TA 1538) and in DNA polymerase-deficient *E. coli,* as well as in *Drosophila.* No teratogenic effects of any rate were reported.

Discussion. In light of the recent evidence by the NCI bioassays showing that DCE has carcinogenic properties, it is considered prudent to avoid exposure. The mouse population showed a dose-dependent response that further warrants caution. Although the capacity of DCE to cause genetic change is weak, it has been shown to cause mutations in microbial systems. Taken together, the NCI bioassays showing carcinogenicity and microbial tests for mutagenicity should put DCE in the suspect carcinogen class relative to humans (National Cancer Institute, 1977). With this in mind, it is pointed out that our limited level of sophistication in medical science precludes establishing "absolutely safe" levels of ingestion. Based on the animal data, it is currently the practice to extrapolate dose values to acceptable limits in attempting to protect the public health to the best of our capability.

Using the low dose for mice of 47 mg/kg per day, and using a safety factor of 100% (due to being the lowest dose which causes a carcinogenic response), it is recommended that the maximum level of DCE in drinking water be no more than 21 μg/liter for a 1-week exposure, and that the exposure for 1 month be no more than 2.1 μg/liter. A lifetime dose cannot be calculated with any degree of certainty and is contrary to the principals of protecting public health.

ments received federal funds from EPA to assist in the resolution of a groundwater contamination case. Part of that money was used to publish a weekly newsletter that was mailed directly to all the affected residents. The newsletter provided progress reports and health effects information. It even had a section called "Residents Speak Out," which contained letters from people who were affected by the contamination. This allowed residents to express their concerns or their outrage, and also let them participate in the communication process.

In 1984, because of the number of contamination cases with which we were dealing, we received a federal grant to develop a local groundwater protection program. This may have been due to the fact that our agency was quite a "squeaking wheel." Every time we had a contamination case, we called EPA's Region V for help. They may have finally decided that if they funded us, maybe we could do a better job ourselves and would not call on them as often for assistance.

One of the things that we did with these funds was to develop a slide-tape presentation. It was narrated by a local radio personality and included some music. It turned out to be a very entertaining as well as educational tool. We showed it to various service organizations and in the schools. The whole focus of the tape was to sensitize the community to our growing groundwater contamination problem. Both the newsletter and the slide-tape presentation were very effective tools in communicating health risks to local residents.

In conclusion, I would like to say that a coordinated effort by all the agencies that provide information to the general public is vital to the orderly resolution of health risk cases. The more closely we work with affected citizens and the more personalized we can make the information process, the better informed they will be. For instance, people tend to take notice if they can attend a meeting where an involved official is speaking to them directly and can answer their questions. While the most effective way to communicate is on a one-to-one basis, this clearly cannot be accomplished in every case. Site coordinators placed within a community can be a very effective means of dealing with concerned citizens.

The farther away we get from individual contact, the more room there is for confusion and misunderstanding. A coordinated effort involving competent, informed officials from all levels of government leads to effective risk communication and, eventually, to a better-informed citizenry.

REFERENCES

National Academy of Sciences–NRC. 1977. *Drinking Water and Health*, Washington, D.C., pp. 723–24.

National Cancer Institute. 1977. *Bioassay of Tetrachloroethylene for Possible Carcinogenicity*, CAS #127-18-4, NCI-CG-TR-13 DHEW Pub. 77-813, Washington, D.C.

12

A White House Perspective on Risk Communication

Alvin L. Young

The past two decades have ushered in a shift of almost revolutionary proportions in the study of health and disease. The preoccupation with infectious disease has been replaced with a heavy commitment to the study of chronic, life-threatening illnesses. Increasingly, more investigators have recognized that behaviors that place an individual at risk for developing physical illness seldom occur in isolation from other pathogenic activities. Although the public acknowledges that life-style and disease are related (e.g., smoking may be detrimental to your health), the fear of malign influences in our environment is so widespread today that the general public believes that it is those factors they cannot control that will bring about their early demise. Thus, a major concern is the presence of "unwanted" chemicals in our environment.

In 1984, the National Academy of Sciences noted that:

1. 65,000 chemicals are currently produced in the United States.
2. 12,000 are manufactured in substantial amounts.
3. 500–1000 new chemicals are added to the inventory each year.
4. The vast majority benefit society and improve the quality of our lives.
5. There are 30 laws regulating the use of chemicals in the United States (National Research Council, 1984).

Public concern has shifted away from the visible, demonstrable problems associated with environmental pollution and instead has focused on the small, invisible problems relative to "potential impact." Despite the fact that, as a society, we are living longer and enjoying a much better health and quality of life than ever before, we have become

Alvin L. Young • Office of Agricultural Biotechnology, U.S.D.A., Washington, D.C. 20250.

consumed with fear and seem obsessed by the risks in our lives. How shall we define risk and how do we communicate about risks?

Risk is a measure of the probability that an adverse effect will occur. In the case of a chemical, it is a function of the dose and of the intrinsic capacity of the material to cause an adverse effect (Wilkinson, 1986). The publication of Rachel Carson's *Silent Spring* rudely awakened the public to the potentially "disastrous" effects of chemicals on human health and the environment. Great changes have occurred in our industrial sector since that time. Two decades of learning and of changing the methods of handling and processing hazardous wastes have passed. Tremendous progress has been made in cleaning up our environment and workplace. Yet public perception and acceptance of these accomplishments can be wiped out in a single event (e.g., the tragic accident in Bhopal, India). As Lundeen (1985) cautioned: "If our industry simply waves the banner of scientific knowledge and ignores existing public perceptions, we will shortly face some unpleasant realities."

It would be ideal if we could clearly define risks—if we could conduct all the necessary research before we ever released a chemical. However, in the real world, no amount of research can eliminate all uncertainties associated with assessing the risks of exposure to potentially hazardous chemicals. No amount of research can eliminate the controversial judgments inherent in any decision about control of chemical exposures. Yet, there are opportunities to reduce scientific uncertainties and to increase the public's confidence that health is protected and that the economic consequences of imposed chemical control are justified. The need for regulation is recognized.

As Wilkinson (1986) said, "We are caught up in a vicious circle which, in attempting to respond to public pressure, regulators are focusing on and 'identifying' increasingly smaller chronic health risks that in turn alarm the public and create more pressure to regulate. At the present time, we are unable to distinguish trivia from more clear-cut health risks." Gough, in his recent book *Dioxin, Agent Orange: The Facts* (1986), noted that "these are bad times for conventional wisdom."

The dioxin controversy has shown us how difficult it is to find solutions to environmental problems. Proposed solutions are costly and, therefore, are frequently opposed by special-interest groups as well as by taxpayers. Research is complex and the risk assessments are not easily explained to lay audiences. Lastly, solutions to many of the environmental problems require national and international cooperation.

Environmental issues have involved the media and publicity, lawyers and litigation, and politics and money. These are the realities associated with difficult scientific issues that have large social components, but they are not solutions. It is only the use of reason and scientific data that can bring about lasting solutions. To that end, a disciplined way of approaching environmental assessment and regulation is critical to the effectiveness and acceptability of the government's program to reduce environmental risks. Similarly, it is critical that we learn how to effectively communicate environmental risks.

With regard to the control of chemicals, Wilkinson (1986) rightly noted that "the major question revolves around how this can be achieved in a sound, common-sense manner that on one hand provides all necessary safeguards to minimize risks to human health and the environment and on the other, encourages industry to conduct the research and development required to continue to produce new materials of real value to society."

The issue is not whether regulations should exist. The benefits of regulation are clear, and the public supports the concept. However, too many unnecessary and unintended regulatory constraints adversely affect innovation, research, development, and product approval. The 1985 report by the President's Commission on Industrial Competitiveness concluded that unnecessary regulation posed potential long-term problems and strong disincentives to innovation. Such regulation contributes to a reduction in the rate of new chemical innovation and to rising research and development costs. The impact of regulation on the innovative stature of the chemical industry in this country cannot be ignored if the industry is to remain competitive in global markets.

Winston Churchill said, "Ten thousand regulations destroy all respect for law." It then follows that a basic requirement of good public policy is to establish the connection between some expenditure and some recognized public good. Risk assessment represents a tool used for regulatory purposes to analyze scientific evidence to evaluate the relationship between exposure to toxic substances and the potential occurrence of disease. The ultimate goal is to have a common, explicit, consistent, scientifically sound approach to quantitative risk assessment. Only then will we be able to say that we have a truly effective platform on which to develop a risk communication strategy.

How does the Office of Science and Technology Policy (OSTP) get involved in all of this? The Office has a charter to "seek to define coherent approaches for applying science and technology to critical and emerging national and international problems and for promoting coordination of the scientific and technological responsibilities and programs of the Federal Departments and Agencies in the resolution of such problems." Thus, OSTP functions to advise the President of scientific and technological considerations regarding the economy, national security, health, foreign relations, the environment, and recovery and use of resources; to evaluate the scale, quality, and effectiveness of the federal effort in science and technology and advise on appropriate actions; to assist the Office of Management and Budget and the agencies in science and technology budget preparation and evaluation; and to assist the President in providing leadership and coordination of the federal research and development programs.

An example of activities of OSTP in the risk assessment arena is its document, *Chemical Carcinogens: A Review of the Science and Its Associated Principles* (Interagency Staff Group on Carcinogens, 1986). In developing this interagency, consensus, peer-reviewed document, we learned that a large number of uncertainties exist in the conduct of a risk assessment. Uncertainties arise because we are forced to make a relatively large number of assumptions and inferences to complete a risk assessment, such as weight of evidence; problems in hazard identification; uncertainties in dose response assessment; and uncertainties in exposure assessment.

Principle 27 of the OSTP carcinogen document noted that the quantification of the various sources of uncertainty involved in cancer risk assessment can be as important as the projection of the risk estimate itself. Without the sources of variability made explicit, it is very possible that the uncertainty associated with the estimates could be seriously underestimated by the risk managers and the public.

Principle 31 of the document noted that, because of the uncertainties associated with risk assessment, a full evaluation of risk to humans should include a qualitative consideration of the basic strengths and weaknesses of the available hazard and exposure data, in addition to any numerical estimations that are made.

Another critical component of risk assessment is assessing exposure. Ignoring the differences between administered and received doses in various animal species and at different dose levels can result in a serious over- or underestimation of low-dose chemical risks to humans. It is the target tissue dose that is most relevant to the toxic effects. The role of analytical chemistry, e.g., the analysis of the toxin 2,3,7,8-tetrachlorodibenzo-*p*-dioxin (TCDD) at less than the parts per trillion level, has affected our understanding of levels of a chemical present at organ sites.

Both the science and the art of toxicology are of central importance to the development of a sound regulatory policy toward chemicals. There is little doubt that the rapid emergence and growth of the discipline of toxicology has been dictated by the demands of the regulatory process. In the rush to regulate, the limitations of toxicology are often forgotten. Precise estimates of risk exaggerate the capabilities of toxicology.

To work toward minimizing risk, we must better understand toxicology: toxicology requirements; acute versus chronic toxicity; new methods; and simulation modeling. In 1983, OSTP commissioned the National Academy of Sciences to assess for us the needs of toxicology research. That report outlined five areas of research needs: (1) to improve the basis for dose and interspecies extrapolation to humans; (2) to predict effects of multiple chemical exposure; (3) to develop cellular and molecular markers of exposure; (4) to develop means to distinguish carcinogens on the basis of modes of action; and (5) to expand the use of existing federal data collection activities (National Academy of Sciences, 1983).

If the necessary research is to be conducted, we must have the funding resources. Accordingly, in fiscal year 1985, the federal agencies committed about $400 million for toxicological research; approximately half of that supported basic research while the remainder supported testing and methods development. Very few dollars are allocated to developing information on risk communication; clearly, social science research is underfunded.

If the public is to accept government decisions on the environment and health, a concerted effort must be made to offer straightforward statements that can be backed up by precise risk assessment statements and fully explained risk management decisions. Note that there is a difference between risk assessment and risk management. The National Academy of Sciences stated that risk assessment is considered to be a scientific process that characterizes the nature of the risk and assesses the probability of its occurrence, whereas risk management is the process whereby an appropriate regulatory decision is reached that will deviate, minimize, or otherwise manage the risk (National Research Council, 1983). It is true that factors other than science must go into the final decisions. Nevertheless, we must avoid the development of a policy that too readily removes well-tested chemicals from commerce and replaces them with alternatives that are perceived to be less hazardous simply because fewer test data are available. No risks are associated with a chemical for which no test data are available.

These, then, are the crucial components of risk analysis and risk communication. To communicate risks, we must have a strong science base (e.g., risk assessment), and we must have policies that are rational and congruent with our national goals. Lastly, we in the federal government must learn to be consistent with the messages we communicate to the public. The job of communicating with the public, so that the public is fully aware of the actions of government, is crucial to the acceptance of actions that impact their health and environment.

REFERENCES

Gough, M. 1986. *Dioxin, Agent Orange: The Facts*. New York: Plenum Press.

Interagency Staff Group on Carcinogens, Office of Science and Technology Policy. 1986. Chemical carcinogens: A review of the science and its associated principles. *Environmental Health Perspectives* 67: 201–82.

Lundeen, R. 1985. Editorial. *Chemical and Engineering News*. December 9, 1985, p. 3.

National Academy of Sciences. 1983. *Report of the Research Briefing Panel on Human Health Effects of Hazardous Chemicals Exposure*. Research Briefings for the Office of Science and Technology Policy. Committee on Science, Engineering, and Public Policy. Washington, D.C.: National Academy Press, pp. 99–100.

National Research Council, National Academy of Sciences. 1983. *Risk Assessment in the Federal Government: Managing the Process*. Committee on the Institutional Means for Assessment of Risks to Public Health, Commission on Life Sciences. Washington, D.C.: National Academy Press.

National Research Council, National Academy of Sciences. 1984. *Toxicity Testing—Strategies to Determine Needs and Priorities*. Steering Committee on Identification of Toxic and Potentially Toxic Chemicals for Consideration by the National Toxicology Program, Board on Toxicology and Environmental Health Hazards, Commission on Life Sciences. Washington, D.C.: National Academy Press.

President's Commission on Industrial Competitiveness (J.A. Young, Chairman). 1985. *Global Competition—The New Reality*. Washington, D.C.: U.S. Government Printing Office.

Wilkinson, C. F. 1986. Risk assessment and regulatory policy. *Comments on Toxicology* 1(1): 1–20.

IV

Case Studies of Government Risk Communication

13

The Newark Dioxin Case

James R. Marshall

In November 1980, the Environmental Protection Agency's Office of Research and Development published a report (Dioxins—EPA-600/2-80-197) that summarized the then-current literature on dioxins, their formation, sources, routes of human exposure, and the like. An appendix listed companies that manufactured products that might form dioxins as byproducts. About 50 of these were classified as I or II—products most likely to produce dioxins—and about 125 as class III—dioxins less likely but still possible. This list subsequently became the basis for EPA's National Dioxin Strategy.

In April 1983, New Jersey's Governor's Science Advisory Board reviewed this EPA report and advised sampling the class I sites located in that state. One of these sites was a former Diamond Shamrock plant on the Passaic River in Newark's Ironbound district, a mixed industrial and residential area. In the 1960s, this plant manufactured herbicides, including Agent Orange, for the Defense Department. A sample taken on the former plant site by New Jersey's Department of Environmental Protection (DEP) showed more than 600 parts per billion (ppb) of 2,3,7,8-tetrachlorodibenzo-*p*-dioxin (2,3,7,8-TCDD), the dioxin isomer of greatest concern. At DEP's request, the EPA Region II field investigation team (FIT) took nine more soil samples from the site, and one control sample. The tests confirmed high levels of 2,3,7,8-TCDD, with results ranging from 60 to greater than 1200 ppb. Subsequent reanalysis showed one sample, from beneath the former reactor, to have over 50,000 ppb.

IMMEDIATE PROBLEMS

This site was on the banks of the Passaic River in a densely populated mixed industrial/residential/commercial area. Private homes and a large produce distribution center

James R. Marshall • Office of External Programs, U.S. Environmental Protection Agency, Region II, New York, New York 10278.

were located within a few hundred yards of the front gate. Operating industries were immediately adjacent. Heavy traffic, both truck and rail, passed close by the site and into and out of the Ironbound district.

Concern about the presence of chemicals in the neighborhood was already high among residents of the Ironbound area because of recent spills and fires. An activist committee had been formed and was represented by an attorney formerly employed by the DEP.

It was essential for EPA and DEP to determine quickly to what extent the dioxin contamination may have spread off the site and what risks existed for the residents, nearby workers, and the food handling operation as a result. It was also essential to communicate quickly and directly with these affected publics and with the press, and to enlist the aid and cooperation of local officials. It was important to determine what health effects, if any, might have appeared among local residents or former workers at the site.

FIRST STEPS

Governor Kean of New Jersey decided to take an early direct role in communicating the problem. On June 2, 1983, the day following confirmation of EPA's tests, he held a press conference at which he announced the test results, and EPA announced plans for an immediate off-site screening to determine whether significant migration had occurred. The Governor made available temporary alternate housing (a downtown YMCA) for the 25 to 30 families in the site's immediate vicinity and ordered the produce distribution center closed.

That same day, EPA, DEP, and the State Department of Health met with Newark officials to enlist the city's aid in identifying and contacting residents and businesses in the area, and in providing police, fire, and community relations support. The city was able to provide community relations professionals familiar with the neighborhood and able to speak Spanish and Portuguese. That afternoon and evening, the Governor toured the community and met informally with the residents.

To get a quick indication of any off-site migration, particularly as it might affect the residents, EPA's FIT collected 31 samples the following day. These consisted of vacuum cleaner bags from 17 families, 4 street sweepings, 2 soil samples, and air conditioner filters from the 2 adjoining industries.

Because press and community interest was very high, EPA and the state agencies established the following procedures:

1. A daily press briefing was conducted at the site by EPA's Deputy Regional Administrator, which included demonstrations of sampling techniques and protective gear.
2. Community relations teams drawn from EPA, DEP, and the city of Newark developed fact sheets and conducted door-to-door visits of all affected residents as far in advance of the sampling teams as possible.
3. A DEP official visited all industries in the neighborhood.
4. The State Department of Health established an information trailer at the produce center.

5. A public meeting presided over by the Mayor of Newark was held with residents of a public housing development in the affected area and the city made available a vacant apartment in this development as a community relations command post.

On June 7, the Governor was able to hold another press conference at which he released the results of EPA's 31 off-site tests. These showed little off-site migration: one home showed 1.1 ppb; one industry showed 1.2 ppb; one soil sample showed 5.8 ppb; and the rest were either nondetectable or too masked with other compounds to detect dioxin. The Governor continued the State's offer of temporary relocation, but no residents availed themselves of the opportunity.

It was now apparent that an immediate public health threat did not exist off-site. However, further investigation was needed. In consultation with DEP, the Governor's Science Advisory Board, the State Department of Health, and the federal Centers for Disease Control (CDC), EPA's field investigation team developed an extensive off-site testing program and began to carry it out on June 13. The program covered a 4000-foot radius and consisted of four phases: areas of human habitability (including the 800-unit public housing project, a church, and a school); open spaces (parking lots, a park and public pool, and street corners); transport routes (roads, rail lines, and storm sewers); and the river (sediments and fish).

This testing program took several weeks and required intensive community relations preparation and frequent press briefings. Priority treatment was accorded to analysis of the samples, and all results were made public as soon as quality was assured.

SUBSEQUENT DEVELOPMENTS

The off-site testing did not turn up significant contamination of residential areas. However, low levels (1 to 3 ppb) around the swimming pool necessitated its closing and cleaning, and low levels on some of the streets leading away from the site led to an extensive vacuuming and cleaning. Similarly, positive hits for dioxin on some portions of the rail lines were remedied by covering with tarpaulins and/or ballasts pending permanent cleanup. Diamond Shamrock hired a contractor to lay tarpaulin over exposed soil on the plant site to prevent further migration pending the final remedy.

The sampling program also turned up a secondary source of contamination—a scrap metal dealer several blocks from the plant site, where surplus vessels and equipment from the plant had been disposed of after its shutdown. Today, all off-site contamination, including materials from the scrap metal dealer, has been consolidated and contained at the former plant site, and DEP is negotiating terms of the final remedy with Diamond Shamrock.

In summary, the following techniques were found to be effective in communicating the risks at this site to the affected publics and in fostering a cooperative and understanding atmosphere during the sampling and cleanup operations:

1. Early high-level involvement (the Governor, his commissioners, and EPA's Deputy Regional Administrator).
2. Recognition that priority had to be given to sampling the residential areas.

3. Involvement of outside experts perceived as objective (CDC and the Governor's Science Advisory Board).
4. Immediate release of data.
5. Involvement of local officials and agencies.
6. Frequent detailed briefing of the press and recognition of their needs (good visuals).
7. Frequent one-on-one contact with affected residents, with information and discussion available in their language of choice.
8. Advance information about sampling and cleanup activities.
9. Avoidance of large public meetings in favor of small, individual, or group sessions (only one large meeting was held and it was nonproductive and confrontational).
10. Availability of a sufficient number of press and community relations specialists.

The following communication problems were encountered:

1. Lack of good informational handouts on dioxins.
2. Lack of consensus on acceptable exposure levels for 2,3,7,8-TCDD, a problem that persists.
3. Existence of community interests with an agenda bigger than the contamination from this site. The community group ultimately took DEP to court in a successful effort to require full disclosure of all information related to this and other Ironbound sites. This resulted in a residual mistrust of the government agencies that was never completely resolved.

14

A Landfill Case in California

Raymond R. Neutra

This case describes a neighborhood problem in California that was one of the worst headaches for the California State Department of Health Services but now has developed into a most satisfying relationship with a local community. It illustrates that society's outrage increases with the visibility and concentration of the population at risk.

BACKGROUND

In the late 1960s, an insurance company bought up a large tract of hills in West Covina, about half an hour's drive east from Los Angeles. The local community activists claim that the insurance company was related to the BKK Corporation, a consortium of companies that dealt with waste. A garbage dump was started in West Covina. There were few houses close by, and there was moderate opposition to the dump. However, within the next 5 or 10 years the dump began receiving hazardous waste.

This 40-acre area is shaped like a bowl formed by a range of hills. It was the main repository of hazardous waste for the Los Angeles area, with truck after truck of hazardous waste driven through this community. Eventually, developers were allowed to build houses right up against the dump site. Indeed, in a gesture almost of irony, one of these little developments has a road called "Aroma Drive."

Aromas were present because the practice at the dump was to mix various chemicals with the garbage. The notion behind this was that organics such as vinyl chloride, trichlorethylene, and benzene would comingle with the banana peels and other garbage and bacteria would break down the chemicals. Liquid wastes would be absorbed by the garbage and everything would be covered with soil at the end of the day. However, bacterial decomposition of garbage produced methane, which migrated to the surface and carried

Raymond R. Neutra • California State Department of Health Services, Berkeley, California 94704.

with it a variety of organic chemicals. The odors created by this process were best characterized as repulsive.

COMMUNITY COMPLAINTS

By the late 1970s, more and more citizens complained about these odors and requested information on the health implications of airborne exposures. The company paid an engineer at a local university to do a study. The assessment was that the airborne exposures were not very dangerous.

But citizen pressure to study the situation more adequately led in 1981 to the discovery that vinyl chloride was present in the gases coming off that site into the adjacent neighborhood, and it exceeded the state ambient air standard of 10 parts per billion, which had been set a few years before on the basis of the level of detectability. Further dumping of vinyl chloride was barred from the site, but people in the community then wondered what other chemicals were in the ambient air and continuing to be dumped there.

By 1983, further analysis revealed a variety of substances in the ambient air at the site, including at least nine that are considered to be potential human carcinogens. These were vinyl chloride, perchlorethylene, trichlorethene, vinylidene chloride, chloroform, ethylene dichloride, benzene, chlorobenzene, and trans-1,2-dichloroethene.

A public meeting was held during which our agency presented a risk assessment for ambient air vinyl chloride levels for the area. The assessment concluded that, compared to another area a few miles away where some of the chemicals also had been found at detectable levels, the upper bound estimate of the excess lifetime risk from seven years of exposure (1976–1983) near the BKK landfill was approximately on the order of 5 in 100,000. Therefore, state epidemiologists did not expect to see any added cases of cancer in this population.

This determination was made in a setting where we had not developed an ongoing relationship with the several constituencies in the community, largely because we did not have the resources to pay the necessary attention to the problem. We felt that epidemiological studies were unlikely to be productive and, at the same time, we did not have the resources to do anything near that site. Consequently, we adopted the usual bureaucratic mode, which meant that after a while we avoided talking to the most strident and demanding people.

The report had been mailed to the community before the meeting. Some citizens attacked us at the meeting because they found a long list of things to criticize about the document, including every typographical error and one graph that deviated slightly from the figures in the text. Every time someone read off any one of those errors, the audience applauded and cheered; this went on for about half an hour. There was an accusation that we had purposely chosen a comparison area that had higher levels of pollution than their area so as to minimize their risk. Many citizens expressed the belief that we had tinkered with the results and conducted the assessment in such a way that the site would not be closed down.

At this point, much of the community living near the dump had an image of our agency as a duplicitous group of people who were absolutely not to be trusted. We had made the mistake of not trying to create a mechanism for communicating regularly with the community's several constituencies. Nor had we been communicating regularly about these health risk issues with the company that owns the dump. We had not acknowledged the legitimacy of the outrage of this community trapped next to these odors and whatever chemicals accompanied them. Our unresponsiveness must have appeared to them as negligence, for they had no way to assess our competence, to assess the reliability of the data that we were presenting to them, or to assess us as people.

METHANE EMERGENCY

Subsequent to that meeting, several other events occurred that made the situation even worse. In the summer of 1984, after we had become aware of the problem of methane migration through the soil, our hazardous waste engineers began checking houses in the area near the dump to see whether methane was migrating. Other issues then arose that took precedence and the inspections had to be discontinued. A month later, however, we were notified by the local gas company that while checking gas meters they had measured methane near a home at a level close to the explosive level.

The agency and the fire chief got together quickly and confirmed that methane was present near the first ring of houses around the dump, and 19 homes were evacuated. The next question was, if methane is present, is vinyl chloride also present at unacceptable levels?

The decision was made not to allow people back into their homes until (1) the methane was no longer an explosion danger and (2) it could be guaranteed that there was no danger from the various carcinogens that might be present. Thus, an ambitious sampling plan was initiated.

This decision created a terrible debacle because the laboratory was not able to process all this information in a timely fashion. Furthermore, one contracted laboratory turned out not to have the proper quality assurance so some of the sampling had to be repeated.

The owners of the site had already installed a gas collection system, which they improved so that the methane problem was solved within about a month. Meanwhile, we still were not able to identify the levels of carcinogens in their homes. Therefore, it took from July until about the end of the year before the information on the situation was available and people could return to their homes.

COMMUNITY COMMUNICATION PROGRAM

The EPA Community Relations Program set up a regular mechanism to meet with the most concerned and active community groups. Once this communication was established, all kinds of health issue questions were raised, and demands for health studies and toxicological explanations were made. The EPA personnel came to us and told us that we were the only people who could respond to the situation, short of the people across the continent at the Centers for Disease Control. They advised us to get together with the people in the community and at least talk to them.

About that time, some resources were freed up and a change of personnel occurred.

Another employee and I were assigned to the problem, and we made the commitment then that we were going to talk to constituencies in this community and establish constructive relationships.

At our first meeting with the community after that, we announced several things. One was that, unbeknownst to them, the agency had been carrying out a cancer registry-based study of the community. The study had been going on for two years, but it had not been announced because it was going slowly and we had wanted to wait until it was finished. However, there had been unforeseen delays.

We had also set up an advisory committee to review the results of the study when it was completed. This committee was a subcommittee of a standing State Advisory Committee, which was augmented by local physicians who we contacted because they petitioned the director of the agency to close the landfill. We thought that this would be adequate community input.

However, one part of the community, the "Coalition of West Covina Homeowners," let us know in no uncertain terms that this was not adequate community input. They did not know who the physicians were. There are 60,000 people within a mile of this site and probably 50 to 100 of them were the most worried about the health effects and had been following the issue for the last seven years. The physicians who reviewed our study were not known to this group; therefore, their assessments were not accepted by them.

Another group had been named by the local City Council to review progress on the site—a mixture of people from the Chamber of Commerce and concerned citizens from the neighborhood near the landfill. There also is the City Council itself, many of whose members tend to be quite sympathetic to the site owners, who give millions of dollars in taxes to the city. The various groups do not talk to each other much, yet all of them have an intense interest in this issue. There was no one organization to which one could go to reach all of these people.

In short, we saw that we had a problem in releasing our just-finished study, which showed no excess cancer around this site and had been reviewed by an advisory committee composed of people who were not particularly trusted by the concerned community.

COMMUNITY INPUT

To receive more input on the study, we agreed to send a preliminary copy of the report to several of the most active and concerned people. People trusted by the community's different constituencies were chosen. We had the understanding that they would look at the draft report, after which we would release it and make it available in the public library. We would then discuss the report with these individuals and hold a public meeting about it. We also allowed these representatives to sit in on the advisory committee meeting as it discussed the draft report.

The report was a very complex epidemiological study. After it was presented, one evening was spent with the community group answering their questions from about 7:00 p.m. to 1:00 a.m. The next day, we presented the study to the City Council.

Finally, a community meeting was held at which the study was formally presented. After the meeting, some of the activists came up and gave me a thick stack of paper filled with criticisms of the study. They told me they had many criticisms and had considered bringing them up at the meeting, but because they thought our agency basically had done a credible job, they wanted instead to present these points to us privately.

In the interim between the time the study was released to the community and the time we first met with them, we also had several other meetings in which we listened to their demands for health assessments. Their demands were extensive but understandable. They wanted an assessment of what people had been exposed to, a list of the chemicals that were present, and a toxicological description of what was known about the chemicals as well as all possible interactions. They wanted a registry to be set up of people who had lived around the site so that it would be possible to follow them for their lifetimes. They also wanted targeted medical examinations, including tests for body burdens and for subtle physiological indicators of physiological damage.

Our agency considered their requests and responded by saying that what they had proposed amounted to a multimillion dollar study and therefore was not feasible. At that time, EPA made available $150,000 to a contractor who spent a year producing five phonebook-sized volumes that summarized data about all the substances to which the community might have been exposed. The conclusion was that much is known about groundwater that nobody drinks, but every other mode of exposure was really inadequately characterized; nonetheless, our estimate was that probably it was not a large exposure. At the community's request, a review of birth certificate data is under way.

What our agency has done is acknowledge the legitimacy of the community's outrage at the exposures they have had. We have given them a chance to judge our biases and our competencies. And we have given them a substantial role in suggesting what needs to be done. We do not always agree with them, but we feel that many of their suggestions have been reasonable and we have carried them out. In doing all these things, we have established an ongoing and valuable relationship with this community.

15

Phosphorus Release in Miamisburg, Ohio

Allan D. Franks

At 4:30 p.m. on Tuesday, July 8, 1986, 15 cars of a 44-car CSX Transportation freight train derailed near downtown Miamisburg, which is in southwest Ohio, not far from Dayton. A tanker car containing white phosphorus caught on fire when holes in the side allowed air to enter (the material self-ignites upon contact with air).

Because of the potential for human health problems, a general evacuation was ordered by city officials at 5 p.m. The evacuation involved all of Miamisburg, some area businesses, a shopping mall, and several nearby communities; in all, some 30,000 persons.

The staff at the Ohio Environmental Protection Agency (Ohio EPA) initially heard of the accident through the media. The agency's Emergency Response Team was sent to the scene immediately and CSX formally notified the agency at 5:45 p.m. Key agency personnel were then called and asked to return to work. I was sent to the Governor's office to help coordinate initial communications and assess the incident.

At 10:30 p.m., Governor Celeste visited the site and ordered all appropriate state agencies to assist. This included the Ohio EPA (in emergency response and communication), the Disaster Services Agency (in coordination), the Public Utilities Commission (in coordination), the State Fire Marshall's Office (in fire assistance), the Ohio State Patrol (in aerial surveillance), the Ohio Department of Health (in health issues), and the Department of Agriculture (in yard and garden concerns). By early morning on Wednesday, most agency representatives had arrived.

The head of the Ohio State and Local Government Commission was asked to coordinate the efforts of the various state agencies and I was asked to serve as the State's spokesperson on the scene. The staff at the Ohio EPA district office in nearby Dayton and at the central office in Columbus also handled media calls.

On Wednesday morning, the situation was fairly stable. The water being pumped onto the burning car was holding down the smoke, other control options were being

Allan D. Franks • State of Ohio Environmental Protection Agency, Columbus, Ohio 43266-1049.

discussed, and some people were allowed to return home. However, the situation changed that afternoon. A second car containing sulfur was lying next to the burning phosphorus car, and health officials were concerned about the possible formation of hydrogen sulfide. To prevent this from happening, an attempt was made to move the phosphorus car. When this was done, new leaks occurred.

A meeting of local city/county officials only was held at 4 p.m. to discuss options. The State was excluded from this meeting, even though the Director of the Ohio EPA personally asked that staff be allowed to attend. A press conference was called for 6 p.m. to announce that a special foam might be used to control the fire. At 6:05 p.m., on live television, the fire reignited and a huge cloud of smoke erupted from the tank car. A second evacuation was then called.

When the wind shifted, the command post was moved. The wind continued to shift during the night and the command post had to be moved again. Problems occurred when the media could not find the new command posts and when some reporters decided to stay at the site.

On Thursday, a decision was made to allow the fire to burn itself out. Because nobody was certain how much phosphorus remained in the tank, it was impossible to predict when the fire would actually be out. By Saturday morning, the fire had dwindled and fire personnel were able to pour sand in the car and extinguish the few remaining flames. The evacuation was lifted and people returned home. The ensuing cleanup took approximately two months.

COMMUNICATIONS

Initially, communication at the scene was difficult at best. People were hard to find, few telephones or walkie-talkies were available, and information was hard to verify. Later, a formal Emergency Operation Center (EOC) was set up with equipment and desks for all key agencies. A state hotline was set up and staffed around the clock with personnel from the various state agencies. Hundreds of calls were received and directed to the appropriate agency person.

The news media was the most used communication tool. Media from throughout Ohio and other nearby states covered the event hourly from about dawn until midnight, with one TV station videotaping continuously, 24 hours a day. The degree of sophistication ranged from fledgling reporter to the network press.

A local radio station used a two-hour talk show to allow people to ask questions. Staff from the state hotline were asked to assist in answering questions and concerns. Most of the questions dealt with health, both human and animal, and agricultural problems (gardens, grass, shrubs, etc.). Staff members at Ohio EPA offices and a hotline in Columbus also received calls.

Gaps in information occurred early because of the initial confusion and lack of knowledge. There was limited knowledge about who was doing what and what was actually happening. The local fire chief and city manager were clearly in charge of the operation, but with seven state agencies, numerous local officials, and various federal agencies on the scene, it was hard to coordinate information. This situation improved by the third day and was in good operation by the fourth.

Messages were communicated in several ways. Personal interviews of officials by the media were frequent. Meetings were held often on an as-needed basis. Portable telephones were used extensively and the local chapter of the "ham" radio operators proved to be invaluable. With stations around the county, they were especially helpful in communicating weather information.

Anytime a few hundred strangers are gathered together, each with his or her own responsibilities, a difficult situation can develop. This happened in this case initially but was resolved over time. Turf battles over who should be in charge, who should be included in meetings, or who should talk to the media were all issues that had to be resolved.

PUBLIC RESPONSE

The public responded in pretty much the typical fashion: some people were not worried at all and chose to remain in their homes; some were angry; some were frustrated; and most were scared. Their concerns ranged from personal health, to pets, to gardens, to homes, and to loved ones. Consequently, their questions involved these issues, and it was fortunate that experts from the various agencies were on hand to try and respond.

Most of the evacuees handled the situation well. Overall, the news media did an excellent job of conveying information objectively and without some of the hysteria often associated with this type of story. Because of this, panic never really set in.

Most involved agencies or personnel held interviews; it is hard to tell who was viewed as the most credible. The fact that single spokespersons were designated and items were discussed before they were released probably helped credibility most of all. Conflicting information was released in only a few instances and was corrected as soon as possible.

OUTCOMES

When the fire was put out on Saturday, everyone was relieved and glad to go home. While most people seemed satisfied with the huge effort that had taken place, some were looking for someone to blame. Various suits were filed during and after the incident and are still unresolved. The railroad fully admitted its responsibility and set up a claims office on the day after the initial incident. They have paid several hundred claims.

After the incident was over, a general sense of accomplishment pervaded most of the involved agencies. Thousands of person-hours had gone into the effort, and everyone was relieved that no serious injuries or deaths had occurred. The initial differences among the agencies had been resolved, and by the end, the different groups had a real "team" feeling because they had worked together to successfully deter fear and panic in the community.

16

Individual Notification of Workers Exposed to 2-Naphthylamine

Paul A. Schulte

One of the areas of risk communication in which researchers from the National Institute for Occupational Safety and Health (NIOSH) are involved can be classified under the rubric of individual worker notification (Schulte and Ringen, 1984). This type of risk communication pertains to informing surviving workers of the findings of retrospective cohort mortality studies. Over the past 25 years, both government and private organizations have conducted a variety of retrospective cohort mortality studies. The question has arisen as to whether the subjects of these studies should be individually informed of the results.

A retrospective cohort mortality study involves identifying a cohort of workers, following that cohort of workers, and evaluating the mortality experience within the cohort by comparing it with reference mortality rates; a measure of that comparison is the standardized mortality ratio. This type of study is usually a records search with no direct contact with living members or next of kin of deceased members of the cohorts.

NIOSH's early involvement in worker notification stems from a 1977 Senate subcommittee hearing where the directors of NIOSH and the National Cancer Institute (NCI) were asked why the federal government failed to individually notify the subjects of these studies about their potential risk. Consequently, in 1979, NIOSH began to investigate the issue of individual worker notification. There was little information about how to decide whom to notify or how to do it. A pilot project was initiated to examine the problems that resulted from the individual notification of members of a cohort of workers in Augusta, Georgia, who manufactured textile dyes and had exposure to aromatic amines, most notably 2-naphthylamine and benzidine (Schulte et al., 1985a).

The cohort studied involved 1385 plant workers who were employed between 1940 and 1972. In tracing the cohort, it was found that the individuals were dispersed over 30

Paul A. Schulte • National Institute for Occupation Safety and Health, Cincinnati, Ohio 45226.

states; however, most still remained within the Southeast. Despite intensive efforts to locate members of the cohort, 22% were not located. The tracing mechanisms included the Social Security Administration, the Internal Revenue Service, State Bureaus of Motor Vehicles, and some credit tracing organizations. From a vital status follow-up of the cohort, it was assumed that 1094 of the workers were still alive (eligible for notification) and, of these, that 798 were in and around the Augusta area. A screening program was conducted for these 1094 individuals, with a 77% participation rate. Special methods were employed to screen individuals who lived outside of a 50-mile radius of the Augusta area (Schulte et al., 1985a).

Of these 1385 people, 13 were identified as having bladder cancer (Schulte et al., 1985b). Three of the cancers were identified from death certificates, seven individuals were under treatment by community urologists, and three cases were identified in the first phase of the screening program. Since that time, two other cases of cancer have been identified. The cohort had approximately a four-fold risk of bladder cancer, but some subsets of the cohort had a much greater risk; the highest was among black workers with over 10 years of employment. These individuals had a 111-fold risk of bladder cancer (Schulte et al., 1985b).

The primary lesson learned from the Augusta experience is that individual worker notification is not just a simple process of sending a letter to a former worker about some potential employment risk (Schulte et al., 1985a). It requires initiating a large, diverse, and complex process whereby a variety of information is involved, and the following data are needed: personnel records, epidemiological findings, information to locate the cohort, appropriate information about the cohort to develop the message to be sent and methods to deliver it, information regarding the substance or substances to which the cohort is exposed, and relevant information for the workers and their physicians. Workers who are notified also have concerns about medical surveillance, particularly medical screening; how to obtain appropriate information to relay to their personal physicians; psychological and legal counseling needs; and financial concerns (Schulte, 1985). In the Augusta experience, some of the workers would not participate in the screening program for fear that any health problems that were detected would be too costly to treat. Some individuals needed economic, psychological, or legal support in order to cope with their risk status.

Three issues can become barriers to individual worker notification (Schulte, 1986). The first is that epidemiological risk information is group-specific, i.e., the experience of one group is compared to that of another group. These data do not address the experience of an individual within the group. A determination cannot be made about whether the risk information that is derived from the cohort is applicable to individual members of the cohort. From a public health point of view, members of this cohort are at high risk. Individuals who have had occupational exposure to the substance in question are likely to have some increased risk, but researchers cannot predict the exact rate of increase.

The second barrier is that in many of the mortality studies, the deceased members of the cohort, on whom researchers have based the ascertainment of risk and conducted the mortality determination, may have been those who had the most exposures or were the most sensitive to the substance. Therefore, the workers who have survived and are notified are not necessarily at the same risk; yet the researchers would be sending these individuals notification that they are at risk, based on a study of the deceased coworkers. To avoid this barrier, each study needs to be evaluated on a case-by-case basis.

The third barrier to worker notification involves questions about the truth of the study findings. For example, when researchers evaluate many cause-of-death categories, as in cohort mortality studies, they may find some results that are statistically significant by chance alone. A means of dealing with this problem would be to compare the study findings with other external findings to ensure consistency and to use statistical techniques to adjust for multiple comparisons (Schulte, 1985).

In 1983, NIOSH staff developed the following questions to be used as criteria for worker notification:

1. Was the study positive or did it demonstrate a statistically significant standard mortality ratio (SMR) greater than 100?
2. Was the study conducted with methodological integrity?
3. Was the study statistically significant after adjusting for multiple comparisons that might occur in the study?
4. Was there a true risk in this cohort relative to some other comparison group, such as the national population (Schulte, 1985)?

With these criteria in mind, three different risk groups were identified. Groups with an absolute risk of less than 1 in 1000 were classified as warranting notification if the study was conducted properly. Groups with a risk between 1 in 1000 and 1 in 100,000 were classified as requiring additional criteria; within that risk zone, a criterion for relative risk also would be considered. A relative risk greater than 300 was selected because it was generally large enough to avoid the influence of random variability. The third category involved groups with an absolute risk of death of greater than 1 in 100,000. In this group, a relative risk of ten-fold (i.e., an SMR greater than 1000) would also be required.

In 1985, the NIOSH Board of Scientific Counselors was asked to investigate the problem of worker notification and the Board convened a subcommittee (NIOSH, 1986). The subcommittee did not support the idea of statistical significance as one of the driving forces for worker notification. Also, the subcommittee preferred to use a concept of attributable risk rather than relative risk and absolute risk. The subcommittee developed three options for notification based on the following levels of risk: lowest, medium, and highest. Notification activities were devised pursuant to each of those risk levels.

The first option was designed for the lowest risk category (an attributable risk of less than or equal to 25% an SMR greater than 133, and an absolute risk smaller than 1 in 100,000). A very generalized type of notification would be required for the lowest risk group through companies, unions, and posted reports.

The second option was designed for the medium risk category (an attributable risk greater than 25% but less than 50%, an SMR between 133 and 200, and an absolute risk between 1 in 1000 and 1 in 100,000). Notification for the medium risk group would use the same options as above and also would include an alert to notify local newspapers, the media, and appropriate public health agencies.

The third option was designed for the highest risk group (an attributable risk of 50% or greater, an SMR of greater than 200, and an absolute risk greater than 1 in 1000). Notification activities for this group would require locating the cohort and providing individual notification for workers, as well as support programs for these individuals.

In summary, individual notification procedures for risk factors should be based on a firm scientific foundation and reflect the relative importance of the risk. It is not sufficient to consider the notification process as merely a communication or dispatch about risk status. The initiation of individual notification activities should be approached as a process with component stages. A group that is notified about their relative risk moves through time with a variety of needs based on their risk status. Risk communicators must anticipate the consequences of their communications to increased risk groups. The consequences of risk notification should not be used as an excuse to avoid communicating pertinent risk information but rather as an inspiration for initiating the process correctly.

REFERENCES

Report to the Director of NIOSH from the Subcommittee on Individual Worker Notification, NIOSH Board of Scientific Counselors, May 20, 1986.

Schulte, P.A., and K. Ringen. 1984. Notification of workers at high risk. An emerging public health problem. *American Journal of Public Health* 74(5): 485–91.

Schulte, P.A. 1985. The epidemiologic basis for the notification of subjects of cohort studies. *American Journal of Epidemiology* 121(3): 351–61.

Schulte, P.A., K. Ringen, and W. Gullen, et al. 1985a. Notification of a cohort of workers at risk of bladder cancer. *Journal of Occupational Medicine* 27(1): 19–28.

Schulte, P.A., K. Ringen, and G. Hemstreet, et al. 1985b. Risk assessment of a cohort exposed to aromatic amines—initial results. *Journal of Occupational Medicine* 27(2): 115–21.

Schulte, P.A. 1986. Problems in notification and screening of workers at high risk of disease. *Journal of Occupational Medicine* 28(10): 951–57.

V

The Risk Communication Process

17

Helping the Public Make Health Risk Decisions

Baruch Fischhoff

Making risky decisions is difficult, both for reasons of which we are aware and for those of which we are unaware (Fischhoff, 1988). Many decisions are fairly routine. It is rare to see someone transfixed, unable to decide whether to cross the street, put on a seat belt, or add some table salt. Through trial and error, we have figured out the right way to act and thereby avoid making these decisions deliberatively. When we develop these rules of behavior for ourselves, they become habits; when society provides them, they become traditions. Life becomes difficult with decisions such as those that risk analysts must make, where one must think the decision out from the beginning and get it right the first time, either because the action has irreversible consequences or because the feedback that life provides is so poor that there are no clear indicators to prompt mid-course corrections. How to respond to possible leaks from a local landfill, to the storage of World War II nerve gas in one's county, to the health effects of shellfish or olive oil or of a spouse's smoking—these are all tough decisions.

Those who have looked at how people make such decisions, and even simpler ones, find pitfalls in every aspect of the decision-making process. Looking at the options people consider, the consequences they weigh, the facts they believe in, the terms they use, or the integration rules they depend on for putting it all together, in each case one finds vagueness, incompleteness, and sometimes even outright error. Some of these problems seem to come from ignorance about specific issues, but many come from people not knowing how to organize their work. Decision theory never appears on most people's curricula and, where it does, it is often so formalized as to make little contact with intuitive thought processes (i.e., the "how" of people's thinking).

There are few simple, "off-the-rack" messages about decision making. Helping people make risky decisions requires, as one says on the West Coast, figuring out "where they are coming from." This requires a lot of detailed empirical work (Fischhoff et al., 1983).

Baruch Fischhoff • Department of Engineering and Public Policy, Carnegie-Mellon University, Pittsburgh, Pennsylvania 15213.

A specialist in risk communication might be willing to make a best guess at the solution to a risk communication problem. Such specialists know some things that others do not and have a set of somewhat different intuitions. However, like all quick advice, those best guesses call for *caveat emptor*, *caveat vendor*, and, in this case, "*caveat publis*." If you take an incompletely elaborated idea, apply it without thorough pretesting, neglect grounding it in a comprehensive analysis of the recipient's situation, and omit the sort of evaluation needed for fine tuning and mid-course corrections, then we look bad and you look bad and, worst of all, the public looks bad. It takes two to communicate. If we have not gotten our message across, then we ought to assume that the fault is not with our receivers (Fischhoff, 1985a).

As an example of a possible misdirection of our own making, a while ago we suggested that telling people about a technology's safeguards could backfire by making it easier for lay people to visualize all the things that could go wrong. That fit then-current (and even now-current) psychological theory and is probably right as far as it goes. However, much more is going on in most risk communication situations than the simple creation of mental images. All communication is conducted on several levels with complex effects (Slovic et al., 1980).

This prediction would not, for example, account for the apparent successes of the chemical industry's Community Awareness and Emergency Response (CAER) program. Although no empirical studies have been conducted, people in industry involved with the program suggest that they shared our intuition when they started to tell the neighbors of chemical plants about possible risks and intended precautions. Although there was some initial alarm, things seem to have worked out amicably in the long run.

A psychologist's analysis of this success points to several possible reasons. One is simply that there was a long run. The chemical industry had the kind of extended interaction with the lay people needed to learn their concerns and language. A second possible reason for success is that the content of the industry's message happened to match the public's concerns. The public wanted to know what was going on at the plant, what steps were being taken to protect them, and what to do if things went wrong. A third possible reason is that much of the message concerned concrete actions and operations rather than the esoteric number games of risk analysis. Unfortunately, concretizing things is not an advantage that one can enjoy when decisions actually do depend on the question "how risky (or beneficial) is it?" rather than "how does it work?" A fourth possible reason for success is that there is relatively little conflict of interest between the parties in this case. Everyone wants the neighbors to get away safely from an accident. Finally, the professional job done by the Chemical Manufacturers Association in preparing materials probably provided a good place to start, even if it was done without explicit empirical testing.

A descriptive analysis of "where the public is coming from" is needed for a number of reasons. One is to establish what people care about, so that there is some chance that they will listen to communicators and think that we care about solving their problems as well as our own.

A second reason for descriptive analysis is to identify the relationship between our problem and theirs. Sweden in the early 1980s discovered that it had a domestic radon problem. In keeping with Swedish customs and institutions, the authorities disclosed what they knew, while the building industry quickly and voluntarily provided subsidies for home remodeling. To the authorities' dismay, there was little panic. Some people increased their ventilation and heating, but most decided to think about it for a while. Ola Svenson (who was one of the remodelers) and I had some contact with the authorities. Of the things that we suggested, what they seemed to find helpful (or at least therapeutic) was the juxtaposition of simple decision trees offering crude descriptions of their problem and that of the public (Svenson and Fischhoff, 1985). The authorities' decision tree involved such options as alternative standards for allowable radon concentration and consequences like enforcement costs, aggregate national health risk, and housing availability. By contrast, the residents' decision tree included such options as whether to measure their own radon levels at all and whether to move (leaving the problem to someone else). Their consequences were, of course, all personal.

A third reason for studying how lay people think about a problem is to understand their basic terms of reference. One result of risk perception research is discovering the differing definitions given to terms like "risk" (or "safe" or "voluntary" or "exposure") by different lay people and even by different experts. Not speaking one another's language is an effective barrier to communication.

A fourth reason for studying others is to rein in our own intuitions. It is startling, and disheartening, for social scientists to see how readily and confidently others will speculate about human behavior (i.e., our turf) when they would not dare to do so without hard data in their own area. One now-classic case from the 1950s was the failure of "fear appeals" designed to persuade people, for example, to brush their teeth by showing them grisly pictures of the consequences of unhealthy behavior.

To give a personal example of an errant speculation, I recently had an idea for explaining very small probabilities to people. Why not describe a low probability as the conjunction of several jackpot spinner events, each of which is unlikely? One could use abstract spinners or ones showing concrete events, like the probability of a landfill leaking, the probability of toxins getting into your water, and the probability of a resulting health effect. It sounded to me like a great idea, but it did not work. Despite a fairly diligent effort, I could not find a presentation for which the notion of conjunction was intuitively clear (i.e., so that the probability attributed to all three events occurring was at least smaller than the probability attributed to each of them).

One example of the kind of detailed empirical work needed to prepare communications for a public health risk problem is provided by a recent project designed to help women decide what to do about the threat of sexual assault (conducted by Fischhoff, Furby, and Morgan). What women need to know is (1) which protective strategies most reduce the risk of being assaulted at the smallest price in personally valued consequences (such as time, freedom, self-esteem, money), and (2) what to do if actually assaulted, again in terms of one's personal values. What do women find? They find large quantities of confident, conflicting, and categorical advice, telling all women what they should do (Morgan, 1986). A woman might natually ask, who are these experts? How do they know? Are they speaking to me?

We have explored in detail how women (and also some men and experts) think about these decisions in order to communicate more effectively about the risks and what can be done about them. The set of possible action options that we found is enormous, unstructured, and ill defined. A review of the advice literature yielded some 700 different strategies that have been recommended. Our interviews produced another 400 strategies, different enough that one could make some case as to why each strategy would have effects different from those of the others. Many strategies were so imprecise that it is hard to know what they mean (e.g., resist verbally). Few individuals, however, seemed aware of a substantial or representative subset of the overall set of over 1100 strategies. In such a situation, the risk communicator's initial task would be to develop a conceptual framework for talking about these options that would make sense to women and make contact with the research literature into strategy effectiveness (which is itself afflicted with an ill-structured option space).

A review of the advice literature showed that rather few consequences were considered overtly other than: being raped, escaping without being raped, suffering other injury, and promoting self-esteem. Our interviews, however, found many other things on women's minds—and even on the minds of experts—that somehow had not found their way into the recommendations. Here, the communicator's task is to bring potentially relevant consequences to women's attention in a way that will enable them to begin to think about such things as, "how much of an increase in the chance of escape without rape would justify a 10% increase in the chance of other serious injury?" It seems esoteric (not to mention awful) to make such trade-offs, but they are implicit in these (and many other) health risk decisions. Any progress that people can make in thinking clearly is to their benefit—and to ours as communicators. Conversely, it is incumbent on us to find ways to make clear the trade-offs implicit in the advice that we experts give them.

Regarding the facts of sexual assault, what women need to know is how undertaking each strategy affects the likelihood of incurring each consequence. Ideally, these effects would be known for every kind of situation, assailant, and woman. The research is hard, and the literature is sparse. In aggregate, it provides much less precision in its estimates than one would hope. In addition, much of the research is performed and communicated without consideration for women's decision-making needs. Most studies concentrate on significance levels, whereas what women need is reliable information on effect size. They need to know not only whether a strategy makes a difference but how much of a difference.

A second form of insensitivity to women's decision-making needs is that few studies collect data on the temporal order of strategies and consequences. As a result, although it appears that greater physical resistance by women is associated with greater violence by men, we do not know which causes which. (It appears that women resist physically because they are being hurt, more than men becoming violent when women resist.)

A third form of insensitivity can be found in studies that advise women to respond differently to different kinds of assailants, without considering whether women can even make such diagnoses under real-life conditions. Moreover, these studies seldom discuss the prevalence (or "base rates") of the different kinds of assailant in the population, an essential piece of information for making any diagnosis. Finally, some studies actually make the "base rate fallacy," concluding, for example, that pleading is more effective than fighting because, among women who escape, 80% do the former and only 20% do the latter (Furby and Fischhoff, in press).

In our studies, we compare women's beliefs with those held by experts and with those beliefs that can be substantiated by the literature, as a prologue to determining what risk information needs to be communicated. Our criterion for deciding what needs to be told is a rough value-of-information analysis. It leads one to place the highest priority on communicating information that will have the greatest contribution to women's choice of option. A complicating factor is that the best estimate of the truth may lie somewhere between the estimates produced by different studies, each with its biases, and the estimates that women hold intuitively.

The final step in this approach to designing risk communications is somehow to help women put all these pieces together to reach a personally relevant decision. It would be ideal if more citizens could get the sort of professional counseling for their critical decisions that is available for corporate and government decisions. In this project, more modest alternatives are being explored and matched to the amount of effort that a woman might want to devote to this topic and to the modes of delivery available for reaching women.

Although the details will differ, other serious problems may demand something like this level of intensity in order to find out what risk communication is needed. Where the resources are not available, then even some simple analysis, like our little Swedish radon trees, might help ensure a more comprehensive and pertinent approach. Other partial solutions to communication problems can be found in the technical literature on judgment and decision making (e.g., how to express uncertainties) (Fischhoff et al., 1987). In principle, we would not have to evaluate individual communications if we had a robust set of empirically evaluated principles for constructing communications. In practice, we have a way to go. In the interim, it is important to remember that inappropriate risk communications can have serious health consequences (including undue alarm, panic, and apathy). From a public health perspective, one should be no more willing to expose the public to an untested message than to an untested drug.

A precondition for such an analysis of communication needs is having a comprehensive picture of the problem. Over the last couple of years, I have talked to various groups of journalists working the risk beat about how to tell risk stories to the lay public. An unsurprising theme in the reporters' responses has been that they feel that they can do a fairly good job of telling these risk stories. A more surprising theme has been that they report having trouble getting the story, in the sense of figuring out the full set of possible options, consequences, and sources of uncertainty that need to be considered. If they could get a glimpse of each, then they could use their skills to ferret out better information. However, as nonspecialists, they cannot work on issues that are not mentioned. Their complaint is that experts tend to talk about those pieces of a risk puzzle that they feel most comfortable with or most responsible for. When lay people or reporters get different pieces of an issue from different sources, then they are likely to respond inconsistently and to look bad.

One thing that I have taken to doing in these talks with journalists or citizen groups, and in the papers that I have written for them, is providing interrogatory schemes to ensure that the experts reveal all significant missing pieces of the puzzle (Fischhoff, 1985b,c). One such scheme, which I think is going to be of particular interest in the future, is used for determining just where judgment enters an analysis. That is, where do the data end and educated guesses take over (Fischhoff, in press; Fischhoff and Cox, 1986)? And, therefore, how much must the definitiveness of an analysis's conclusions be qualified? On the one hand, U.S. weather forecasters show an excellent ability to assess the limits of their own knowledge in their probability of precipitation forecasts (Murphy and Winkler, 1984). On the other hand, the historical record of particle physicists' confidence in their estimates of the value of physical constants suggests consistent overconfidence, like much of what has been observed in more mundane laboratory studies (Henrion and Fischhoff, 1986).

Would that risk analysts had created such an historical record, allowing us to evaluate the validity of the judgments used in their risk analyses. We ought to be as willing to scrutinize our own risk perceptions as we are those of the public.

REFERENCES

Fischhoff, B. 1985a. Managing risk perceptions. *Issues in Science and Technology* 2(1): 83–96.

Fischhoff, B. 1985b. Protocols for environmental reporting: what to ask the experts. *The Journalist* (Winter): 11–15.

Fischhoff, B. 1985c. Risk analysis demystified. *NCAP News* 4(1): 30–32.

Fischhoff, B. 1988. Judgment and decision making. In *The Psychology of Human Thought*. Ed. R. J. Sternberg and E. E. Smith. New York: Wiley.

Fischhoff, B. Forthcoming. Judgmental aspects of risk analysis. In *Risk Assessment: The State of the Art*. Ed. V. Covello and M. Merkofer. New York: Plenum Press.

Fischhoff, B. and L. A. Cox, Jr. 1986. Conceptual framework for benefit assessment. In *Benefits Assessment: The State of the Art*. Ed. J. D. Bentkover, V. T. Covello, and J. Mumpower. Dordrecht, The Netherlands: D. Reidel, pp. 51–84.

Fischhoff, B., P. Slovic, and S. Lichtenstein. 1983. The "public" vs. the "experts": perceived vs. actual disagreements about the risks of nuclear power. In *Analysis of Actual vs. Perceived Risks*. Ed. V. Covello, G. Flamm, J. Rodericks, and R. Tardiff. New York: Plenum Press, pp. 235–49.

Fischhoff B., O. Svenson, and P. Slovic. 1987. Active responses to environmental hazards. In *Handbook of Environmental Psychology*. Ed. D. Stokols and I. Altman. New York: Wiley.

Furby, L., and B. Fischhoff. In press. Rape self-defense strategies: a review of their effectiveness. *Victimology*.

Henrion, M., and B. Fischhoff. 1986. Assessing uncertainty in physical constants. *American Journal of Physics* 54(9): 791–98.

Morgan, M. 1986. Conflict and confusion: what rape prevention experts are telling women. *Sexual Coercion and Assault*, 1(5): 160–68.

Murphy, A. H., and R. W. Winkler. 1984. Probability forecasting in meteorology. *Journal of the American Statistical Association* 79: 489–500.

Slovic, P., B. Fischhoff, and S. Lichtenstein. 1980. Informing people about risk. In *Product Labeling and Health Risks*, Report No. 6. Ed. L. Morris, M. Mazis, and I. Barofsky. Cold Spring Harbor, NY: Banbury Center, pp. 165–81.

Svenson, O., and B. Fischhoff. 1985. Levels of environmental decisions: a case study of radiation in Swedish homes. *Journal of Environmental Psychology* 5(1): 55–67.

18

Scientific Uncertainties and How They Affect Risk Communication

Dale Hattis

The past several years have seen a great increase in demand from the judiciary (Aqua Slide 'N' Dive Corp. v. CPSC; Industrial Union Dept. v. American Petroleum Institute; American Petroleum Institute v. OSHA) and executive agencies (Ruckelshaus, 1983) for both

1. More assessment of risks and the expected benefits from potential control measures in quantitative form.
2. "Better science" in the assessment of all kinds of risks to public health and safety.

The simultaneous demands for greater scientific rigor and more extensive and detailed quantification have challenged the capabilities of traditional risk assessment methodologies drawn from toxicology, statistics, and engineering, among other disciplines. To quantify the expected frequency and consequences of low-probability events that are not susceptible to direct measurement, a variety of predictive modeling approaches have been used—depending in many cases on analogies, indirect inferences, and professional judgment for key assumptions and data.

For those cases in which risks/bad consequences are directly measurable, and one can predict the results of different interventions to control risk on the basis of validated past experience, one hardly needs an analyst; an accountant will do. But whereas the scientist can select a narrow corner of the universe for study where the available tools have

---

Dale Hattis • Center for Technology, Policy and Industrial Development, Massachusetts Institute of Technology, Cambridge, Massachusetts 02139. This paper is an adaptation of an extended essay titled "What's Wrong with Quantitative Risk Assessment?" in *Quantitative Risk Assessment* (1987, ed. R. F. Almader and J. M. Humber, New Jersey, Humana Press, pp. 57–105).

a good chance to uncover new information, the risk assessor must follow the chain(s) of causation of a particular hazard (and the efficacy of control options) through whatever number of twists and turns they happen to take in the real world. There is often a need to trace a complex causal pathway through the following steps:

1. Regulatory rules, enforcement, and compliance.
2. Actual operating procedures of a particular technology that give rise to discharges.
3. Environmental transport and transformation via various media to the sites where hazardous substances come in contact with people.
4. Complex behavioral processes of eating, breathing, and so on, that lead to absorption.
5. The series of transport, metabolism, reaction, and repair processes that mediate dose–response relationships, and their variability among diverse individuals in the exposed population.

The risk analyst is faced with this task regardless of how much may be known about each of the transitions in the sequence. This combines with the necessity, within the context of decision-making, to make choices about risk. Doing nothing about a problem is, of course, also a choice. However, the choice not to complete the analysis and reserve judgment until more information is available is generally more costly than it is in the basic science context, where the only penalty may be in a somewhat more extended effort to repeat and confirm specific experimental findings.

The appropriate rules for theorizing in risk assessments have not yet been fully worked out. Even less established are ways of fairly assessing and communicating the uncertainties in our assessments of risk. This chapter will first discuss some of the difficulties with current practices in simply analyzing the uncertainties in risk assessments, and will then address some communication issues that exacerbate these difficulties.

TECHNICAL ANALYSIS OF UNCERTAINTIES IN RISK ASSESSMENTS

While the need to make quantitative judgments under uncertainty may often appear new and troubling to technical specialists in areas central to health and safety risk assessment, similar problems have been the subjects of extensive study in the decision analysis and management sciences literatures. Certain cognitive heuristic processes and resulting biases in the perception of probabilities have been well characterized (Tversky and Kahneman, 1974; Fischhoff, 1982; Wallsten and Budescu, 1983), and there have been concrete proposals for methods to reduce these known biases (Winkler, 1967; Lichtenstein and Fischhoff, 1980; Alpert and Raiffa, 1982; Kahneman and Tversky, 1982). Two specific biases appear especially relevant to risk assessment:

1. Overconfidence in the reliability of subjective predictions—assignment of too narrow confidence limits to uncertain quantities.
2. Neglect of general distributional information on the "prior" probabilities of

various outcomes, in favor of even very weak information bearing on the likelihood of those outcomes for the specific case under study.

A classic example of the latter bias is an experiment in which people were asked to judge whether an individual was an engineer or a lawyer. If the people were given no narrative description of the individual, they correctly used information on the proportions of lawyers and engineers in the general population in judging the probability that an unknown person was a lawyer. However, they completely ignored this distributional information if they were given even a highly ambiguous description of the individual (Tversky and Kahneman, 1974):

> Dick is a 30-year-old man. He is married with no children. A man of high ability and high motivation, he promises to be quite successful in his field. He is well liked by his colleagues.

Given such a description, respondents tended to say that there was a 50–50 chance that he was an engineer, even if they knew that there was a 70%–30% split of lawyers and engineers in the population.

One direct analogy in carcinogenesis risk assessment is that, in deciding whether to judge a chemical to be carcinogenic, it is rare for toxicologists to systematically consider information on the frequency of positive carcinogenicity findings in structurally related chemicals. This is true even when available data on the chemical of interest come from questionable experiments. (For such cases, the structural group information may be the best available basis for judging the likelihood of activity.)

Another example is that in fitting alternative dose–response curves to carcinogenicity data, biostatisticians tend to treat a wide variety of curves as having the same inherent likelihood (Gibson, 1983; Ozga et al., 1984; Grinstaff and Cook, 1984), so long as they can be made to fit the data equally well. Large differences between simple maximum likelihood estimates of risk based on the array of models used by Occupational Safety and Health Administration (OSHA) have recently been cited as a reason for OSHA to defer control action on formaldehyde (Bureau of National Affairs, 1985). However, some mathematical formulations have very strong foundations in the theory of cancer mechanisms, whereas others are simple mathematical constructs that have no known linkages to causal processes. An appropriate Bayesian analysis* should accord much higher likelihood to the former types of models than to the latter.

Recent experience suggests that the first kind of bias listed above (assigning too narrow confidence limits to subjective assessments of probability) can be reduced by

*It should be acknowledged that the whole Bayesian approach suggested here is highly controversial among academic statisticians, specifically because it (1) admits of a role for subjective judgment of the likelihood of circumstances/outcomes for which there are no observations of actual frequencies, and (2) because of some technical difficulties and ambiguities in specifying "priors" [see, for example, the "paradox" cited by Seidenfeld (1979), p. 12]. There is a whole school of "frequentist" thought, pioneered by the celebrated R. A. Fisher, which has sought to derive an appropriate procedure for inferring the probability density function for an unknown parameter entirely from empirical measurements of that parameter—without using any "prior" information on the expected distribution of the parameter's value in the absence of the measurements (e.g., Hacking, 1965). These efforts do not appear to have succeeded (Seidenfeld, 1979, pp. 219–222). Therefore, it seems that at the most basic methodological level, a purist of the frequentist school could not appropriately claim to produce estimates of the likelihood of any risk (or any other unknown quantity) from any imaginable empirical data.

calibration exercises (Lichtenstein and Fischhoff, 1980; Alpert and Raiffa, 1982). An additional possibility is that analysts could adjust experts' expressed subjective probabilities in the light of this phenomenon. The second type of bias (neglect of general distributional information) can be addressed by a five-step procedure suggested by Kahneman and Tversky (1982):

1. Selection of a reference class.
2. Assessment of the distribution for the reference class (defining the "prior" probabilities of outcomes).
3. Intuitive estimation of outcomes from the case-specific information.
4. Assessment of the predictability of outcomes from the case-specific information.
5. Correction of the intuitive estimate from case-specific information using the prior information.

If adopted, such a procedure would make some of the judgmental elements in a risk assessment transparent to both the analysts themselves and to reviewers, but might carry with it some added danger that the analysts would be accused of prejudice in the formation of their prior and case-specific judgments of likelihood.

Interesting as the Tversky/Kahneman suggestions may be, it is by no means clear that they address all, or even a very large fraction, of the uncertainties in current risk analyses. Uncertainties take a number of forms and arise at more than one level (see Table 1). It may not always be entirely straightforward to do a simple sensitivity analysis or even

Table 1. Examples of Uncertainty in Risk Assessments[a]

Model uncertainties. Arising from possible errors in the form or completeness of the mathematical formulation used to represent causal processes producing damage, such as:

- The damage pathways analyzed do not represent all potentially important modes of failure or damage.
- Failure to appreciate possible common-mode failures of parallel or redundant systems.
- Inappropriate aggregation or needless disaggregation in the system model. Inappropriate aggregation occurs, for example, in ecosystem modeling when "compartments" with different kinetic properties are treated as if they had similar kinetic properties—a "U.S. Freshwater" compartment might erroneously lump rivers (in which materials are purged to the sea within one year) with lakes (in which incoming toxic material may persist for extended periods). Inappropriate aggregation can also occur when inhomogeneous data are grouped together for analysis.
- Inappropriate attribution of cause and/or neglect of important causal determinants: A + B (unrecognized) causes C. Subsequent model predictions will make erroneous estimates of C from information on A alone.
- Inappropriate definition of system boundaries (where to stop in tracing ripple effects).

Parameter uncertainties. Arising from possible errors in the expected values of specific parameters (components of a causal model) or probability density functions used to describe the estimated errors in those parameters, such as:

- General misestimation (usually underestimation) of uncertainties of individual parameter estimates.
- Misperception of the likely form of uncertainties in specific elements (e.g., normal versus long-normal; unimodal versus multimodal).

[a]Some of the same general categories of uncertainties that appear in this table are discussed in more detail in Vesely and Rasmuson (1984).

to devise a Monte Carlo simulation procedure to estimate the overall probability density function for risk in the light of uncertainties of diverse types. However, the procedure outlined above would be an improvement over current practice. At present, it seems that in current risk assessments, when some quantification of uncertainties is offered at all, what is quantified is some derivative of simple experimental sampling error. Unfortunately, that is generally a trivially small proportion of the uncertainty in the overall analysis and therefore tends to be quite misleading (Mendez et al., 1980).

DEFINING THE QUESTIONS FOR ANALYSIS

Difficulties also exist in conceptualizing the questions for analysis in risk assessments and in expressing results in appropriate forms. Holdren (1982) in an excellent and very readable article expresses the general set of problems of these types and their relationship to policy considerations:

> Whether you prefer an energy source that slightly increases the chance of nuclear war or one that poisons one in ten thousand of its users depends on your personal preferences and aversions. Such choices are not the province of analysts: they belong properly to the public, which expresses its preferences through the political process. But many analysts tend to make these choices on the public's behalf, intentionally or unintentionally, by omitting those hazards that they have decided are uninteresting, too difficult to quantify, too speculative, or too likely to be "misinterpreted." Such omissions hide the analysts' values in the way the assessment is conducted and presented, thus biasing the outcomes.

The Holdren quotation above strongly suggests that analysts should assess and report all potential effects of alternative policies so that the appropriate societal decision-makers (and members of the constituencies they are supposed to represent) can apply their preferences to an unbiased, unweighted assemblage of the technical "facts." As a practical matter, however, the time and resources available for performing analyses are limited. Even if, in reasonably short order, one can compile a reasonably comprehensive list of potential consequences of alternative risk control policies for (1) diverse initiating events or discharges, (2) diverse damage pathways, and (3) diverse effects, as an analyst, one must make some choices about where to focus the analytical efforts to reduce the uncertainties that exist at the beginning of the study. How should the analyst allocate effort between, for example, well-established effects of relatively low consequence and poorly established effects of relatively great consequence?* These choices must be based on judgments about where analytical efforts can in fact reduce uncertainties and about the relative importance of reducing specific uncertainties to the degree anticipated. The former is arguably a technical (albeit itself highly uncertain) judgment, but the latter must unambiguously involve application of some value framework. It means anticipating what

*Simplification (including censoring) of technical information is an integral part of the processes by which experimental science itself is practically conducted, as has been elegantly documented in a recent empirical study by Star (1983) of a group of working neuroscientists.

information will turn out to be important for the purposes that the risk analysis is intended to serve. Holdren can fairly ask that these judgments be disclosed to the ultimate consumers of the information, but he cannot really ask that judgments not be made.

As it happens, a host of other operational choices of a similar character are involved in actually doing an analysis including:

1. Should the analyst be trying to find "best estimates" of risks, the likelihood and consequences of "worst case" scenarios, "conservative" upper bounds on risk, or to define the entire probability density function of valued outcomes?
2. Should the analyst take pains to uncover and disclose the distribution of the risk among the population? A 10^{-6} risk of death from a specific hazard for an aggregated group might translate into 10^{-2} for a particularly at-risk subset. Holdren (1982) cites possible differences in the distribution of risk between rich and poor, the medically susceptible and the population as a whole, and between those who have a voice in the acceptance of risk and those who do not.

In each case, I would suggest that the general criteria the analyst should apply would be those of relevance for foreseeable decisions the audience might wish to make based on the risk information. If it seems reasonably likely that more accurate information of a particular type or on a particular topic could influence the choice of risk control options, then the analyst should seek to provide that type of information as part of the analysis. If the analyst knows of a category of information that would have a good chance to influence choices (if it were available) but that cannot be provided, that fact should be disclosed. Otherwise the analysis in its incomplete form may be given more weight than it should in decision-making. In this way, the analyst can help avoid what Holdren accurately cites as a tendency to "confuse things that are countable with the things that count."

EXPRESSING THE RESULTS OF RISK ASSESSMENTS

Another way to express the ideal goal for communicating risk information is that the summary of results should allow the diverse members of the audience to apply their own value standards and yet make as informed a choice of whether to accept the risk as if the affected parties themselves had gone through the process of fully analyzing the risk information. This includes communicating the uncertainty of the information and/or reasonably likely worst case scenarios.

This is all about getting at the issues. It is fundamental to any good policy analysis, and it is not a simple problem. Furthermore, it typically must be accomplished through an iterative process of questioning and answering—where what is known about which unknowns are most relevant is to a large degree a function of existing information about both the technical "facts" and the potential significance of those facts for specific decisions. For the purpose of performing this iteration, it is helpful for the analyst to have some opportunity for interchange with the decision-maker(s) (or other audience) who are to be informed by the results.

Unfortunately, while there is a very substantial field of research documenting the difficulties and inaccuracies people have in understanding the relative magnitudes and consequences of the risks caused by different hazards (e.g., Slovic et al., 1980; Von Winterfeldt et al., 1981), there does not appear to have been a great deal of systematic study of practical ways to create more accurate risk perceptions. This task may be even more difficult when the risk information must be communicated indirectly via the news media. Although at least some types of probabilistic information in numerical forms have become commonplace in the public media in recent years,* it is fair to assume that in many cases both journalists and members of their audience may have difficulty in correctly interpreting quantitative information on low-probability risks.

Beyond the problems that arise from simple misunderstanding, the traditional journalistic goal of telling a single "story" in brief capsule form (answering "who, what, when, where, and why") is often complicated when the information conveyed must be heavily qualified, or when numerical conclusions must be communicated with very wide bounds of uncertainty (Tichenor, 1979; Friedman, 1983). Experts sometimes complain that the press sensationalizes risk information (*The Morning Call*, 1983; *Editor and Publisher*, 1983), and this may make some reluctant to face the task of communicating with members of the press.

The notion that the analyst should strive to communicate information in the most helpful way possible for decision-making by the audience may seem straightforward enough. However, when we start to consider how to make this criterion operational, significant difficulties quickly appear. In particular, the honesty of the analyst will be under constant scrutiny as to whether he or she is being too "helpful" to the audience in reaching one type of policy conclusion on the basis of the data rather than another.

First, some modes of expression can be misleading in implying inappropriate causal models. If we were to take the number of head injuries that occur in major league football every year and divide it by the number of showers taken, we could calculate that there are some specific numbers of head injuries per shower. That would be literally correct, but the implication that most of the injuries occur while showering—or were in some way causally connected to showering—is quite false, as would be the implication that showering safety should receive priority attention in reducing football injuries.

Another example of the possible introduction of policy bias by the terms of reference used involves the degree of aggregation used in expressing the results. Consider a risk expressed as 10^{-6} per individual per lifetime for all U.S. citizens. It is approximately mathematically equivalent to say that the hazard will cause 0.008 death per day in the United States, or 3 deaths per year, or 200 deaths over a 70-year lifetime for current U.S. citizens. However, I suspect that these different formulations convey appreciably different notions of the magnitude of the problem. The 10^{-6} and 0.008 numbers are relatively hard for the mind to grapple with and may, if anything, call forth associations with the number

*For example, weather forecasters have been expressing the probability of precipitation in percentage terms since 1965 (Wallsten and Budescu, 1983). Also, it is now very common to see the results of public opinion polls accompanied by at least some vague statement of the "uncertainty" in the poll results.

of deaths from lightning one might expect. They seem small. Expressing the risk as 3 deaths per year calls forth in our minds an association with a bad traffic accident—a tragedy, but not so significant or remarkable that it would seem to warrant attention on the first page of the *New York Times*. By contrast, the 200 deaths per lifetime calls forth associations with a major airline disaster or the bombing of the U.S. military barracks in Beirut, subjects that have been the focus of headline attention.*

Another distinction that appears in this example is between aggregate risks for the nation and individual risks. Expressing risks in individual terms focuses attention on the policy issue, "Is it fair or appropriate for this individual (or type of individual) to be required or permitted to assume *x* level of risk?" On the other hand, expressing risk results in national aggregate terms focuses attention on the policy issue, "Is it reasonable for society as a whole to expend the resources required to avoid this amount of expected harm?"

The same type of phenomenon comes into play in the expression of the uncertainty of the results. There is no particular reason why a raw statement of the probability density function for different levels of risk from a particular exposure should be different from agency to agency or audience to audience (e.g., there could be a 5% chance that the risk was less than 10^{-9}, a 50% chance that the risk was less than 10^{-6}, and a 95% chance that the risk was less than 10^{-3}). However, the particular form used for summarizing such uncertainty may be more or less relevant for choices under a specific statute or by a specific audience. Under a risk/benefit balancing type of statute, the full probability density function for all sectors of the exposed population may be relevant to the decision-maker's choice, whereas only an "upper confidence limit" (at some defined probability level) for a select "sensitive subgroup" within the population may be relevant under a statute that requires the decision-maker to assure that the standard will "protect public health with an adequate margin of safety." If the analyst chooses only one form for expression of uncertainty, he or she is implying that this specific form is the one that is most relevant for decision-making by the audience.

Specific modes for expressing numerical quantities can implicitly draw the audience's attention to some kinds of perspective-giving comparisons, and away from other comparisons. The challenge to the analyst in assisting the audience in making as informed a choice as if members of the audience themselves had done the analysis implies that the analyst must try to anticipate and illuminate the comparisons that are most likely to be helpful in the context of the choice situation faced by the audience, and the values that the audience may wish to bring to the analysis of the options. Part of the analyst's responsibility is to consider how his or her statements will be interpreted, and as much as possible to make sure that the perceptions of the audience are consistent with the actual findings (and uncertainties) of the analysis. This may well require that the results be presented in more than one form.

*The contending parties in risk control controversies have long recognized the effect of the simple size of the number in expressing the concentrations of hazardous substances in various media. For asbestos, one group will express a particular exposure as one fiber per cubic centimeter, whereas another will say there are a million fibers per cubic meter. Discussing dioxin contamination of soil, one group might say there is 0.005 part per million, whereas another might say there are 5000 parts per trillion. It is often not too difficult to infer the general policy position of specific parties from the terms of reference they choose to use.

CONCLUSION

Even if we had good analytical techniques for assessing the "truth" about our uncertainties, and experts well trained in applying them, there would still be a problem. This is because the "facts" about both risks and uncertainties can be arranged in helpful or unhelpful ways relative to a particular decision problem. There are relevant facts and irrelevant facts, and facts that are stated in such a way as to even be misleading. To be useful for any of the several purposes people have in wishing to assess risks, the analysis must be—and be seen to be—the result of a reasonably impartial application of standards of inference to the hazy subject matter. However, the terms we choose for communicating both our main findings and our uncertainties generally imply a particular framing of the decision problem for our audience that makes some implicit value-laden assumptions. Like the famous modern painting of a can of Campbell's soup, the very act of selecting a particular object to portray makes a nontrivial statement that this specific object should be elevated to special status relative to the objects not so portrayed. Therefore, risk assessors must be sophisticated in the risk decision/policy area in order to achieve reasonable fairness in communication.

REFERENCES

Alpert, M., and H. Raiffa. 1982. A progress report on the training of probability assessors. In *Judgment Under Uncertainty: Heuristics and Biases*. Ed. D. Kahneman, P. Slovic, and A. Tversky. New York: Cambridge University Press, pp. 294–305.

American Petroleum Institute v. OSHA. 1978. 581 F.2d, pp. 493–503.

Aqua Slide 'N' Dive Corp. v. CPSC. 1978. 569 F.2d, p. 831, 5th Cir.

Bureau of National Affairs. 1985. OSHA denies UAW petition for ETS, announces meeting to gather information. *Occupational Safety and Health Reporter* 14: 580.

Editor and Publisher (Anonymous). 11 June 1983. Press hit on coverage of radiation issues.

Fischhoff, B. 1982, Debiasing, in: *Judgment Under Uncertainty: Heuristics and Biases* (D. Kahneman, P. Slovic, and A. Tversky, eds.), pp. 422–44, Cambridge University Press, New York.

Friedman, S. M. 1983. Environmental reporting: Problem child of the media. *Environment* 25(December): 24–29.

Gibson, J. E. 1983, Risk assessment using a combination of testing and research results, in: *Formaldehyde Toxicity* (J. E. Gibson, ed.), pp. 295–302, Hemisphere, New York.

Grinstaff, G., and B. Cook. EPA Exposure Evaluation Division, 27 March 1984. *Quantitative Cancer Risk Assessment: Formaldehyde*. Memo to Rich Hefter, EPA Risk Management Branch.

Hacking, I., 1965, *Logic of Statistical Inference*, Cambridge University Press, Cambridge.

Holdren, J. 1982. Energy hazards: What to measure, what to compare. *Technology Review* 85(3): 32–39, 74–75.

Industrial Union Dept. v. American Petrol. Inst. 1980. 448 US, pp. 607–22.

Kahneman, D., and A. Tversky, 1982, Intuitive prediction: Biases and corrective procedures, in: *Judgment Under Uncertainty: Heuristics and Biases*, (D. Kahneman, P. Slovic, and A. Tversky, eds.), pp. 414–21, Cambridge University Press, New York.

Lichtenstein, S., and B. Fischhoff. 1980. Training for calibration. *Organizational Behavior and Human Performance* 26: 149–71.

Mendez, W., D. Hattis, and N. A. Ashford. 1980. *Discussion and Critique of the Carcinogenicity Assessment Group's Report on Population Risk Due to Atmospheric Exposure to Benzene*. Report to the Office of Air Quality Planning and Standards of the U.S. Environmental Protection Agency. MIT Center for Policy Alternatives, Publication No. CPA-80-1.

Ozga, G., I. S. Rodgers, B. Fountos, and R. Beliles. 1984. *Preliminary Assessment of the Health Effects of Formaldehyde*. Office of Risk Assessment, Directorate of Health Standards Programs, Occupational Safety and Health Administration.

Ruckelshaus, W. D. 1983. Science, risk, and public policy. *Science* 221: 1026–28.

Seidenfeld, T., 1979, *Philosophical Problems of Statistical Inference*, D. Reidel, Boston.

Slovic, P., B. Fischhoff, and S. Lichtenstein, 1980, Facts and fears: Understanding perceived risk, in: *Societal Risk Assessment: How Safe Is Safe Enough*? (R. C. Schwing and W. A. Albers, Jr., eds.), pp. 181–216, Plenum, New York.

Star, S. L. 1983. Simplification in scientific work: An example from neuroscience research. *Social Studies of Science* 13: 205–28.

The Morning Call (Allentown, PA), 23 June 1983. AMA claims dioxin is focus of a witch hunt.

Tichenor, P. J. 1979. Teaching and the "journalism of uncertainty." *Journal of Environmental Education* 10(Spring): 5–8.

Tversky, A., and D. Kahneman. 1974. Judgment under uncertainty: Heuristics and biases. *Science* 185: 1124–31.

Vesely, W. E., and D. M. Rasmuson. 1984. Uncertainties in nuclear probabilistic risk analyses. *Risk Analysis* 4: 313–22.

Von Winterfeldt, D., R. S. John, and K. Borcherding. 1981. Cognitive components of risk ratings. *Risk Analysis* 1: 277–87.

Wallsten, T. S. and D. V. Budescu. 1983. Encoding subjective probabilities: A psychological and psychometric review. *Management Science* 29: 151–73.

Winkler, R. L. 1967. The quantification of judgment: Some methodological suggestions. *Journal of the American Statistical Association* 62: 1105–20.

19

Translation of Risk Information for the Public: Message Development

Elaine Bratic Arkin

The development of messages that will inform the public about risks to their health and encourage them to take appropriate action is a vital step in the communications process. Because the abstract concept of risk is difficult to explain and comprehend, message development may be one of the most frustrating stages in the process. This frustration is shared by agency officials who are responsible for risk communication and face a public untrained to understand scientific methodology and technical terminology, as well as citizens who want concrete answers and action regarding health risks instead of uncertain responses. Barriers to effective communications include the nature of health risk science, limitations of the media and other communication channels, and public perceptions of risk. Therefore, the message development process must encompass how the public perceives health risk messages, characteristics of the target audiences and selected communications channels, principles for message design, and message testing.

FACTORS AFFECTING THE PUBLIC'S PERCEPTION OF HEALTH RISKS

Issues that affect the communication of complex health risk information to the public sometimes may appear as complex as determining the levels of risk. However, considering how the public perceives health risks prior to message development can help assure that the public will hear and heed the information conveyed. The following factors affect public acceptance of health risk messages:

Elaine Bratic Arkin • The Institute for Health Policy Analysis, Georgetown University Medical Center, Washington, D.C. 20007.

Risk Is an Intangible Concept—The general public does not understand the concept of relative risk, and so personal decisions may be based on faulty assumptions. For example, the public tends to overestimate their risk of accidents, homicides, and other events that frequently make the news and underestimate their risk of less newsworthy but more common health problems, such as strokes and diabetes (Fischhoff, 1985; Slovic, 1985).

The Public Responds to Easy Solutions—The ability to act in order to reduce or eliminate an identified risk can lessen the actual risk and can abate the fear, denial, or mistrust that may result from new risk information. The public is more likely to respond if the call for action is relatively simple (e.g., discontinuing the use of hair dryers that contain asbestos) and less likely to act if the price of that action is higher (e.g., changing occupations). Unfortunately, there may be no risk reduction action possible or the action may be complicated (such as quitting smoking to reduce the risk of cancer following exposure to asbestos).

The Public Calls for Absolute Answers—Risk messages, which describe intangible, often invisible hazards, usually can only predict possible outcomes. The public does not want probabilities; they want concrete information by which they can make decisions. In the absence of firm answers from scientists, the media sometimes will draw an inappropriate conclusion that provides the public with faulty but conclusive information. Also, the contrasting clarity of absolutes may skew an individual's interpretation of personal risk. That is, a 5% risk may be perceived as an unacceptable level of risk for the individual who wants a 100% guarantee of safety; yet a 75% risk may appear more acceptable than it should when presented to an individual who compares it to a 100% risk certainty (Allman, 1985). This misperception can turn information intended to reassure the public about a relatively small risk into a new subject for major personal concern.

The Public Reacts Unfavorably to Fear—Frightening risk information, which sometimes cannot be avoided, may result in personal denial or disproportionate levels of hysteria, anxiety, and feelings of helplessness, compounded by an absence of actions that an individual can take to ameliorate the risk.

The Public Wants Personal Control—People desire control over their personal well-being and many environmental health risks represent a loss of control (National Cancer Institute, 1983). Although the public believes that it does not have control over environmental health risks, individuals can control personal health risks; therefore, they are more willing to accept personal risks.

The Public Doubts the Verity of Science—The public knows that scientists can be wrong and recalls incidents such as the swine flu epidemic and Three Mile Island. They may hesitate to believe a scientist's prediction.

The Public Has Other Priorities—New health risk information may not be integrated as one of an individual's priorities. When the National Cancer Institute conducted focus groups with World War II shipyard workers, they found that a future threat of cancer from a long-ago exposure to asbestos paled in comparison with the daily infirmities of this older population (Freimuth and Van Nevel, 1979). Conversely, teenagers, many of whom may never have experienced poor health, may find it inconceivable that they are susceptible to future illness, regardless of their exposure to risk.

Individuals Are Not Personally Susceptible—The public has a strong tendency to underestimate their personal risk. One survey found that 54% of respondents believed that a serious illness couldn't happen to them and considered their risk to be less than that of the general public, regardless of their actual risk (National Cancer Institute, 1983; Yankelovich et al., 1978–79).

The Public Holds Contradictory Beliefs—Even though an individual may believe that "it can't happen to me," he or she can still believe that everything causes cancer. Many people believe that there is no way to avoid cancer "when your time comes" and no need to alter personal behavior (National Cancer Institute, 1983; Yankelovich et al., 1978–79). Also, the belief that everything causes cancer can contribute an unwarranted imbalance to perceptions of news regarding carcinogens.

The Public Lacks a Future Orientation—The majority of Americans believe that it is better to live for the present than to worry about tomorrow (Yankelovich et al., 1978–79). Members of the public, especially those in lower socioeconomic groups, have difficulty relating to the concept of the future, and environmental health risks foretell of outcomes far in the future. Focus group participants who convened to help plan a cancer prevention program said that it would take an actual health scare or seeing a health problem in a friend or loved one to make them alter their own behavior (National Cancer Institute, 1983).

The Public Personalizes New Information—New risk information is frequently described in terms of its effect on society (such as predicted morbidity and mortality rates). The individual needs to translate that information into personal risk to understand it and translation of information offers an opportunity for misinterpretation and misjudgment.

The Public Does Not Understand Science—Technical data, risk models and methodology, the variables involved in calculating risk, and the fact that science is not static but evolves and changes over time tend to be poorly understood by the public. Therefore, many individuals lack the basic tools that are required to understand and interpret risk information.

Although public perceptions of science and health risks make message development a challenge, the extensive body of research on public perceptions provides guidance for formulating messages. This knowledge, combined with a profile of target audiences, decisions about appropriate channels for message delivery, and a clear statement of the issue or problem to be addressed, can help direct message development and help avoid "bad science" in communications program planning.

PLANNING MESSAGES: DETERMINING THE TARGET AUDIENCE

There is not one "public" but rather diverse interests, needs, concerns, and priorities among different segments of the public. Message development, while not an insurmountable problem, is difficult. Clearly, no one message is appropriate for various audiences with different levels of knowledge and different media habits.

Prior to message development, the public must be divided into manageable groups according to risk, media exposure, attitudes, knowledge, and behaviors, or other characteristics to help define an appropriate message. Target audiences may be defined by demographic characteristics (e.g., age, sex, occupation, risk/exposure, or education) or by psychographics (such as personality traits, interests, opinions, or cultural and life-style characteristics) to help identify appropriate appeals. The process of defining target audiences can help clarify the information to transmit, the channels for message delivery, and the specific needs of the target audiences.

For example, when the Office on Smoking and Health planned an antismoking campaign, they separated cigarette smokers into target audiences by age, and identified the rationale for each age group continuing to smoke. They tailored the basic "don't smoke" message for each audience, changing it to "it isn't too late to lower your risks" (for middle-aged men), "smoking isn't cool" (for teenagers), and "smoking can harm your baby" (for pregnant women) in order to address the reasons for smoking in each group. The rationale for smoking and the perceived "benefits" gained were identified through market research, in this case by asking members of each audience group why they smoked.

The segment of the public that is most likely to be at risk (for occupational and other societal risks) is the blue-collar worker. This lower socioeconomic group also is likely to be less well educated, less likely to comprehend abstract information, and less likely to have the flexibility to change personal behavior or life-style (including occupation) to avoid further risk. Out of necessity, short-term priorities often replace any future orientation. As a result of having less personal control over life, this group also is more likely to be fatalistic (Union Carbide Corporation, 1977). This audience is generally harder to reach and influence with risk messages.

PLANNING MESSAGES: MARKET RESEARCH

Market research information exists about many aspects of the public's health behavior. Existing sources of market research information on the public's health behavior include published survey data from research sponsors (e.g., major corporations concerned with public attitudes toward the environment); survey research firms (e.g., Gallup, Harris, and Opinion Research); and market research studies conducted to provide information about public attitudes, buying and consumption patterns, and media habits for marketing and advertising agencies. Both published and unpublished survey reports are available from government agencies.

However, sometimes data are unavailable or out of date and it is necessary to conduct audience research prior to message development. This investigation can involve large, statistically significant numbers of respondents or a few representatives who are typical of the group to be reached. Agencies frequently rely on the latter (qualitative research) because it is faster, less expensive, and, for federal agencies, less likely to require Office of Management and Budget clearance.

PLANNING MESSAGES: CHANNEL SELECTION

Once target audiences have been defined, it is necessary to choose the communication channels that are most likely to reach the audiences and most appropriate for the kind of information to be relayed. Channel selection might include a mix of mass media (television, radio, newspapers, and magazines), interpersonal communication (e.g., peers, family members, and health professionals), and community groups (employers, health departments, and schools). Each channel offers different benefits and requires a different message design (although not necessarily different messages) to fit the channel.

The mass media can transmit news quickly to a broad audience but cannot alone be expected to motivate people to change their behavior. The mass media are the public's primary source of information but may be less trusted than more intimate sources of information. Media channels may focus too much attention on new information that affects limited segments of the population; may increase the chances for miscommunication of complex or controversial news; and may communicate incomplete information (i.e., omit information that explains what should be done about a risk). Loss of control over how the information is communicated sometimes is a trade-off for broad and rapid transmission.

Program planners should remember that the purpose of mass media is to entertain, not educate. Therefore, if the complete message is too complicated or simply not considered interesting enough for general consumption, the risk communication program planner is obligated to design a message that is appealing in order to use the mass media. Mass media offer many opportunities beyond the news, including entertainment programming (e.g., topical issues presented on popular dramatic television programs), public affairs and interview shows, editorials, and health and political columns.

Interpersonal communication channels can place risks in a more familiar context. These channels are more likely to be trusted and influential (especially physicians, friends, and family members of the target audiences). However, development of messages, materials, and links for interpersonal channels requires time-consuming and often costly development. Influence through interpersonal contacts requires familiarity with the message; therefore, it may more appropriately follow long-term exposure to and acceptance of media messages. Similarly, community channels, including schools, employers, and community organizations, can reinforce and expand on media messages and offer instruction regarding how to act to reduce risks or how to become involved in appropriate decisionmaking. The establishment of links with community institutions and organizations can shortcut the development of interpersonal routes of influence within the target audience. Interpersonal and community channels are two-way models that allow discussion and clarification, encourage motivation, and reinforce action.

Use of as many channels as possible will increase the repetition of the information and improve the chance of the audience hearing the information a sufficient number of times to absorb and remember it.

MESSAGE CONSTRUCTION

The purpose of communicating new information influences message design. Information may be designed to convey new facts, alter attitudes, change behavior (such as encouraging protective action), or encourage participation in decisionmaking. These purposes sometimes overlap; often they are progressive. The public must receive, understand, believe, agree, and act accordingly in order for the persuasion to work. Regardless of the purpose, messages must be developed with consideration of the desired outcome. The following factors that help determine public acceptance should be considered before messages are drafted:

1. Clarity—Messages must convey information clearly to assure the public's ability to make informed personal choices (if necessary) and to limit the chances for misunderstanding or even inappropriate action. Clear messages contain as few technical, scientific, and bureaucratic terms as possible, and eliminate information that the public does not need in order to make necessary decisions. Readability tests, which take approximately 15 minutes to conduct, can help determine the reading level required to understand the drafted material and help writers to be conscientious about the careful selection of words and phrases.
2. Consistency—In an ideal world, all messages on a particular risk topic would be consistent, lessen the confusion and mistrust of science, and increase the probability of public understanding. In the real world, unfortunately, consistency on a risk issue is difficult when experts legitimately can interpret new health risk data differently, and consensus among government, industry, and public interest spokespersons with regard to the interpretation of new data is unlikely.
3. Main points—The message designer should clarify the most important points for the public to comprehend and ensure that those points are stressed, repeated, and not hidden within less important information.
4. Tone and appeal—A message should be appropriately reassuring, alarming, challenging, or straightforward, depending on the desired impact on the target audience. Messages can be presented in either a positive or negative manner, and public decisions can be influenced by the choice of the presentation style.
5. Credibility—The spokesperson or source of the information should be trustworthy and consistent. The spokesperson should be able to present the message convincingly and in a clear manner.
6. Public need—For a message to break through the information clutter with which the public lives, messages should be based on what the public perceives as most important and what they want to know, rather than what is most important or most interesting to the originating agency.

MESSAGE TESTING

Prior to final production, messages should be pretested with the target audiences (and in some cases with channel "gatekeepers") to ensure public understanding and other intended responses. Even if risk messages are carefully drafted, there is only one way to find out whether the target audience will understand, believe, and follow the advice: ask representatives of the target audience.

Qualitative research should be conducted in the early stages of message development, before full funds have been committed to program development, so that the messages can be changed if necessary. Testing can be useful at the concept development stage, once target audiences and message strategies have been determined, and prior to message development. Contact with target audience members at this stage, most frequently through focus group discussions, can help determine appropriate message appeals (e.g., fear arousing versus factual); spokesperson (e.g., a scientist, public official, or member of the target audience); and appropriate language (determined by noting the group's use of language).

Testing of drafted materials prior to final production (through focus groups, written questionnaires, or personal interviews) permits identification of flaws prior to final production. For example, a self-test designed to identify personal health risks and methods to reduce risks was greeted with enthusiasm by the target audience. They found the test interesting and informative. However, they could not understand the scoring system at the end of the quiz; therefore, they could not determine their personal health risks. As a result of this pretest, the scoring system was simplified prior to the printing and distribution of several million copies of this booklet.

Completed information materials also may be tested prior to beginning a new phase of a preexisting program. The National High Blood Pressure Education Program produces new public service announcements each year. Prior to beginning each new production phase, spots from the previous year are tested to determine whether hypertensives recognize, like, and identify with them. Based on test results, themes may be used for several years to help ensure message recall or new themes may be developed.

Pretesting can be used to assess an audience's comprehension, the message's believability, personal relevance, acceptability, and other strong and weak points. Different pretesting methodologies should be selected depending on the purpose of the testing, the sensitivity of the subject, and the resources available for alternate testing methods (National Cancer Institute, 1984).

This investigation is especially important when developing sensitive or potentially frightening messages or when presenting complex new information to the public. For example, a current Kent cigarette campaign features silhouetted figures engaged in sports activities accompanied by the message, "The experience you seek." Some people interpreted the figures as ghosts, which unwittingly reinforces the efforts of the antismoking community. Although the campaign was tested, the advertising agency may not have been aware of how reluctant individuals can be to discuss sensitive subjects such as death or to strongly disapprove of materials being tested. A different test design, additional testing, or greater awareness of public reaction to health-related issues may have saved the company public embarrassment and expense (*The Wall Street Journal*, 1987).

Such testing research does not provide answers that can be projected to the public as a whole; it is conducted to provide insights into the thinking and behavior of the target audience and to help refine message strategies and choose appeals most likely to be successful. Therefore, pretesting must be conducted with care, analyzed by professionals who are familiar with testing and with the subject matter, and used in conjunction with (not instead of) professional judgment.

In addition to the appropriateness of the message, a pretest can be structured to test the length of copy, appeal of graphics and charts, credibility of sources, and presentation style or information format. For example, the Public Health Service developed a series of booklets on nutrition, smoking, and other health-related subjects for low-income women. Although the draft booklets were tested to reveal any confusing or incomprehensible information, the tests revealed that despite the simplicity of the information, the booklet was too long and boring to read. The information was redesigned as a less expensive, more attractive series of fact sheets (Arkin, 1985). Pretesting materials prior to final production can help avoid costly mistakes in terms of agency resources as well as public understanding, health, and well-being.

THE NEED FOR PUBLIC EDUCATION

The public wants guidance regarding health risks (National Cancer Institute, 1983). They are confused by all of the government health warnings (Yankelovich et al., 1978–79). They want to be allowed to make risk-related decisions but do not feel qualified to do so (Union Carbide Corporation, 1977). The public needs to be able to interpret risk information, weigh contradictory information, accept science as it progresses and changes, and seek additional information necessary for decisionmaking.

An informed public is more likely to be able to identify the strengths and weaknesses of risk measures and new risk information, relate the information to their personal situation, and avoid the comparison of dissimilar risks. The public needs to be taught to accept the uncertainties of science and to understand the concept of relative risk and the methods used to predict risk.

Different government agencies have the responsibility of informing the public about different kinds of risk information. However, in an era of diminishing resources and pressing priorities, it is unclear whether any specific agency has the responsibility for providing the public with the context for understanding risks they may face individually or collectively. Furthermore, there are compelling reasons why an agency should not undertake broad-scale public education. Education could raise public expectations for more information, services, and policies at a time when many government agencies are facing budget and staff reductions, internal political pressures, and bureaucratic inertia.

Yet there is an obvious and compelling need for public understanding that is apparent each time there is new information to communicate. An informed consumer would be better prepared to focus on the real issues surrounding new risk information, even if those issues included the need for abatement services or a public role in policymaking.

Public education has been called a long-term goal; yet it appears that short-term problems preclude tackling this goal. However, the dilemma of how to design effective messages and communication strategies for an uninformed public will continue until the public is provided with a context for integrating new risk information into its own base of knowledge.

REFERENCES AND SELECTED BIBLIOGRAPHY

Allman, W. F. 1985. Staying alive in the 20th century. *Science 85* 6(8): 30–37.

Arkin, E. B. 1985. *Designing Effective Mass Media Materials for Health Promotion*. Paper presented at the Marketing and Health Promotion Conference, Ohio University, Athens, Ohio.

Cohen, A., M. J. Colligan, and P. Berger. 1985. Psychology in health risk messages for workers. *Journal of Occupational Medicine* 27(8): 543–591.

Covello, V. T., D. von Winterfeldt, and P. Slovic. 1986. Communicating scientific information about health and environmental risks: problems and opportunities from a social and behavioral perspective. In *Uncertainties in Risk Assessment and Risk Management*. Ed. V. Covello, A. Moghissi, and V. R. R. Uppuluri. New York: Plenum Press.

Fischhoff, B. 1985. *Perceptions of Risk Perceptions*, unpublished.

Freimuth, V. S., and P. Van Nevel. 1979. *The Role of Gatekeepers in the Asbestos Awareness Campaign*, National Cancer Institute, unpublished.

Higbee, K. L. 1969. Fifteen years of fear arousal—research on threat appeals: 1953–1968. *Psychological Bulletin* 72(6): 426–444.

Jacobs, J. A. 1982. News from health research: toward a better understanding. *The Journal of School Health* 52(10): 614–618.

Kasperson, R. E. 1986. Six propositions on public participation and their relevance for risk communication. *Risk Analysis* 6(3): 275–281.

National Cancer Institute. 1982. *National Survey of Public Knowledge, Attitudes and Practices Related to Cancer* (Phase One), unpublished.

National Cancer Institute. 1983. *Public Attitudes and Behavior Regarding Cancer Risk and Prevention*, unpublished.

National Cancer Institute. 1984. *Pretesting in Health Communications*, NIH Publication No. 84-1493.

Sharlin, H. I. 1986. EDB: a case study in communicating risk. *Risk Analysis* 6(1): 61–68.

Slovic, P. 1985. *Risk Perception and Risk Communication*, unpublished.

The Wall Street Journal, January 15, 1987. Ads for Kent cigarettes spark lively debate about ghosts.

Union Carbide Corporation. 1977. *An Analysis of Citizen Attitudes Toward Cancer Risks*, unpublished.

Weinstein, N. D., and P. M. Sandman. 1985. *Radon Risk Communication Symposium: Generic Findings*, Contract C-29190 for the Office of Science and Research, New Jersey Department of Environmental Protection.

Wilson, J., R. M. Romano, and J. Stein. 1985. Public perception of cancer risk and prevention: implications for physicians. *Maryland Medical Journal* 34(1): 63–66.

Winsten, J. 1985. Science and the media: the boundaries of truth. *Health Affairs* 4(1): 5–23.

Yankelovich, Skelly, and White. 1978–79. *Family Health in Era of Stress*, The General Mills Family Report.

20

Reaching Target Audiences with Risk Information

James D. Callaghan

The development of an effective communications strategy for almost any purpose depends on both the nature of the message and the nature of the audience that is the target of that message. An assessment of these two factors is necessary before communications channels can be considered. In communications programs that deal with risk, the following groups are most often the target audience: the science and/or medical community; federal, state, or local government administrators; legislative bodies; regulators; the media; a specific community; and the general public. In specific situations there are always a number of subgroups, but for general purposes these will serve to illustrate the appropriate means of communication.

The selection and priority ranking of the audiences depends on the nature of the message and the type of action that it encourages. For instance, if the object is to get people to stop eating some commonly sold food item, the general public is the most crucial audience. If the prime need is some sort of legislative or regulatory prohibition or restriction, then of, course, the major target is the body with the power to take that action. Again, if the risk is to worker health, the target becomes the workers and those who are in a position to institute protective measures.

Two additional points can be made about the different audiences. First, the methods used to reach the general public will reach (in one way or another) all of the audiences on a target list. Second, although the media are usually considered a channel through which to reach an audience, in risk situations that involve complex and highly technical issues, they often must be educated before they can be accurate channels.

James D. Callaghan • Consultant, New York, New York 10028. The author is a retired senior vice president of Hill and Knowlton, Inc., where he was the director of the firm's Division of Scientific, Technical and Environmental Affairs.

THE MESSAGE IS KEY

Formulation of the message in risk situations requires a special point of view. Because of the nature of the subject, effective communication demands maximum accuracy and a minimum of gimmickry. In most situations, the aim is to convey a body of information that warns of a risk while at the same time suggesting some remedial action.

This communications effort is unlikely to occur in a vacuum. With the exception of natural disasters, epidemics, and such rare issues as radon contamination of homes, risk communications tend to "gore someone's ox." Thus, the communication often occurs in an adversarial situation.

The initiators of a risk story must be very careful not to lay traps for themselves in the first statements. It is important that there be strong scientific backup for the message—that the proposed action match the severity of the threat—and that reality not be stretched for dramatic effect. For instance, in the debate on saccharin and health, the Food and Drug Administration's (FDA's) claim that the artificial sweetener was causing 1200 cases of bladder cancer a year presented an easy target. All that was needed to instill doubt was an explanation that this extrapolation was really zero to 1200 cases and that zero was just as likely as 1200. In addition, it was noted that the FDA extrapolation was based on a use of saccharin five times the current level. This is a small point, perhaps, but if enough small points are assembled, they can cripple the credibility of a risk communicator.

Another key point is to make sure the same information is being conveyed to all audiences. The language, types of forums, and amount of detail may vary from audience to audience, but the information should not. If the caveats that surround most scientific information are identified in the beginning and put in context, the communications task will be easier when opposition arises.

REACHING THE SCIENTIFIC AND/OR MEDICAL COMMUNITY

The scientific or medical community is often an important audience in risk issues. Members can become powerful allies in a communications effort if they are motivated and armed with useful information. They are also often sources of information for the media, advisors to state and local government, and have the ear of the people. This community can be reached through the special media that serve the various disciplines, existing forums and conferences, special conferences, personal communications, and impartial data bases.

Nearly every medical and scientific discipline is served by one or more journals. These are valuable publications for studies dealing with risk and for letters that provide a rapid means of flagging a risk. The provision of material or personal visits may spur editorial support for a particular point of view.

Another important channel to the scientific community is the semitechnical press. These publications provide brief reports, roundups, and straight news that are relatively jargon-free and journalistic in tone. They are excellent outlets for risk information and offer an opportunity to provide more detail than the general press will take. Their existence also makes a point about the scientific community. Its members do indeed prefer getting their information in simple English and then going to the sources if they need to know more.

Scientific conferences provide the opportunity to present papers on risk issues, but this represents only one of the many communications possibilities available at such meetings. These sessions provide the opportunity to set up peer meetings and hold press conferences for both the general and semitechnical press. Printed proceedings can carry the information and views far beyond the meeting rooms to the broader scientific community. Additional mailings by an interest group can provide an even larger audience for the message. Special conferences can focus on specific risk issues.

When a risk issue is embroiled in controversy, it is often helpful to develop new scientific newsletters or bulletins that can convey current developments, provide in-depth analysis of various studies, and offer properly labeled opinions. One such newsletter developed to discuss the ozone depletion issue provided the only continuing source of valid scientific information during the time of greatest controversy on that problem. It became a "bestseller" in academia, with many chemistry professors requesting large numbers for use in the classroom.

Other communication methods that have seen success include traveling seminars that bring a body of information to organizations such as state and local medical societies; cooperative communications efforts with medical and/or scientific professional societies; and provision of the basic scientific data behind whatever action is being recommended to well-known scientists who might be motivated to speak out on the issue.

The language of scientific communications remains, for the most part, exceedingly formal and technical. It is frequently denser than necessary and can profit from the editing efforts of a professional communicator. A sound professional writer can usually add clarity to a scientific paper without distorting it and by doing so make the information accessible to a much broader audience.

COMMUNICATING WITH GOVERNMENT

Methods that have worked well in developing understanding and cooperation from state and local governments have included:

1. Development of information packages that consist of a position statement in lay language backed up by the appropriate research information. This is for use with officials such as state health commissioners, heads of local EPAs, legislators with a strong interest in health issues, and others with the power to act or inform.
2. Personal presentations to individuals or groups in government by a scientist or a group of experts.
3. Concentration of information efforts on a particular key official who might, if convinced, carry the message to other important arms of the state or local government.

All of these methods have as a common thread the willingness to provide at the start the in-depth information that allows state officials to support a particular position on the basis of their own evaluation. They are treated as equals and asked to be partners in action rather than followers. Federal agencies often withhold information from their state counterparts because of a fear of leaks. This creates enormous problems for state agencies and officials, who are most likely to receive the follow-up calls from the media or a frightened citizenry. Often, the withholding of information and the resultant chaos turn state agencies into allies of those who might oppose federal action on a particular issue.

THE MEDIA AS AUDIENCE

The media have a good deal of trouble with risk information. They generally are less interested in understanding it than in reporting who caused the risk and what is being done to reduce it. They also can be keenly interested in any political controversy that surrounds a risk issue.

Public understanding of how risk is determined, both generally and in specific instances, is a key to resolving the controversy that swirls around so many of the proposed actions associated with these problems. The media can be helpful in developing that understanding, but first they themselves must understand how risk is determined. Getting them to understand often involves "force-feeding."

One method that works well involves bringing the experts to the media for in-depth discussions of a particular issue. This is provided as background with the objective of developing understanding rather than producing a story. In most cases, however, a story does result that is helpful to the risk communicator's point of view.

Another method that is used both in conjunction with visitation by the experts and alone is the comprehensive background paper. This paper is used to present the basic science and studies involved in a particular issue in lay language and is an effective way of explaining what information underlies a particular position.

REACHING COMMUNITIES

When a risk issue affects a small group such as a community or a specific work force, the communications can be more tightly focused and involve more personal communications. Open meetings, although they require considerable handling skills on the part of the moderator, can work well in getting across a risk message or a suggestion for a particular course of action. They are particularly valuable in providing the instant feedback that indicates if the message is effective and what follow-up communications may be needed. This technique has potentially disruptive aspects, but it can act to clear the air by allowing people to vent their emotions, and it establishes an openness that is important to credibility. Most importantly, it sets the stage for a continuing dialogue and smaller group cooperative efforts.

Workers can be reached through union and company publications, through plant meetings, and through training and information efforts that can include the use of videotapes, printed materials, and classroom instruction.

COMMUNICATING TO THE GENERAL PUBLIC

Most often, the general public is reached through the filter of print and broadcast media, which can lead to distortion, oversimplification, and, perhaps, a loss of the primary points in a risk message. When the message is simple and straightforward, most conventional public relations methods will suffice to get the story across, including press conferences, news releases, interviews, video and audio clips, media hotlines, etc. But when the issue is cloudy and controversial, it is necessary to develop believable ways to get the information out with minimal filtering. Methods useful in doing this include:

1. A media tour of experts aimed at hitting radio and television talk shows, radio call-in programs, and other major public forums. These kinds of programs allow spokespersons to say what they want in the way that they want.
2. Op-ed page newspaper articles. A good job of writing on a hot topic such as risk, under an expert byline, is not hard to sell to op-ed page editors.
3. Bylined magazine stories. These are much the same as op-ed page articles and, as in the case with op-ed pieces, the articles can be reprinted and mailed to audiences of special significance.

RESEARCH

Market research can be valuable in identifying audiences' awareness of a risk or issue, and thus aid in the honing of a message. It is particularly valuable with influential or decisionmaking groups and can supply information about why these people feel as they do. Such research has often identified gaps in knowledge that are easily filled. On the other hand, a study may show that emotional biases are so strong that no amount of information or persuasion will work.

In general, it would be helpful to know more about how people receive messages about risk, especially risks that are not immediately threatening. It also would be useful to determine if the enormous amount of risk information that has been issued over the past decade has had a sort of numbing effect on the way people react to dangers.

Another area of research that could help improve communications would be information on whom the public is most likely to believe when it comes to announcing risk. The current wisdom is that scientists make the best spokespersons when they can be taught to speak simple English. They usually bring with them the authority of a degree that indicates they have some relevant knowledge and usually can supply the backup information necessary to make a message convincing.

Many risk communications program strategies have relied heavily on the use of experts or third party spokespersons who are convinced of the need for a certain course of action. These types of spokespersons have three qualities that render them invaluable in carrying a risk message: they can get a hearing before any type of audience; people tend to believe them; and they are least likely to distort the message. A major problem with using scientists as spokespersons is that often they are too busy to participate in the program.

However, their willingness to participate in communications is often a signal that the risk in question is serious.

To summarize, reaching target audiences with credible risk messages depends on a few key factors. The message must be technically accurate and the information it contains must be conveyed consistently. Appropriate channels must be used to carry the message to the targeted audience. Special communication efforts should be considered to reach the scientific/medical community, the involved state and local governments, and the media. Finally, and perhaps most importantly, the spokesperson chosen to convey the risk communication should be someone who is perceived by the target audience as impartial and knowledgeable. Incorporating these practices into a risk communication strategy will help to ensure that the intended message will successfully reach and be heard by the target audiences.

21

Evaluating Risk Communication

Roger E. Kasperson and Ingar Palmlund

This chapter inquires into the potential and limits of evaluation as a component of risk communication programs in diverse institutional settings. We begin by discussing the roles of institutional setting and government in risk communication. Then we ask why risk communication programs need to be evaluated and what assessments may contribute. We next inquire into the ways in which implicit models and paradigms of risk communication influence the way we think about objectives and approaches. We examine the evaluation process for insight into effective means for organizing and conducting the assessment. Finally, we propose specific criteria to guide the evaluation of risk communication programs.

INSTITUTIONAL SETTING

Risk communication is all about us. It enters our lives in a multitude of forms, sometimes in the imagery of advertising, sometimes in a whisper in the back row of a public hearing, sometimes in a local corporation's formal statement. Sometimes it fails to say anything, as in certain multivolumed and impenetrable technical risk assessments. Even when government is the risk communicator, the objective is, alternatively, to inform, to incite to action, to reassure, to co-opt, or to overpower. This suggests not one risk communication problem but many. It also suggests that evaluating risk communication is fraught with difficulty because the meaning of success—or, for that matter, failure—will be elusive.

What is certain is that the institutional setting of risk is important. Risks of concern and controversy characteristically involve asymmetric distributions of responsibility and

Roger E. Kasperson and Ingar Palmlund • Center for Technology, Environment, and Development, Clark University, Worcester, Massachusetts 01610.

power. Risk in the doctor's office is intensely personal, and regulatory agencies have generally avoided intrusion on the sanctity of the doctor/patient relationship. The risk communication problem here is to change long-standing patterns of behavior and for individuals to assume greater responsibility for personal health decisions.

Risk in the workplace occurs in a setting where the risk generator is also the risk manager, and where the risk bearer has few options for avoiding the risk. Here the risk communication problems are many: How to encourage the full informing of risk when such information may stimulate labor problems or subsequent legal action? How to encourage workers to learn about risk when they usually can do little in the short run to change the basic risk conditions? How to raise worker consciousness about actions that can be taken to limit and prevent risks in the long run?

Risk in the community setting is different still. Here the individual is beset by multiple and conflicting sources of information and uneven access to local and distant authorities.

Whatever the institutional setting, government is frequently called on to intervene in risk issues. The challenge is nearly always fraught with conflicting goals and diverse interests.

GOVERNMENTS AND RISK COMMUNICATION

In most cases, risk communication occurs outside the scope of governmental influence and control; indeed, risk communication is part of the social processes that only in certain instances creep into governmental agendas. The conflict of interests between risk generators and risk bearers is the milieu in which government mediates disputes, formulates norms for determining acceptable risk, and fashions measures to reduce risk.

Governments initiate risk communication for three main reasons: to determine the range where a lack of consensus prevails as to the acceptability of risks; to mediate among conflicting interests or to persuade those concerned that the actions decided on by government are appropriate and equitable; or to induce the general public to act individually or collectively to reduce its risk.

To communicate means either to impart information (i.e., a one-way process) or to have an interchange of ideas whereby more than one party actively gives information. Requirements that consumers of pharmaceuticals or workers be provided with information about risks are examples of one-way communication. Environmental impact statements or public inquiries on major installations affecting the physical environment, the public discussion of such evidence, and the public hearings regarding regulatory measures concerning risk management are two-way communication processes.

Governmental programs for risk communication involve both form and content. Such programs may aim only at establishing the forms of communication that should be observed by risk generators in their interaction with risk bearers. An example of this is the requirement in Sweden that a safety committee be set up in each workplace that has more than 50 workers, with participation from both employers and employees, as a forum for handling occupational risks. Governmental programs for risk communication may also aim at establishing only the content of risk communication, leaving to others the definition of appropriate forms. Requirements that drivers know about and comply with traffic rules for highway safety is an example of this. Typically, however, governmental involvement in risk communication concerns both form and content, as in the mandatory labeling of pharmaceuticals.

The role of government in communicating risk becomes especially important during emergencies and crises. Major industrial accidents—such as those at the Three Mile Island nuclear power plant, the pesticide factories in Seveso, Italy, and Bhopal, India, and the 1986 accident at the nuclear power plant at Chernobyl—are challenges to any governmental bureaucracy. In such emergencies, government is expected to provide the correct interpretation of what is happening, to create conditions for preventing harm and provide relief for those at risk, and to compensate for material and physical loss. For governments not used to sudden disasters, but accustomed to ample time for planning and carefully considered action, this is an unusual situation.

Risk communication is often a direct invitation or an incitement to action by those exposed to risk. When government communicates risk without also providing advice on remedies or opportunities for protection, it creates an incentive for converting risk situations into political campaigns. Risk is not only an objectively verifiable element of a situation; it is also a culturally defined phenomenon that reflects the distribution of power, the political atmosphere, and societal values and conflicts.

Evaluation of government programs often aims at investigating how faithfully specific rules, objectives, or directives have been implemented. In such evaluations, the investigator can retain the politically defined intention or assess how the results correspond with what was desired by various political interests. If the aim of the evaluation, however, is to decide which programs—public or private—best contribute to solving the problem at hand, the situation becomes one of policy formulation. Policies are expressions of the intentions or rationales that guide people's behavior in specific situations. Evaluation in situations of policy formulation requires a conscious search for clear objectives, an open declaration of the values used in measuring success, and an assessment of the different activities that may synergistically contribute to the problem to be solved.

PURPOSES AND MOTIVATIONS: WHY EVALUATE RISK COMMUNICATION PROGRAMS?

The urge to evaluate is rooted in a view of human progress as a trial-and-error process. Evaluation, however, is a matter of values, of political agenda, and perhaps of taste. Therefore, evaluation depends critically on who orders the assessment, how the risk communication problem is constructed, and what measuring rod is used. These depend, in turn, on the motivation for evaluation. In the discussion to follow, we identify five distinct motivations for evaluation.

Evaluation as Commodity Marketing

Many risk communications have a product, service, or idea to market. The commodity is often a government or industry risk management program, such as the Environmental Protection Agency's Superfund program or a post-Bhopal Union Carbide, seeking to restore its credibility as a manager of health and safety. Evaluation here becomes an indispensable tool for the organization to assemble documentation that efforts are working and merit continued support, and that government goals and the public interest are being met. Organizations tend to be very resistant to information that runs counter to organizational goals, so that selective use, or distortion, of information emerging from evaluations is not uncommon (Wilensky, 1967). Throughout, this self-evaluation tends to serve the central purpose of solidifying, justifying, or extending the risk management or technology program.

Evaluation as Mandated Accountability

In mandatory accountability, evaluation is a *pro forma* means of verifying compliance with requirements placed on the organization by the external environment. These evaluations can be used to modify and further develop the risk communication performance. Affirming that material safety data sheets (MSDSs) are being used as a means of complying with the rule of the Occupational Safety and Health Administration on hazard communication is one example. In other cases, the evaluation itself may be either a requisite for program continuation or a part of regulatory compliance.

Evaluation as Program Development

Frequently, the organization is uncertain about its performance, threatened by failures or outside criticism, or involved in decisions concerned with allocating scarce resources. The scope of the evaluations can include the revision of implementing strategies or even goal reassessment. Evaluation tends to be more open-ended and to make greater use of independent, outside evaluators. The risk communicator may be more open to information critical of organization performance, unless the core of organizational activity is at stake. This type of evaluation is, therefore, more likely to be found in newer organizations whose programs are still in flux or the more peripheral programs in well-established organizations.

Evaluation as Safety Valve

When confronted by crisis in their risk management and communication programs, organizations seek ways of diverting public pressure and gaining time to marshal resources and to formulate responses. Stimulated by such motivation, evaluation has not only a factual but also a symbolic role—in demonstrating interest in what went wrong, in seeking solutions, in making concessions to outside critics, and in allocating blame and responsibility. Since legitimacy is frequently at issue, the institutional process and the composition of the evaluators become essential. Evaluation, as the Challenger and Kemeny Commissions suggest, may also provide opportunity to resolve internal conflicts.

Evaluation as War Tool

This motivation for evaluation is the converse of commodity marketing. A higher level of bureaucracy, a legislative oversight committee, or an external opponent may seek to weaken or destroy a particular organization or to dissolve its risk management program. Sometimes the evaluation is conducted by the hostile party; other times an external, and unfriendly, evaluator is enlisted. The process of evaluation, providing the opportunity for "leaks" to the media, can be as important, and damaging, as the evaluation product itself.

These differing motivations will largely determine how managers define risk communication problems, how they conceptualize success, and how they use the results. Thus, the purposes of evaluation need to be clear.

IMPLICIT PARADIGMS

Different approaches to evaluation have evolved over time. Here we describe several of the major types and suggest how they enter into the underlying assumptions and substance of evaluation programs. They are essentially implicit paradigms of risk communication that are sometimes complementary, sometimes conflictual.

Information Systems

One common approach to communication research arises from the field of information systems, in which interest focuses on such concepts as sender, receiver, messages, information channels, channel density, target audiences, and information overloads. These concepts have enjoyed wide use in communication engineering, which structures the communications process as (1) the communication source, (2) the message, (3) the communication channels, and (4) the receivers. The source relates to the attributes of the sender of information (e.g., credibility). The message involves the specific package of information used to accomplish a particular purpose; it may be factual or emotional in appeal and may use or avoid symbols. As noted earlier, in risk situations, the intent may be to incite to action, warn, inform, or reassure. Lee (1986) notes that message variables include such factors as emotional versus logical presentation; fear appeals; message style; implicit versus explicit conclusions; placing explicit conclusion first versus last; how opposition arguments are addressed; and where the message is pitched.

Communication channels include not only, prominently, the mass media, but other interpersonal and intergroup networks as well. The receivers are those for whom the messages are designed, alternatively the risk bearer, the risk manager, or the general public. Variables of the receiver include prior experience with the risk, group membership, education, and personality. Evaluation, in the information systems context, tends to focus on four components—source, message, channel, and receiver. The assumption is that the key to success is the timely and efficient flow of messages from source to receiver, along diverse channels, with as little loss of information as possible.

Marketing

The marketing approach to risk communication consists of a diverse set of methods and strategies that have evolved in advertising and marketing products to consumers. In this view, risk communication is not conceptually distinct from the selling of soap.

Central concepts, which include consumer information processing and market segmentation, have been reviewed by Earle and Cvetkovich (1984).

Research on consumer information processing recognizes the various limitations that exist for prospective consumers of information. The difficulty of consumer choice, for example, relates to the number of alternatives that exist and the extent to which information formats facilitate comparisons. The amount of time available for processing information suggests that some media are preferable to others. The information format chosen can either facilitate or impede the amount and type of information processing.

The concept of market segmentation recognizes the basic fact of individual differences in interest and need. The goal of segmentation is to produce the most efficient groupings of people (i.e., disaggregation of the market) so that marketing may target its message to particular consumer groups.

Much of this risk communication paradigm derives from the "dos and don'ts" emerging from the practical experience of advertising and marketing, as suggested in Lesly's guides for effective communication (Lesly, 1982).

Psychometric Research

If information systems highlight message flows and marketing approaches emphasize consumer behavior, then psychometric studies center on the "receiver," now characterized as an individual coping with alternative decision situations and making judgments based on perceptions and values. The psychometric paradigm uses psychophysical scaling and multivariate analysis techniques to produce quantitative representations, or "cognitive maps," of risk attitudes and perceptions (Slovic et al., 1986). Within this paradigm, people are asked to make quantitative judgments about the existing and desired riskiness of different hazards and the desirable level of regulation for each. These judgments are then related to such issues as (1) attributes of the hazard (e.g., voluntariness, dread, knowledge), (2) benefits accompanying the hazard, (3) number of deaths caused by the hazard in a disastrous year, and (4) the seriousness of each death from a particular hazard relative to death from other causes (Slovic et al., 1986). This work has led to important conclusions, as recently articulated by Baruch Fischhoff (1985), directly relevant to risk communication efforts:

1. To cope with decision and information overloads, people simplify.
2. Once people's minds are made up, it is difficult to change them.
3. People remember what they see. For most people, the primary sources of information about risk are what they see or hear in the news media and what they observe in everyday life.
4. People cannot readily detect omissions in the evidence they receive. As a result, their risk perceptions can be manipulated.
5. People disagree more about what risk is than about how large it is. Lay people and risk managers use the term "risk" differently.
6. People have difficulty detecting inconsistencies in risk disputes. As a result, risk communication needs to provide people with alternative perspectives.
7. People have difficulty evaluating expertise.

The Cultural Hypothesis of Risk

This approach to risk begins with the premise that different institutional cultures exist with their own characteristic views of the world, or cultural biases, including viewpoints on risk and danger (Douglas and Wildavsky, 1982). Underlying this notion of cultural bias is the premise that in order to steer through the daily social maze, an individual's ideas must be generally consistent with the social constraints on interactions arising from organizational and institutional contexts. Thus, individuals structure their world views in ways that are consistent with their shared, daily social experience. It has been argued (Rayner, 1984; Rayner and Cantor, 1987) that there may be as few as four basic ways of structuring a world view, according to what has been termed the "grid" and "group" variables of organizational life. Grid refers to the degree of constraint that exists on individual interaction; group refers to the range of social interaction. These dimensions can be used to generate different prototypical visions of social life. Seen this way, risk is a way of classifying a whole series of complex interactions and relationships between people, as well as between man and nature (Rayner, 1984). This perspective on risk has generated a number of propositions relevant to risk communication:

1. Culture is the coding principle by which hazards are recognized. The community sets up the individual's model of the world and the scale of values by which different consequences are reckoned grave or trivial (Douglas, 1985).
2. A polymorphous definition of risk is needed that encompasses purely societal concerns about equity as well as concerns about the probability and magnitude of adverse consequences.
3. Technology options must be debated on the explicit basis of trust and equity rather than on rival estimates of quantitative risk.
4. Different institutional cultures engaged in controversies over technological risk have great difficulty in understanding the fears and objections of others.

Public Participation

Since the early 1960s, new expectations for the right of citizens to know and to participate in public decisions that affect their lives have become quite apparent. This change in social responsibilities has its roots in the civil rights, antiwar, consumer, and environmental movements. In Europe, the Seveso accident had far-reaching implications for the European Community in the form of the Seveso Directive, which imposed obligations for both the assessment of risk and its communication to responsible authorities and the public. In the United States, the Occupational Safety and Health Administration's hazard communication rule has set new expectations, and responsibilities, for informing those at risk. The 1987 Superfund amendments not only expand hazard communication responsibilities but substantially increase local participation on hazard assessment as well.

Experience with public participation over several decades has afforded a variety of insights into both the nature of the obstacles and realistic expectations of what is possible. A recent analysis (Kasperson, 1986) has identified a number of different propositions, emerging from several decades of public participation research, for formulating risk communication programs. These include:

1. Conflicts emerging in public participation often center on means/ends differences in expectation. Citizens will see programs as an invitation to share power, to participate in defining ends. The agency managers, by contrast, will see it as having only an instrumental function, a means to, say, realize established health and safety objectives.
2. A lack of early and continuing involvement of the public is a characteristic source of failure.
3. The believability of risk information is clearly related to institutional credibility and trust.
4. Effective public participation depends substantially on the development of indigenous resources and the technical means to act on and assess increased knowledge.
5. Members of the public differ in arenas and scope of involvement, suggesting the need for differing communication strategies.
6. Although a large array of participation exists, current knowledge, especially about risk communication, does not allow for successful prediction as to which forms of participation are likely to be most effective under different conditions.

RISK COMMUNICATION IN SWEDEN IN THE WAKE OF THE CHERNOBYL ACCIDENT

On April 28, 1986, headlines in the Swedish newspapers warned that something was wrong with one of the nuclear reactors in the Stockholm region. The news the following day revealed that the radioactivity had emanated from a nuclear reactor failure in the Soviet Union.

The following day, the headline in one of the major newspapers was 2,000 DEAD IN THE ACCIDENT, THE SOVIET UNION ASKS FOR HELP, coupled with NO DANGER IN SWEDEN in smaller print. That was the first communication from the Swedish National Radiation Protection Institute (SSI) concerning the risks following the Chernobyl accident.

During the following days, measurements of radiation showed values at a level about 10 times higher than the natural radiation from the ground in an area along the northeastern coastal region. That was a level, however, far below the point at which emergency measures would be deemed necessary. Authorities advised that the drinking water could be used as usual but that people should not use rainwater. Some independent physicians recommended that parents not allow small children to play in sand or mud puddles for a few days. No special recommendations regarding animals were necessary, according to SSI. Milk had been measured for radioactivity, but no high values had been encountered. The SSI also announced that it would not be necessary to take iodine tablets. So people gathered for their Valborgsmass festivities and traditional May 1 national holiday without apparent worry about radiation hazards.

But soon other orders were forthcoming. Farmers were forbidden to release their cattle for grazing until the regions where they lived had been classified as safe. Milk showing high levels of radiation had to be poured on the ground. Farmers were told to cut their grass but not to store it in heaps. The farmers organizations protested that compliance with the rules would mean considerable loss for the farming community. Eventually, the government promised full economic compensation to the farmers for extra costs due to the prohibitions. Gradually, through May, the restrictions on grazing cattle were lifted, first in the southern regions, then gradually further north as values from radiation measurements got lower.

The SSI also soon warned that people should avoid eating the traditional spring food, young nettles, as well as rhubarb and other leafy vegetables. Later it was detected that meat from cattle and reindeer in the regions of heavy fallout had been contaminated so that it could not be allowed on the market, which meant an erosion of the economic basis for the ethnic Lapp minority. By the end of May, some areas around the town of Gaevle in Sweden had some of the highest levels of radioactive cesium (137,000 becquerels) in Western Europe. While no acute damage to humans was involved, cancer and genetic damage rates are expected to increase slightly over the long term.

The Swedish governmental agencies in charge of the assessment and communication of risks generally did a good job under the circumstances. Their stance seemed to aim at avoiding unnecessary anxiety while openly informing the public about what they knew. The authorities did what they could to make the technical information comprehensible, comparing radiation levels from the fallout to those experienced during X-ray examination. Most people responded with a quiet sadness, but some had the following criticisms: Kiev had lower levels of radioactivity than Sweden. Yet why were women and children evacuated from Kiev but not from Gaevle? Why were the Swedish people initially informed that there was no danger, when later the government decided on many restrictions on grazing cattle? Were they hiding something? Questions also arose in the media and in the Swedish Parliament.

The Chernobyl accident carries a number of lessons in risk communication. Early reassurances in risk events may not always be the best strategy for a government, but balancing warning and reassurance appropriately is difficult. Openness and candor are critical if trust is to be built. Providing the contexts so that information can be interpreted may be as important as the risk data themselves. A single source of authoritative information helps to prevent confusion.

THE PROCESS OF EVALUATION

Simplified models of organizational decisionmaking envision a sequence of activities, typically including a statement of objectives, a search for information and options, formal decisionmaking, implementation, evaluation, and feedback. In this context, evaluation has the same function as it does in experimental research—to assess the value of the experiment that has been performed. When government or other interests intervene to disseminate information or to initiate a dialogue with risk bearers over health and environmental impacts, the experimental research analogue breaks down. Science is no longer the objective, the role of the analyst changes, and evaluation takes on political meaning. Evaluation of risk communication should include the following considerations.

The Formulation of Objectives

Which are the stated and which the real purposes of evaluation? As noted above, the motivations for evaluation are diverse. Assessing efficiency, i.e., carrying out programs in a cost-effective manner, is one common objective. Investigating effectiveness, i.e., the accomplishment of goals regardless of cost, is another.

The Locus of Evaluation

Should the evaluation be organized in-house or should external evaluators be brought in? Generally, the ethics of auditing prohibit the persons responsible for the accounts from auditing their own performance. In organizational activities, separating these roles and minimizing potential conflict of interest is no less important. However, much depends on the organizational motivation for the evaluation. An external evaluation can be very helpful if the goal is commodity marketing. Such an evaluation may bring new knowledge or valuable perspective, thereby redefining the problem or offering new solutions.

However, if the administrator of the risk communication program opposes the evaluation it is likely that the evaluation will have little overall impact. The program administrator has many reasons to resist outside evaluation. Risk communication is a highly uncertain activity with high visibility and political stakes. The simple fact of the matter is that we know relatively little about how best to communicate complex risk issues. The external evaluator typically has little first-hand knowledge of the trials and tribulations of the risk communication practitioner.

Evaluations located in-house have their own advantages and prices. The internal evaluator is highly knowledgeable about the organization, program, and constraints. However, the evaluation runs the risk of being partial and distorted, so as not to threaten agency or department goals. Data may be suppressed or selectively interpreted. While in-house evaluation may be more closely geared to agency goals and cognizant of constraints, it may also be safely ignored. In short, differing loci of evaluation shape the evaluation and its ultimate impact.

Timing

Whether an evaluation is foreseen and planned before the activity (*ex ante*) to be evaluated starts, or undertaken after the fact (*ex post*), is extremely important. Characteristically, evaluation is retrospective. The timing of an evaluation may coincide with budgetary review to determine if the risk communication program is an appropriate reason for expenditure of funds. The evaluation may seek to document the agency's risk management program, or it may serve as a map for avoiding the mine fields of wrong turns in the communication process. *Ex post* evaluation involves a number of serious problems:

1. Relevant data may no longer be available, particularly if the need for evaluation was not anticipated at program inception.
2. Participants or risk bearers may be difficult to locate.

3. Evaluation may not be available in time to correct program deficiencies.
4. The purpose of the evaluation may influence the results.
5. Program managers may be suspicious of an evaluator who arrives after the fact to assess a program in which he was not involved.
6. Changes in program operation or impacts may be difficult to discern after the program is completed (Morgenstern et al., 1980).

It can be argued, correspondingly, that *ex ante* (planned, ongoing) evaluation also has its problems, particularly in the intrusion of the evaluator and the potential disruption that could occur. The essential point is that evaluation should be used to inform, and improve, the communication process as it unfolds. A well-founded evaluation effort will also incorporate baseline data obtained at the beginning of the process so that changes can be accurately assessed.

Training and Monitoring of Evaluators

Too often overburdened program staff carry out the evaluation effort, with little training in evaluation and little monitoring of their performance. For many of the staff, evaluation will be less important than communicating the risks, and they will allocate their scarce time and resources accordingly (Comfort, 1980b). Searching evaluation requires that different members of the program reflect sensitively and thoughtfully on their performance. In this way, the evaluation process becomes a central means by which the organization develops the skills of its staff in the performance of risk communication.

The Role of the Individual in Risk Communication

What should be the role of those for whom the risk communication program is intended—the "target groups" in marketing terminology? Should their role be restricted to providing information to the evaluators or should they contribute to the design of the evaluation process and instruments? Differing parties in the risk communication program will clearly ask different questions and desire different kinds of data in an evaluation.

Especially if the risk communication program is designed to be interactive in nature and to serve multiple needs, then public or risk bearer participation in the formulation of evaluation programs seems essential. In all cases, the degree of expressed public satisfaction with the program is one appropriate measure of success.

Boundaries of the Evaluation

We live in a time when the scope of risk is increasingly transnational, sometimes even global, while government remains national. Technology and products are disseminated globally, carrying benefits and risk into a space that is far broader than any government can control. Chernobyl, Bhopal, fluorocarbons, and the 1986 Rhine pollution all suggest the internationalization of risk. If the boundaries of goals and evaluations are drawn too narrowly, comfortable results may ensue but may correspond badly to the real risk problems.

The Measurement Trap

A classic anecdote recounts how a man searching on a dark night for his lost key concentrates on the illuminated circle under the lamppost, since that is where the key would be most easily found. The focus and scope of evaluation are often defined less by what we most need to know than by what can be measured easily or by a favorite measuring tool. Risk communication programs need to be seen, given the current state of knowledge, as exploratory and experimental; in short, as serious research ventures using the most appropriate yardsticks, qualitative as well as quantitative. Learning from experience, then, will require substantial methodological investment and resources, so that thoughtful questions are asked and causality is pursued with determination.

TEN CRITERIA FOR EVALUATING RISK COMMUNICATION PROGRAMS

Based on the discussions above, we propose 10 criteria for evaluating risk communication programs. In doing so, we recognize that such criteria rest on normative conceptions of success in risk management and that debate over such propositions will continue in the coming years.

Needs Appraisal

Risk communication should not be based solely on assumptions by the manager of what risk bearers need to know about risks. Rather, a careful appraisal should be made of the risk bearers' needs and how they might best be met. Such judgments should be based on information from both expert and lay opinion. It should also include the identification of groups who are especially affected by the risks and how communication can be tailored to reach them in depth. An explicit formulation of concrete objectives of risk communication is an essential prerequisite for performing an honest evaluation of the results.

Risk Complexity and Social Pluralism

Despite the propensity to convey risk in one-dimensional terms (reduced life expectancy, lifetime fatality risk, etc.), risk, as we know, is multidimensional. Technologies have a broad range of consequences; defining the particular consequence to be assessed is a decision of importance and often a political act. The qualitative attributes of risk—voluntariness, catastrophic potential, and degree of familiarity—affect our responses to them. Then, too, cultural groups define risks differently, attach different values to them, and incorporate them into differing sociopolitical agenda. A primary challenge in risk communication is making complex phenomena understandable to nontechnical people while simultaneously capturing the major attributes of concern to a highly variegated public. In such situations, it is important to err on the side of multiple perspectives, differing characterizations of risk, and richness in communication approaches.

Risk in Context

Technological risk is a complex phenomenon, at once technical, uncertain, probabilistic, and value-laden. Provision of information needs to be accompanied by efforts to assist individuals in comprehending the risk. Types of contextual information include comparisons with other relevant risks (which need to be done with intelligence and sensitivity); comparisons with benefits of the activity or technology; comparisons with regulatory standards or natural background levels, etc.; and comparisons of ways in which the risk can be reduced and what it would require in resources. Invariably, individuals also desire, and may demand, full information on the process that generated the risk—why it occurred, what is being done to reduce it, and why this was not done before.

A Management Prospectus

As suggested by Baruch Fischhoff (1985), risk managers should develop a protocol that ensures that all relevant information concerning the risk management program is communicated to the public. Such a prospectus would include how the manager sees the facts, what options the manager is legally empowered to consider, what the manager considers to be the public interest, how the decision was (or will be) made, and with what envisioned results. A well-thought-out treatment is greatly preferable to speculation on such matters by the mass media or piecemeal construction of the picture over time. Prompt provision of such information will also head off fears that the agency is withholding relevant facts or has hidden motivations.

Timeliness

Risk communication should be timely, meaning that it should occur early enough in the process to alert the individual to the risk so that any available actions can be taken to avoid it or to minimize its consequences. The common error is for risk managers to withhold information until late in the process, when information and evidence are more complete and control strategies and supporting rationales more fully developed. It is possible, however, for communication to be premature, thereby eliciting unwarranted fear or unnecessary protective actions. Repeated overreactive warnings to evacuate in the face of a predicted natural hazard (e.g., an earthquake) or industrial accident (e.g., a chemical release) may result in decreased credibility and, thus, increased risk.

Iterative Interaction

Although there may be special circumstances in which risk communication involves only a single transaction or message, multiple or continuous interaction is nearly always necessary to ensure a flow of relevant risk information. Interaction implies the two-way flow of information, with learning by all those participating in the process. Very few risk communication programs build in the means to listen to or to initiate public response, which should be a requisite to developing the communication program and gauging its effectiveness.

Empowerment

Risk information unaccompanied by power and the means to act on the expanded knowledge is ultimately frustrating. Clearly, it reduces the incentive to acquire risk information and causes the audience to ask "If I can't do anything about it, why are you telling me?" Wherever possible, risk communication should be embedded in a broader approach that empowers those at risk to act in their own protection or to influence those who act in their behalf. The effectiveness of the Swedish information program on workplace hazards is connected in no small part to worker participation in risk management programs. Similarly, the recent success in community consideration of a monitored retrievable storage facility for radioactive wastes in Tennessee was associated with the power the community of Oak Ridge was able to assume.

Credibility

Success in risk communication depends heavily on the confidence individuals place in the sources of information. Credibility is multidimensional, involving perceived competence, commitment to public health and safety, and caring about those who bear the risks.

Ethical Sensitivity

The current risk communication initiatives that have been started by a broad array of institutions assure that a great many campaigns will soon be in place and that experience will grow rapidly. Safeguards are needed that reflect thoughtful deliberations on the ethical issues involved, including:

1. Identification of unintended adverse consequences in programs and structured means for avoiding them.
2. Respect for the autonomy of the individual and avoidance of paternalism.
3. Recognition of potential self-interest or bias in the institution acting as risk communicator.
4. Respect for the rights of those bearing the risks so that programs will be responsive to them.
5. Means to ensure that risk communication will be compassionate and respectful of those addressed by the communication.
6. Avoidance of undue worry and fear.
7. Assurance that agency staff will have the right to refuse to engage in unethical conduct.

To assure that these ethical issues are addressed, the creation of codes of conduct for risk communicators would be helpful.

Resiliency

Given our limited understanding of risk communication, false steps and approaches are nearly certain. A well-designed risk communication program should therefore assume surprises and failures, and plan accordingly. Programs should include conflict among information sources; unforeseen events; potential blockages in information channels; inadequate identification of interested groups and citizens; unidentified value structures and community agenda; higher levels of distrust than assumed; and substantial departure in expert and lay risk judgments. The objective of attempting to anticipate failure should be to make the communication process resilient, so that accurate information gets through, sensitivity is developed, interaction occurs, and credibility grows in the face of adversity and the unexpected.

CONCLUSION

Communicating risk is an emerging major activity of institutions responsible for managing risks. It requires a sensitive balance between providing factual information on risk and avoiding undue anxieties. Evaluation provides a central means for assuring appropriate goals, content, and outcomes of such programs. Such evaluation will have the potential for both good and harm, and requires clear criteria by which success can be measured, the good maximized, and the harm avoided. Most of all, evaluation must be taken seriously as a central part of risk communication programs, and not merely an activity to conduct if sufficient funds are left when the program is ended.

REFERENCES AND SELECTED BIBLIOGRAPHY

Abt. C., ed. 1976. *The Evaluation of Social Programs.* Beverly Hills: Sage Publications.

Agarmala-Rogers, R. 1977. Why is evaluation research not utilized? *Evaluation Studies Review Annual*, Vol. 2. Beverly Hills: Sage Publications, pp. 328–33.

Baram, M. 1984. The right to know and the duty to disclose hazard information. *American Journal of Public Health* 74(4): 385–90.

Comfort, L. K. 1980a. *Evaluation and Effectiveness in Educational Policy.* Elmsford, NY: Pergamon Press.

Comfort, L. K. 1980b. Evaluation as an instrument for educational change. In *Why Policies Succeed or Fail.* Ed. H. M. Ingram and D. E. Mann. Beverly Hills: Sage Publications, pp. 35–57.

Cuthbertson, I. D. 1983. Evaluating public participation: an approach for government practitioners. In *Public Involvement and Social Impact Assessment.* Ed. G. A. Daneke, M. W. Garcia, and J. Delli Friscoli. Boulder, CO: Westview Press, pp. 101–109.

Deutscher, I. 1976. Toward avoiding the goal-trap in evaluation research. *The Evaluation of Social Programs.* Ed. C. Abt. Beverly Hills: Sage Publications, pp. 97–119.

Douglas, M. 1985. *Risk Acceptability According to the Social Sciences.* New York: Russell Sage Foundation.

Douglas, M., and A. Wildavsky. 1982. *Risk and Culture: An Essay on the Selection of Technological and Environmental Dangers.* Berkeley: University of California Press.

Earle, T. C., and G. T. Cvetkovich. 1984. *Risk communication: A marketing approach*. Paper prepared for the NSF/EPA Workshop on Risk Perception and Risk Communication, Long Beach, California.

Fischhoff, B. 1985. Managing risk perception. *Issues in Science and Technology* 2(Fall): 83–96.

Homenuck, P., J. Durlak, and J. Morgenstern. 1978. Evaluation of public participation programs. In *Involvement and Environment*. Ed. B. Sadler. Edmonton: Environment Council of Alberta, pp. 103–19.

Ingram, H. 1973. Information channels and environmental decision making. *Natural Resources Journal* 12(1): 159–169.

Ingram, H. 1976. The politics of information: constraints on new sources. In *Water Politics and Public Involvement*. Ed. J. C. Pierce and H. R. Doerksen. Ann Arbor, MI: Ann Arbor Science, pp. 63–73.

Kasperson, R. E. 1986. Six propositions on public participation and their relevance for risk communication. *Risk Analysis* 6(3): 275–81.

Kasperson, R. E., and J. X. Kasperson. 1983. Determining the acceptability of risk: ethical and policy issues. In *Risk: A Symposium on the Assessment and Perception of Risk to Human Health in Canada*. Ed. J. T. Rogers and D. V. Bates. Ottawa: Royal Society of Canada, pp. 135–55.

Lee, T. R. 1986. Effective communication of information about chemical hazards. *The Science of the Total Environment* 51(May): 149–183.

Lesly, P. 1982. The changing evolution of public relations. *Public Relations Quarterly* 27: 9–15.

Morgenstern, J., J. Durlak, and P. Homenuck. 1980. Making the evaluation of public participation programs feasible. *Public Participation in Environmental Decision Making: Strategies for Change*. Ed. B. Sadler. Edmonton: Environment Council of Canada, pp. 121–39.

Ontario Crafts Council and the College, University and School Safety Council of Ontario. 1983. *A Personal Risk Assessment for Craftsman and Artists*. Toronto: The Councils.

Rayner, S. 1984. Disagreeing about risk: the institutional cultures of risk management and planning for future generations. *In Risk Analysis, Institutions, and Public Policy*. Ed. S. G. Hadden. Port Washington, NY: Associated Faculty Press.

Rayner, S., and R. Cantor. 1987. How fair is safe enough? The cultural approach to societal technology choice. *Risk Analysis* 7(1): 3–13.

Rosenthal, R. A., and R. S. Weis. 1966. Problems of organizational feedback. In *Social Indicators*. Ed. R. A. Bauer. Cambridge, MA: MIT Press.

Sandman, P. M. 1985. *Getting to Maybe: Some Communication Aspects of Siting Hazardous Waste Facilities*. Trenton: Hazardous Waste Advisory Council, New Jersey Hazardous Waste Facilities Siting Commission.

Sharlin, H. I. 1985. *EDB: A Case Study in the Communication of Health Risk*. Washington, D.C.: HIS Associates.

Slovic, P., B. Fischhoff, and S. Lichtenstein. 1986. The psychometric study of risk perception. In *Risk Evaluation and Management*. Ed. V. T. Covello, J. Menkes, and J. Mumpower. New York: Plenum Press, pp. 3–24.

U.S. Environmental Protection Agency and U.S. Centers for Disease Control. 1986. *A Citizen Guide to Radon: What It Is and What to Do About It*. Washington, D.C.: U.S. EPA and U.S. DHHS.

Weinstein, N. D. 1979. Seeking reassuring or threatening information about environmental cancer. *Journal of Behavioral Medicine* 2(2): 125–139.

Weiss, C. 1972. *Evaluation Research*. Englewood Cliffs, NJ: Prentice-Hall.

Wildavsky, A. 1972. *Evaluation as an Organizational Problem*. Working paper, No. 13. London: Centre for Environmental Studies.

Wilensky, H. L. 1967. *Organizational Intelligence*. New York: Basic Books.

Appendixes

A

Inventory of Government Risk Communication Programs

Vincent T. Covello, David B. McCallum, and Maria Pavlova

AGENCY FOR TOXIC SUBSTANCES AND DISEASE REGISTRY (ATSDR)

Overview of Risk Communication Activities

Background The Agency for Toxic Substances and Disease Registry (ATSDR) is part of the Public Health Service. The ATSDR's two program offices are the Office of External Affairs (OEA) and the Office of Health Assessment (OHA). Under the directive of two areas of the mission statement of ATSDR, the agency provides consultation and technical assistance to federal, state, and local agencies on public health and scientific matters related to Superfund and develops and implements training programs for state health departments to increase the departments' capacities to carry out health assessments.

Message

- Superfund-related issues

Subjects

- Public perceptions of health risks from potential or actual exposures to chemicals at Superfund sites
- Effective communication about health concerns and risks

Vincent T. Covello • Center for Risk Communication, Division of Environmental Sciences, School of Public Health, Columbia University, New York, New York 10032. *David B. McCallum* • The Institute for Health Policy Analysis, Georgetown University Medical Center, Washington, D.C. 20007. *Maria Pavlova* • U.S. Environmental Protection Agency, Region II, New York, New York 10278.

Target Audiences

- General public
- Federal, state, and local agencies
- Health professionals

Communication Channels/Programs

- The ATSDR communicates through the following channels:
  - Emergency response program
  - Health education program
  - Health assessments program
  - Literature inventory/dissemination program
  - Exposure and disease registries
  - Toxicological profiles
  - Worker health and safety program
- *Program on Risk Communication and Risk Perception* is currently being developed to
  - Inform the public and health professionals about the nature and magnitude of risks involved with potential or actual exposures to chemicals at CERCLA and RCRA sites
  - Understand the concerns and information needs of health professionals and the public

Information Resources

Public Information Office
Agency for Toxic Substances and Disease Registry
1600 Clinton Road
Atlanta, GA 30333
(404) 454-4631

Research/Planning/Evaluation

The ATSDR conducts research in the form of on-site work, which is performed in response to specific requests and petitions. Currently, ATSDR is planning the following projects in research and communication:

- Program for public education that will involve evaluation, aided by Rutgers University
- Registries of health effects toxics and toxic profiles, with a component aimed at the lay public

AGRICULTURAL RESEARCH SERVICE (ARS)

U.S. Department of Agriculture

Overview of Risk Communication Activities

Background The U.S. Department of Agriculture (USDA) was created by an act of Congress in 1862. The original mission of USDA was defined as research and the education of people with regard to food production and protection. Currently, this department has 26 agencies providing a wide range of activities. Some USDA-originated services have become the foundation for newer federal agencies such as EPA and FDA. The Agricultural Research Service (ARS) is the major research agency of USDA; its mission covers most subjects related to agriculture, such as food production and protection, human nutrition, toxic substances, and environmental issues. Research-based information frequently becomes part of the data base used for regulatory action.

Messages

- Research
- Public education

Subjects

- Food production and protection
- Human nutrition
- Toxic substances
- Environmental issues

Target Audiences

- General public via USDA network
- USDA agencies
- Local health officials and personnel

Communication Channels/Programs

- *Public information* is channeled through communications and information exchange between ARS and USDA Extension Services and local health officials.

Research

The ARS conducts research on food production and population protection, specifically

- Prevention of soil erosion
- Diversification of farm production
- New methods to control pests

- Technology to ensure food wholesomeness
- Water quality
- Environmental protection

Information Resources

Office of Cooperative Interactions
Agricultural Research Service
Beltsville, MD 20705
(301) 344-2734

CENTERS FOR DISEASE CONTROL (CDC)

Overview of Risk Communication Activities

Background The mission of the Centers for Disease Control (CDC) is to prevent unnecessary morbidity and premature mortality and to improve the quality of life. The CDC provides epidemiological and laboratory expertise, services, and training to local, state, national, and international disease and injury prevention efforts. In addition, CDC is the lead agency for assuring the implementation of the 1990 Objectives for the Nation in the areas of immunization, sexually transmitted disease control, surveillance and control of infectious diseases, fluoridation and dental health, injury prevention, and occupational safety and health.

Message

- Protection of public health

Primary Subjects

- Disease prevention
- Injury prevention
- Health promotion

Secondary Subjects

- Occupational, environmental, and chronic disease
- Infectious disease
- Immunization
- Sexually transmitted disease
- Improvements in health practices and behaviors

Target Audiences

- General public

- Health professionals
- Public health workers

Communication Channels/Programs

- *Conferences and training programs*
  - Health laboratory practices
  - Infectious and chronic diseases
  - Epidemiology
- *Programs to assist the public health community* in the surveillance, investigation, analysis, prevention, and control of environmentally induced health problems
- *General health education* through collaboration with other agencies and organizations and prevention and control efforts
- *National programs on infectious diseases* to improve identification, diagnosis, prevention, and control
- *Cancer control projects* through cooperative agreements with state health departments
- *Morbidity and Mortality Weekly Report (MMWR)* to increase awareness of disease-related epidemiology

Information Resources

Centers for Disease Control
Office of Public Affairs
Building 1
1600 Clifton Road, NE
Atlanta, GA 30333
(404) 329-3286

Research/Planning/Evaluation

The risk communication goals of CDC include:

- Information and education
- Behavior change and protective action
- Disaster warnings and emergency information
- Joint problem solving and conflict resolution

Evaluation is a component of many of the programs and occurs as a function of the process of program implementation. Other communications-related research within the CDC seeks to identify areas of need for more information and types of appropriate communication.

CONSUMER PRODUCT SAFETY COMMISSION (CPSC)

Office of Information and Public Affairs

Overview of Risk Communication Activities

Agency Background The U.S. Consumer Product Safety Commission (CPSC) is an independent regulatory agency activated in 1973 by the Consumer Product Safety Act. Congress directed the Commission to "protect the public against the unreasonable risks of injuries and deaths associated with consumer products." Since 1973, CPSC has worked to prevent injuries and deaths by:

- Working with industry to develop voluntary safety standards
- Issuing and enforcing mandatory standards, where appropriate
- Banning products for which no feasible standard would adequately protect the public
- Obtaining the recall or repair of products that present substantial hazards or imminent hazards to consumers
- Conducting research on potential hazards
- Conducting information and education programs

Under the Consumer Product Safety Act, Congress granted the Commission authority to issue and enforce safety standards prescribing performance requirements, warnings, or instructions for use of consumer products. The Commission also regulates products covered by four acts previously administered by other federal agencies: the Flammable Fabrics Act, the Federal Hazards Act, the Poison Prevention Packaging Act, and the Refrigerator Safety Act.

Messages

- Consumer protection
- Product safety

Subjects

- Chemical hazards associated with acute effects (burns, poisoning, death) and chronic effects (cancer, birth defects, neurotoxicity)
- Fire/household hazards
- Hazards from electrical/mechanical/children's products

Target Audiences

- The public as consumers
- Other regulatory agencies
- State and local governments
- Private organizations concerned with product safety

Communication Channels/Programs

- *Office of Information and Public Affairs* develops, implements, and evaluates a comprehensive national public affairs program to promote product safety by educating the public as consumers and by encouraging behavior change and protective action through:
  - Print and audiovisual materials for public dissemination
  - Networks of national organizations, state and local governments, and business and consumer groups
  - News releases and public service announcements
  - Articles for national magazines and weekly newspapers
  - News conferences
- *Public Information Services* include
  - Hotline
  - Commission response to incoming correspondence
  - Conferences and symposia
  - Recalls and alerts
  - Media relations
  - Daily Newslog
  - Freedom of Information activities

Research

- Data sources include the National Electronic Injury Surveillance System (connected to hospital emergency rooms) and data from death certificates
- Information efforts evaluated to demonstrate effects in consumer awareness, behavior change, and reduction of deaths and injuries
  - Pre- and posttest
  - Questionnaires
  - Statistics from multiple sources

Information Resources

Office of Information and Public Affairs
Consumer Product Safety Commission
Westwood Towers
5401 Westbard Avenue
Bethesda, MD 20207
(301) 492-6580

Communication Research/Planning/Evaluation

Information gathered from the National Electronic Injury Surveillance System (connected to hospital emergency rooms), consumer complaints, news clips, and death certificates serve to identify problem areas for CPSC attention. Other risks are identified through CPSC's Substantial Product Hazards Program, through which industry is required to report possible substantial product hazards. Consumer complaints about potential hazards also are used by CPSC to identify products for future investigation.

Evaluation efforts have been required of CPSC information campaigns by U.S. Senate and U.S. House of Representatives oversight committees. Some of the most recent evaluations and problems of evaluation are summarized in a December 1985 memorandum addressing the issue of effectiveness of information programs. CPSC has evaluated its information efforts to demonstrate their effect on consumer awareness, behavior change, and reduction of deaths and injuries.

Although the impact of information efforts is hard to quantify, CPSC measures behavior change through consumer questionnaires. Results indicate, for example, that consumers do install safety devices (smoke detectors, GFCIs, or grab bars) or eliminate hazards (replace frayed cords). CPSC also uses pre- and posttests to measure changes in consumer awareness.

FOOD AND DRUG ADMINISTRATION (FDA)

Health Affairs

Overview of Risk Communication Activities

Background The Food and Drug Administration (FDA), within the U.S. Public Health Service, was created with the Pure Food and Drug Act of 1906. It has jurisdiction over food, pharmaceuticals (including cosmetics), and medical equipment, including both diagnostic and therapeutic devices. The use of these diverse products is regulated by the FDA through direct investigation of their safety and effectiveness and promulgation of standards affecting contaminants (in food, cosmetics, and drugs) and emissions levels for radiation equipment. Protection of the consumer from hazardous chemicals and radiation is the overall objective of the various FDA programs. The Office of Public Affairs and the Press Office convey information about the FDA activities and decisions. The FDA itself is a regulatory agency; these offices are nonregulatory.

Messages

- Consumer protection
- Product safety

Subjects

- Hazardous chemicals and radiation
- Food
- Pharmaceuticals, including cosmetics
- Medical equipment, diagnostic and therapeutic

Target Audiences

- General public
- Manufacturers
- Health care professionals
- Federal agencies

Communication Channels/Programs

- *Educational programs* warn consumers of adulterated, mislabeled, or illegal products
- *Risk assessment boards* determine the seriousness of a situation. Possible actions include:
  - Recall of a defective product from the market
  - Notification or safety alert about a medical device
  - Seizure—action taken to remove product from commerce
  - Injunction—civil action taken against individual or company in an attempt to stop continued production or distribution of products
  - Prosecution—against individual or company
  - Disposition—final order entered by a court to conclude case involving prosecution or injunction
  - *Research and quality control programs* ensure the safety and efficacy of drugs, biological and medical devices, and registration of blood banks and promote quality, nutritional adequacy, and integrity of the nation's food supply
  - *Surveillance and inspection* of manufacturers are conducted to monitor compliance with regulations
  - *Published materials* include magazines, monthly news columns, scientific publications, letters to physicians, letters to manufacturers, pamphlets, and press releases (*FDA Talk Papers*)

Information Resources

FDA Talk Papers are distributed in response to public inquiries. FDA also produces the *Consumer Magazine* regularly. For information on specific publications, contact:

Health Affairs
U.S. Food and Drug Administration
5600 Fishers Lane
Room 1495 (HFY-1)
Rockville, MD 20857
(301) 443-6143

Research/Planning/Evaluation

The FDA deals with a whole spectrum of risk, from short-term (e.g., Chernobyl) to chronic exposure (e.g., risk associated with use of tampons; package tampering). The agency disseminates information through press releases, journal articles, interagency programs, and speeches and television appearances. The FDA sponsors workshops on many topics and has response groups to address specific issues. These activities, as well as much research, are often in response to events such as testing products for approval or developing more efficacious means of reaching and protecting the public. As such, FDA has no formal evaluation mechanism for their communications programs, but they use feedback from these activities to help plan future efforts.

HEADQUARTERS, U.S. AIR FORCE

Directorate of Engineering and Services
Environmental Division

Overview of Risk Communication Activities

Background The U.S. Air Force education program was developed as a response to concern about the management and disposal of hazardous wastes on and around Air Force base installations. Improper practices, although inadvertent, led to contamination of the environment: liquids and dissolved chemicals leached into groundwater used for drinking and for agriculture; contaminated dust and vapors polluted the air; and erosion and flooding washed contaminated soil into waterways. Toxic waste materials migrated from the source, Air Force bases, to the surrounding areas. The Air Force, as a large industry and landowner, recognized its responsibility for some of these problems. In 1980, therefore, the Air Force implemented the Installation Restoration Program (IRP) to clean up health-threatening hazardous waste sites on military installations.

Message

- Protection of the public
- Protection of the environment

Subjects

- Groundwater and soil contamination
- Air pollution
- Waterways
- Migration of toxic waste

Target Audiences

- Military
- Civilian workers
- Populations adjacent to Air Force installations

Communication Channels/Programs

- *Installation Restoration Program* was implemented to clean up public health/environmental threatening hazardous waste sites on military installations. The presence of contaminants and remediating waste disposal sites that pose a threat to the public health or environment are identified and confirmed through:
  - Records searches
  - Confirmation and quantification studies

  The program is also responsible for technology development and remedial action including emergency response and simple removals.
- *Public Affairs Officers* operate at each Air Force base to communicate with community leaders and community spokespersons to ensure that public comments are included in technical decision documents involving remediation. Methods of communication tailored to particular audiences include written materials, public announcements, and public activities. The Department of Defense also maintains contact with the Environmental Protection Agency and the Occupational Safety and Health Administration regarding regulations and standards.

Information Resources The main source of information and contact is the public information officer at each separate installation.

Communication Research/Planning/Evaluation

There are no specific measures to evaluate the effectiveness of the programs. Risk communication is based on the data collected with regard to the various phases of the IRP. The problems of communication based on risk data are complicated by the length of time involved in eradicating the dangers; for example, many of the substances that are in the ground descend in a vertical fashion and tend to migrate laterally and upwardly with a half-life of 50 years. The major thrust of risk communication projects and the most difficult aspect of such programs is the conveyance of the idea of probability and the concept of probability in terms the public can understand.

NATIONAL CANCER INSTITUTE (NCI)

Overview of Risk Communication Activities

Agency Background The National Cancer Institute (NCI) was created in 1937 to support research and demonstration programs for discovering the causes of and therapeutic approaches to cancer. In 1944, NCI became one of the National Institutes of Health, with the responsibility for identification of environmental carcinogens, assessment of the relationships between exposure to these substances and cancer incidence, research, and public education.

One of the subdivisions of NCI is the Office of Cancer Communications (OCC), which disseminates to both the public and health professionals a wide spectrum of information on cancer causes, diagnosis, prevention, and treatment. The major information systems of NCI are the Cancer Information Service and the newly introduced Physician Data Query (PDQ) program, which is targeted to practicing physicians.

The NCI's activities, which grow out of identified needs, are aimed at education rather than regulation. The programs serve to support informed choices by the public, cancer patients, and health professionals.

Messages

- Cancer prevention and control
- Risk factors for cancer

Subjects

- Cigarette smoking and other tobacco use
- Diet
- Early detection
- Causes, diagnosis, and treatment of cancer
- Psychosocial aspects of cancer

Target Audiences

- General public
- Cancer patients
- Health professionals
- Special populations

Communication Channels/Programs

- *Cancer Information Service* (CIS) provides information to the public through publications and a toll-free telephone system (1-800-4-CANCER).
- *Physician Data Query* (PDQ) is a data base for physicians treating cancer; it includes the latest information on cancer treatment.
- *Cancer Prevention Awareness Program* includes mass media and health education programs
  - Mass media phase to increase public's knowledge of cancer risk, improve public's attitude toward cancer prevention, and encourage behaviors to reduce risk of cancer.
  - Cancer prevention education projects for specific audiences, such as community activities conducted through the Partners in Prevention, a collaborative effort involving corporations, voluntary organizations, and health care professionals.
- *Patient Education Program* develops and promotes state-of-the-art education and information programs that will enable cancer patients and their families to participate in treatment and care to ensure the best possible quality of life. Cancer patients and their families are the program's primary audience; however, health professionals and the general public constitute an important secondary audience for program materials and activities.

- *Alliances* with other federal, state, and local agencies, private industry, and professional organizations to disseminate cancer prevention and patient education messages and materials.

Research/Evaluation

- Surveys, interviews, content analyses, market research, pretests, and needs assessments
- Evaluation Methods
  - Standards and procedures regarding program objectives, outcome, impact, and costs
  - Pretesting of materials and messages
  - National telephone surveys to track improvement in levels of knowledge
  - Media tracking
  - Special community studies
- Other indicators tracked:
  - Involvement/attendance at media events
  - Number of public inquiries
  - Market research
  - Publication distribution

Information Resources

Good News, Better News, Best News: Cancer Prevention
NCI Monographs
Journal of the National Cancer Institute

For public and health professionals publication lists, contact:

NCI Publications Office
Public Inquiries Section
Building 31, Room 10A24
9000 Rockville Pike
Bethesda, MD 20892
(301) 496-5583

All public materials are free of charge.

The Information Projects Branch of the Office of Cancer Communications is the primary source of information on risk communication programs in NCI.
Contact:

Chief
Information Projects Branch
NCI, NIH
Building 31, Room 4B43
9000 Rockville Pike
Bethesda, MD 20892
(301) 496-6792

The office to contact for scientific information on occupational cancer is:

Chief
Occupational Cancer Branch
NCI, NIH
Blair Building, Room 632A
8300 Colesville Road
Silver Spring, MD 20902
(301) 427-8633

Communication Research/Planning/Evaluation In 1978, in a survey of both workers and the general public, only 28% of respondents felt well informed about cancer risks. The NCI recognizes this information need and conducts an educational program for the public, health professionals, and the media. Through interviews, content analyses, and market research studies, NCI has developed a solid foundation for developing messages for the public.

To understand audiences' information needs, wants, and behaviors, and the perceptions and comprehension of program materials, the Office of Cancer Communications (OCC) uses a step-by-step framework of (1) planning and strategy selection, (2) concept development, (3) message execution, (4) implementation, (5) assessing in-market effectiveness, and (6) replanning and feedback. Communications are formulated for particular target audiences, and specific programs are developed for subgroups.

The Cancer Prevention Awareness Program is evaluated on a number of levels. The NCI develops a set of standards and procedures to assess the program's merits and to provide information about its objectives, process, outcome, impact, and costs. It evaluates program materials and messages using a variety of pretesting techniques before they are put into use. National telephone surveys are conducted throughout the program to track improvement in levels of public knowledge and awareness of cancer prevention. Other evaluation activities, including media tracking studies and special community studies, provide additional information about the success of the program.

More general information on the success of these programs is also tracked by NCI. One indicator is the level of involvement/attendance at media events, meetings, and seminars. Another measure is the number of public inquiries received and publications distributed. Market research studies measure awareness, knowledge, and health practices, and these figures are tallied pre-and postprogram intervention. The measurements can be applied to all programs and used in the design and tracking of new programs.

NATIONAL CENTER FOR HEALTH STATISTICS (NCHS)

Overview of Risk Communication Activities

Agency Background The National Center for Health Statistics (NCHS), Public Health Service, has the overall mission of collecting, analyzing, and disseminating national health statistics through the development and maintenance of comprehensive data systems; conducting research in survey and statistical methodology; and coordinating the

Department of Health and Human Services' health statistics efforts. The Center serves as a focus for national health data and provides the health community, both public and private, with a complete range of data necessary to assess health status and service needs.

Rather than being regulatory, the NCHS activities provide support to other federal and state agencies by compiling statistical data used to develop health policy and public education programs.

Message

- National health statistics

Subjects

- Collection
- Analyses
- Dissemination

Target Audiences

- General public
- Public and private health community
- Federal and state agencies

Communication Channels/Programs

- *Programs to collect morbidity and mortality data* serve as resources for other federal agencies attempting to establish a definite relationship between exposure to environmental factors and disease occurrence. These programs monitor:
  - Health and nutritional status
  - Hospital discharges
  - Ambulatory medical care
  - Births and deaths
- *National Health Interview Survey* obtains information on health through continuous cross-sectional, nationwide surveys of households. This serves as a potential source of information in the area of occupational health.
- *National Health and Nutrition Examination Survey* collects information from the general population on exposures to, body burden of, and health effects of lead, pesticides, carbon monoxide, and cadmium through household interviews and a detailed physical examination.
- Other surveys include National Survey of Personal Health Practices and Consequences; National Medical Care Utilization and Expenditure Survey; National Natality and Fetal Mortality Survey; National Ambulatory Medical Care Survey; National Hospital Discharge Survey; National Nursing Home Survey; National Master Facility Inventory; National Mortality Registration System; National Natality Registration System; and Mortality Surveillance Survey.

- *Public reports* are analyzed and disseminated for a wide range of uses. They are compiled from:
  - Health examinations and tests
  - Interviews/questionnaires
  - Utilization records
  - Birth and death records
  - Health records
- *Educational programs* disseminate statistical data to the public.

Information Resources NCHS provides statistical data to other federal agencies and to the public via its published survey results. For information contact:

National Center for Health Statistics
3700 East-West Highway
Hyattsville, MD 20782
(301) 436-8500

Communication Research/Planning/Evaluation

National programs are planned to obtain information on fertility and to provide more detailed information on the occupations of mothers and fathers.

NATIONAL HEART, LUNG, AND BLOOD INSTITUTE (NHLBI)

Overview of Risk Communication Programs

Background The National Heart Institute was established in 1948. By 1976, the focus and name of the Institute had changed to include heart, lung, and blood diseases. The National Heart, Lung, and Blood Institute (NHLBI)—a nonregulatory agency—conducts and supports fundamental research on the heart, lungs, blood vessels, blood, and diseases that affect them. In the area of risks, the NHLBI is primarily involved in the identification and characterization of risk factors for cardiovascular and pulmonary diseases through epidemiological studies, risk factor intervention studies, and basic research on cardiovascular functions.

In 1972, Congress mandated that the then National Heart and Lung Institute establish a program to disseminate updated information to the health professions and the public regarding risk factors. At the same time, the Department of Health, Education and Welfare (DHEW) mandated the Institute to develop and implement a national program to detect, treat, and control high blood pressure, one of the major factors for cardiovascular disease. In 1976, Congress expanded the Institute's prevention mandate to include the establishment of the Office of Prevention, Education and Control. Its mission is to disseminate information and to develop educational programs designed to reduce preventable heart, lung, and blood disease. These health education efforts primarily address the three major modifiable risks for cardiovascular disease: high blood pressure (hypertension), cigarette smoking, and high blood cholesterol.

Messages

- Prevention
- Risk factor
- Treatment

Primary subjects

- High blood pressure
- Cigarette smoking
- Cholesterol

Secondary subjects

- Obesity
- Physical inactivity

Target Audiences

- Researchers
- Physicians and other health professionals
- Intermediaries such as voluntary health agencies, professional organizations, insurance companies, and employees
- General public
- Patients

Communication Channels/Programs

- Print materials
  - Articles
  - Fact sheets
  - Pamphlets
  - Position papers
  - Patient education materials
  - Resource lists
- Mass media
  - TV and radio public service announcements
  - Infomercials
  - Posters for airports, buses, and subways
  - TV and radio shows
  - Educational print ads
  - Press briefings and responses to press inquiries
  - Networking with communication channels of other organizations
- Programmatic materials and professional education
  - Guidebooks
  - Newsletters

- Slide/speech kits for professional training
- Risk assessment tools
- National and regional conferences
- Materials to assist health professionals to adopt new roles and convey new patient skills for risk factor reduction or control
- A kit for year long activities and publicity about cholesterol, smoking, and high blood pressure as modifiable risk factors; a kit of materials for program use on the local level for publicity and education, awareness, and media projects
- Continuing medical education materials
- Data base and reference collection

- National High Blood Pressure Education Program
- National Cholesterol Education Program
- NHLBI Smoking Education Program

Research/Evaluation

- Surveys of public and professional attitudes and reported practices of cardiovascular disease risk factor reduction.
- Measures of indicators, such as patient visits for high blood pressure and high blood cholesterol, prescribing patterns for appropriate medications, trends in mortality of cardiovascular and lung diseases, changes in prevalence of smoking, and changes in awareness, treatment, and control status of high blood pressure and high blood cholesterol.

Information Resources For high blood pressure, cholesterol, smoking risk factor materials, questions, and professional education materials:

High Blood Pressure, Cholesterol, and Smoking Information Center
4733 Bethesda Avenue
Suite 530
Bethesda, MD 20814
(301) 951-3260

For NHLBI cardiovascular/pulmonary disease publications:

Information Services Section
Communications and Public Information Branch
National Heart, Lung, and Blood Institute
Building 31, Room 4A-21
Bethesda, MD 20892
(301) 496-4236

For mass media materials:

Communications and Marketing Section
Communications and Public Information Branch
National Heart, Lung, and Blood Institute
Building 31, Room 4A-21
Bethesda, MD 20892
(301) 496-4236

Research/Planning/Evaluation

NHLBI conducts basic scientific research as well as research on the public it serves. Ongoing survey research provides information on knowledge gaps and behavior of the public and health professionals regarding health risks. This research aids in planning future activities and programs; it also serves to evaluate current and past programs.

The progress of NHLBI's risk reduction/education programs has been evaluated and measured in a number of ways. Public surveys show substantial gains in knowledge related to high blood pressure, high blood cholesterol, and cigarette smoking as modifiable risk factors for cardiovascular disease. Furthermore, awareness, treatment, and control rates for high blood pressure have increased. Visits to physicians for high blood pressure and high blood cholesterol tests have risen dramatically. Physicians have begun treating patients at lower levels of blood cholesterol. Age-adjusted death rates for heart disease and stroke have declined significantly since the inception of the National High Blood Pressure Education Program—39% for heart disease and 53% for stroke. This progress is thought to be attributed, at least in part, to the efforts of NHLBI's risk factor reduction programs, which are composed of professional education, patient education, and public education. Public service announcements (PSAs) are an important element of public education. Repeated Louis Harris polls have found that PSAs on television and radio are cited as the most frequent source of information for the public about health, second only to physicians. In addition to outcome evaluation, NHLBI pretests the elements of its media campaign with members of the target audience.

NATIONAL INSTITUTE FOR OCCUPATIONAL SAFETY AND HEALTH (NIOSH)

Overview of Risk Communication Activities

Agency Background The National Institute for Occupational Safety and Health (NIOSH) is a prevention-oriented research institute with two overall goals: to produce significant information by identifying and conducting research on occupational safety and health hazards and their control and to transmit this information to those who need to know in order to protect the worker and control work-related disease and injury. Section 20 of the Occupational Safety and Health Act of 1970 mandates NIOSH to conduct research, and Section 21 mandates NIOSH to conduct training and education. NIOSH is specifically authorized to recommend to the Occupational Safety and Health Administration (OSHA) and to the Mine Safety and Health Administration (MSHA) standards for the protection of workers. In all activities, the emphasis is on prevention, intervening before adverse health effects occur. NIOSH is located within the U.S. Department of Health and Human Services, Public Health Service, Centers for Disease Control.

NIOSH is not a regulatory agency. It does develop recommendations for occupational standards based on available research of specific health and safety hazards and the issues related to these hazards, such as engineering control of exposures and personal protection equipment. Regulations based on recommended standards are promulgated by OSHA and MSHA.

Message

- Workplace hazards and risks

Subjects

- Prevention
- Detection
- Evaluation and assessment
- Communication to the public and industry

Target Audiences

- Workers
- Employers
- Industry
- Health professionals
- Federal agencies
- State and local agencies

Communication Channels/Programs

- *Programs for researching job-related injury and disease* that conduct epidemiological and toxicological studies on hazards and risks in the workplace (i.e., occupational injury, respiratory disease, effects of physical agents)
- *Surveillance and evaluation programs* to detect job-related illnesses, exposures, and hazardous agents
- *Guidelines and criteria* to inform workers of workplace hazards and health risks and recommend standards to regulatory agencies
- *Programs to train health professionals* through university education resource centers and research and training grants
- *Programs for public communication* that respond to inquiries and requests from industry and the general public and to distribute information on workplace hazards, health risks, and prevention of adverse outcomes

Information Resources There are seven types of publications disseminated by the Technical Information Branch: criteria documents, current intelligence bulletins (CIBs), ALERT documents, *the NIOSH Pocket Guide to Chemical Hazards*, yearly summaries of NIOSH recommendations, summaries-of-the-current-intelligence bulletins, and technical and special report publications.

In addition to disseminating these documents, the Technical Information Branch responds to inquiries and maintains the NIOSH data base, NIOSHTIC, composed of articles dealing with occupational safety and health that date back to the turn of the century. Altogether there are 136,000 abstracts.

For a list of available publications, contact:

Division of Standards Development and Technology Transfer
National Institute for Occupational Safety and Health
Robert A. Taft Laboratories, C-14
4676 Columbia Parkway
Cincinnati, OH 45226
(513) 533-8000

Communication Research/Planning/Evaluation

Epidemiological and toxicological research in occupational health includes an assessment of the magnitude of the hazard, a qualitative (prior to quantification) assessment of risk, quantification of risk at different exposure levels, and determination of risk estimates for the population at risk. A major issue is that of dealing with inadequate data for risk assessment. NIOSH, as a participant in the Council to Coordinate Environmental Health and Related Programs (CCEHRP), is strongly involved in Department of Health and Human Services efforts to evaluate and communicate risks. The Director of NIOSH is a member of the Governing Council of CCEHRP and Chair of the CCEHRP Subcommittee for Environmental Health Risk Assessment. This subcommittee is charged with the conduct and facilitation of risk assessments, which cut across all of DHHS's responsibilities in environmental health.

An example of research in the area of health risk communication is the field test of a set of guidelines for informing workers of workplace hazards and health risks based on the literature in risk perception, attitude change, and reading education. The effects of this intervention will be measured through pre- and postmeasurements of worker knowledge and through observation of changes in worker conformance with safe work procedures as outlined in the revised guidelines.

NIOSH researchers also have pilot tested a worker notification model to evauluate the issues and practical problems involved in individually notifying workers, using a cohort of chemical workers in Augusta, Georgia, at increased risk for occupationally induced bladder cancer. The results of the project indicate the efficacy of worker notification. In addition, guidelines have been developed providing criteria for successful notification programs.

NUCLEAR REGULATORY COMMISSION (NRC)

Overview of Risk Communication Activities

Agency Background The Nuclear Regulatory Commission (NRC) was created as an independent agency by the Energy Reorganization Act of 1974, which split the Atomic Energy Commission and created the NRC and the Energy Research and Development Agency, which later became part of the Department of Energy. In general terms, the mission of the NRC is to protect the public and the environment in the civilian and commercial uses of nuclear materials in the United States. The mission of the NRC is accomplished through licensing of nuclear facilities and the use of nuclear materials;

development and implementation of regulatory requirements; and inspection and enforcement activities. The emphasis of this regulation is on nuclear power plants and the by-products of the fission process, although licensing of the use of nuclear materials has been transferred to 29 states.

The NRC is also responsible for licensing the import and export of nuclear facilities, equipment, and materials. The NRC's mission is strictly regulatory in nature.

Message

- Safety issues associated with nuclear materials in the United States

Subjects

- Civilian and commercial uses of nuclear energy
- Regulatory requirements

Target Audiences

- General public through the media
- Nuclear facility personnel

Communication Channels/Programs

- *Public Education Seminars* for media
  - News reporters are instructed in topics pertinent to nuclear power, including safety systems of power plants and radiation and its effects.
- *Response to Individual Letters and Questions*
  - Tailored responses to individual letters and questions from the public on nuclear medicine, industrial radiography, manufacture of radioactive material, the use of radioactive material, etc.
  - Explanatory letters in response to nuclear accidents such as Three Mile Island and Chernobyl
- *Environmental statements* included in regulations

Information Resources

Office of Public Affairs
U.S. Nuclear Regulatory Commission
Washington, DC 20555
(202) 492-7715

Communication Research/Planning/Evaluation

There is no formal evaluation process within the NRC for this form of public education on risk analysis and communication. One indicator of effectiveness is how stories relating to nuclear issues are handled by the press. The media seminars help make the news stories better and more accurate. As the press is better able to understand and evaluate situations, these situations are presented more clearly and accurately to the public. Thus, the public is better able to understand and evaluate the same situations and to make educated judgments.

OCCUPATIONAL SAFETY AND HEALTH ADMINISTRATION (OSHA)

Overview of Risk Communication Activities

Agency Background The Occupational Safety and Health Administration (OSHA) was created within the Department of Labor by the Occupational Safety and Health Act of 1970. OSHA's primary functions are the development, promulgation, and enforcement of occupational safety and health standards. Specifically, OSHA is mandated to

- Encourage employers and workers to reduce workplace hazards and implement new or improved safety and health programs
- Establish separate but dependent responsibilities and rights for employers and workers for the achievement of better safety and health conditions
- Maintain a reporting and record-keeping system to monitor job- related injuries and illnesses
- Establish training programs to increase the number and competence of occupational safety and health personnel
- Develop mandatory job safety and health standards and enforce them effectively

Message

- Occupational safety and health

Subjects

- Workplace hazards
- Monitoring of job-related injuries and illnesses
- Safety and health programs for general industry, maritime, construction, and agriculture
- Occupational safety and health personnel training
- Responsibilities and rights of workers and employers
- Hazard communication

Target Audiences

- Employers/employees
- Chemical manufacturers and importers
- Special populations
- Private sector organizations

Communication Channels/Programs

- *Hazard communication standard* reduces the incidence of chemical source illnesses and injuries through
  - Requirements for chemical evaluation
  - Communication of hazard information to employers and workers
  - Labels on containers
  - Material safety data sheets
  - Employee training
- *Comprehensive health standards* are mandatory standards developed for employers. Twenty-four such standards have been promulgated by OSHA under the Occupational Safety and Health Act of 1970. The agency has also established 400 permissible exposure limits to control employee exposures.
- *Grants and training* enable private sector organizations and special populations, through nonprofit organizations, to develop comprehensive and effective programs to address specific safety and health problems.
- *OSHA Training Institute* provides basic and advanced technical programs of instruction in occupational safety and health to state and other Federal agency personnel, to private sector employers, and to workers and their representatives. The Institute also serves as a repository of all materials developed in the area of occupational safety and health.

Information Resources

Office of Information and Consumer Affairs
Department of Labor/Occupational Safety and Health Administration
200 Constitution Avenue, NW
Washington, DC 20210
(202) 523-8148

Communication Research/Planning/Evaluation

OSHA requires reporting and recording of job-related injuries and illnesses and develops programs to avoid these incidents.

OFFICE ON SMOKING AND HEALTH (OSH)

Public Health Service

Overview of Risk Communication Activities

Background The Office on Smoking and Health (OSH), formerly the National Clearinghouse for Smoking and Health, was established in 1978. OSH's area of concern is the health consequences of tobacco use. The Office provides leadership in education and research and serves as a clearinghouse for public and technical information on smoking and health. OSH maintains a Technical Information Center that contains over 40,000 technical reports on smoking and health. Other functions of OSH include an inquiry and reference service, computer search and retrieval services, and periodic and special publications.

Activities of OSH are nonregulatory in nature, as OSH seeks to educate the public on an important health issue, with the goal of decreasing the incidences and rates of smoking. The OSH program strategies have been built on years of work educating the public about the risks of smoking. According to OSH surveys, there is nearly 100% acknowledgment among smokers that smoking is harmful to one's health, indicating that past and current programs have had an impact on public knowledge.

Message

- Health consequences of tobacco use

Target Audiences

- Smokers
- Potential smokers
- Adolescents
- Pregnant women
- Children

Communication Channels/Programs

- *Technical Information Center* contains over 40,000 technical reports on smoking and health and provides
  - Inquiry and reference services
  - Computer search and retrieval services
- Print and broadcast media
  - Periodic and special publications (including the annual *Surgeon General's Report*)
  - Public service announcements
  - Educational materials, such as a science lab book of experiments to illustrate the hazards of smoking
- Alliances with volunteer organizations (American Heart Association, American Cancer Society, and American Lung Association), and state and federal government agencies to develop and distribute materials

Research/Evaluation

- Pretests of materials
- Attitudinal surveys
- Long-term analyses of smoking trends

- Development of demographic profiles of smokers through biannual random sample surveys. Subjects covered in the survey are:
  - Socioeconomic background
  - Experience with tobacco
  - Knowledge and beliefs about the effects of smoking
  - Attitudes toward quitting smoking

Information Resources OSH serves as a clearinghouse for public and technical information on smoking. For information and publications list, contact:

Office on Smoking and Health
Parklawn Building
5600 Fishers Lane
Rockville, MD 20857
(301) 443-5287

Research/Planning/Evaluation

OSH conducts three types of evaluations of its activities: pretests of educational materials, attitudinal surveys, and long-term analyses of smoking trends. Educational materials (e.g., public service announcements) are pretested with the target audience using focus groups or individual (central location) interviews.

Every two years, OSH conducts a random sample survey of the public's attitude toward smoking. A series of questions are asked of respondents regarding socioeconomic background, experience with tobacco (years of smoking, packs smoked per day, use of snuff, etc.), knowledge and beliefs about the effects of smoking (such as whether air pollution is a greater risk than smoking or whether smoking is less harmful than being overweight), and attitudes toward quitting. As a product of the survey, profiles are prepared on the smoking habits and attitudes of different segments of the population as a basis for developing materials and judging the progress of the OSH program.

OSH believes that a certain and constant level of attention has to be given to the risks of smoking, or else there is recidivism among those who quit and a new pool of smokers that begin. This finding may be due in part to the competition the OSH ads receive from tobacco advertisements. Long-term statistics do show a decrease in smoking since cigarette advertisements on television were banned and since the *Surgeon General's Report on Smoking* was first issued. However, any direct effect of OSH's media campaign on smoking behavior cannot be measured.

U.S. ENVIRONMENTAL PROTECTION AGENCY (EPA)

Overview of Risk Communication Activities

Agency Background In 1970, a presidential order consolidated 15 federal environmental programs into a single Environmental Protection Agency, with the mission to protect and enhance the quality of the environment by establishing and enforcing standards and regulations that ensure the public health and welfare and guarantee that property and ecological systems are safe from damage by environmental pollutants. Much of the enabling legislation authorizing EPA to perform that comprehensive role was contained in the following acts and their various amendments, dating from 1963 to 1981: Clean Air; Clean Water; Safe Drinking Water; Resource Conservation and Recovery; Federal Insecticide, Fungicide, and Rodenticide; Toxic Substances Control; Noise Control; and Comprehensive Environmental Response, Compensation, and Liability (Superfund). In dealing with problems of environmental pollution and exposure to toxic chemicals, radiation, and noise, EPA is responsible for monitoring and analyzing the nation's environment, conducting research and demonstration projects, and assisting in the development and implementation of state and local pollution control programs. As part of its mandate, EPA needs to explain risks so that people understand and can participate in regulatory decisions, and to help people decide whether to take their own mitigating action when the risk is beyond the reach of traditional regulatory tools.

Message

- Environmental hazards that threaten ecosystems or human health

Subjects

- Asbestos
- Pesticides
- Radon
- Superfund site issues
- Other hazardous chemicals and toxic substances
- Other: sulfuroxides (health effects and acid rain), ozone, formaldehyde, lead in air and water

Target Audiences

- General public
- Federal, state, and local agencies
- Health professionals
- Media

Communication Channels/Programs Seminars and conferences; publications; development of education and research centers; and the organization of training programs. These activities are undertaken by individual program offices charged with regulating specific hazards and coordinating risk communication activities:

- *The Office of Toxic Substances* issues chemical advisories aimed at people who use toxic substances, usually in occupational settings.
- *The Asbestos Action Program* distributes information on potential hazards to individuals who have been exposed to or who work with asbestos.

- *The Office of Radiation Programs* warns citizens of the risks from radon in the home and other buildings and directs them on preventive action.
- *The Office of Pesticides Program* provides risk advisory information and training to individuals who work with pesticides and alerts consumers to the risk of pesticides used at home.
- *The Superfund Program* provides fact sheets on risk information and on-site administrative and cleanup activities at Superfund sites to interested citizens.
- *The Drinking Water Office* distributes a booklet on the potential health effects from lead in drinking water, stressing that the only way to determine risk is to have tap water tested.
- *The Title III Program* is developing various materials to assess and interpret the risks in communities from routine and emergency releases of chemicals.
- *The Office of Policy, Planning, and Evaluation* manages a Risk Communication Program that coordinates risk communication activities across the agency's program and regional offices. The Risk Communication Program has four components: methods development, consulting and evaluation for specific risk communication efforts, training, and outreach (which includes a clearinghouse for risk communication information).

Information Resources

Risk Communication Hotline, PM-221
401 M Street, SW
Washington, DC 20460
(202) 382-5606

or

Office of Public Affairs
401 M Street, SW
Washington, DC 20460
(202) 382-4361

Communication Research/Planning/Evaluation

In 1987, EPA recognized the importance of its diverse risk communication activities by setting up a Risk Communication Program (RCP) to coordinate these efforts.

Two components of the RCP are directly concerned with research and evaluation: (1) methods development and (2) problem-specific consulting and analysis.

Much of EPA's methods development occurs under its Risk Communication Research Program, which uses cooperative agreements to access risk communication experts at universities and other nonprofit organizations. Examples of studies now under way include:

- Finding ways to get some convergence between subjective risk perceptions and scientists' risk estimates

- Finding ways to motivate people to find out whether they are at risk from environmental hazards that one cannot see, smell, or feel (such as radon)
- Finding ways to motivate those at risk to take self-protective action against radon in homes and other buildings, household pesticides, lead in drinking water, and so on

Other research and evaluation occur in the context of specific risk communication activities that would be undertaken even in the absence of the Risk Communication Program. The difference is that the RCP adds planning from the outset, so that objectives are clearly defined and an evaluation of effectiveness can be conducted as the activity progresses. Examples include:

- Evaluating the effectiveness of the National Response Team's hazard analysis process to serve as the basis for communicating about chemical risks from emergency releases in the community
- Developing guidance on how to write lay summaries of the toxic profiles that ATSDR must provide
- Evaluating the effectiveness of a message stressing ecosystem risk versus a message stressing human health risk for substances in boat hull paints (with the National Ocean and Atmospheric Administration)

Additional information is available on these and other research and evaluation projects from the RCP hotline (FTS/382-5606).

B

Improving Dialogue with Communities

A Risk Communication Manual for Government

Billie Jo Hance, Caron Chess, and Peter M. Sandman

Billie Jo Hance, Caron Chess, and Peter M. Sandman • Environmental Communication Research Program, New Jersey Agricultural Experiment Station, Cook College, Rutgers University, New Brunswick, New Jersey 08903. Final Report in Research Contract C29444: *Communicating Chemical Risks in the New Jersey Department of Environmental Protection.* Division of Science and Research, New Jersey Department of Environmental Protection.

Preface

The Risk Communication Unit of the New Jersey Department of Environmental Protection (NJDEP), Division of Science and Research (DSR), was established as part of an enviromental management initiative to explore the integration of risk assessment and alternatives for reducing risk with risk communication. The overall program is charged with conducting innovative research on this interactive risk management approach, as well as integrating research findings into the general responsibilities and activities of NJDEP.

DSR established a research contract with the Rutgers University Environmental Communication Research Program to undertake development of a guide to risk communication for government agencies. This manual, *Improving Dialogue with Communities: A Risk Communication Guide for Government,* is complemented by a condensed short version that highlights the major guidelines included in the full manual.

The manual provides guidance to staff within the agency on the value of building risk communication strategies into their own programs. Presented as a sequence of "rules of the road" gleaned from risk communication practitioners in a variety of scientific disciplines, it provides a comprehensive and rational basis for implementation. The manual's premise is that involving the public in the processes of agency decision-making is integral to successful environmental health risk management. A workshop presented by the researchers for NJDEP provided a complement to the manual, as well as an initiation to risk communication for agency management and technical staff.

With the beginning of 1988, the Risk Communication Unit has established a research staff with a full complement of backgrounds in journalism, environmental education, hazard perception research, community development and crisis management. The Unit's current research efforts focus on developing strategies to: involve the public in the environmental decision-making process, including risk assessment; evaluate risk communication efforts; set up risk communication strategies; convey risk probabilities successfully to the public; and improve the traditional public hearing process by making it a vehicle for dialogue between agencies and the public. These activities involve research to develop models of risk communication, using case studies of environmental risks being managed by the agency.

Research efforts such as those in the New Jersey Department of Environmental Protection will lead to the development of effective government policy on the relationship between risk communication and risk management. The staff in the DSR Risk Communication Unit can be contacted for further information on the division's research efforts at: New Jersey Department of Environmental Protection, Division of Science and Research, Risk Communication Unit, 401 East State Street, CN409, Trenton, New Jersey 08625.

Improving Dialogue with Communities: A Risk Communication Manual for Government

SUBMITTED TO:
New Jersey Department of Environmental Protection
Division of Science & Research

BY
Billie Jo Hance
Research Associate

Caron Chess
Associate Director

Peter M. Sandman
Director

Environmental Communication Research Program
New Jersey Agricultural Experiment Station
Cook College, Rutgers University
122 Ryders Lane
New Brunswick, NJ 08903

Let's protect our earth

STATE OF NEW JERSEY
DEPARTMENT OF ENVIRONMENTAL PROTECTION
RICHARD T. DEWLING, Ph.D., P.E., COMMISSIONER
CN 402
TRENTON, N.J. 08625
609 - 292 - 2885

January 1988

Dear Reader:

I am pleased to introduce the New Jersey Department of Environmental Protection's manual on risk communication, Improving Dialogue With Communities: A Risk Commmunication Manual for Government. This manual gives clear-cut guidelines for planning and undertaking effective environmental health risk communication. Intended for use by state agencies, this manual summarizes practical lessons learned from successful as well as unsuccessful efforts to generate two-way communication with affected publics.

The NJDEP is deeply committed to continued improvement in our management of New Jersey's environment. Part of this effort is to work cooperatively with communities to identify and resolve environmental hazards. Today's complex environmental problems have led us to recognize the compelling need to integrate risk communication into the management of environmental health risks. Our goal in New Jersey is to develop ways to effectively involve affected communities in solving environmental problems. I believe the accompanying manual provides practical guidance toward achieving this goal.

I hope you find that this manual can provide immediate as well as long-term applications in your efforts to involve the public in decision-making.

Sincerely,

Richard T. Dewling
Commissioner

100% Recycled

Let's protect our earth

State of New Jersey
DEPARTMENT OF ENVIRONMENTAL PROTECTION
OFFICE OF SCIENCE AND RESEARCH
CN 409, TRENTON, N.J. 08625

ROBERT K. TUCKER, Ph.D.
DIRECTOR

January 1988

Dear Reader:

The New Jersey Department of Environmental Protection (NJDEP) Division of Science and Research (DSR) made a conscious decision to include risk communication as an integral part of its overall program to investigate environmental health risk assessment. To some, this was a bold initiative. Historically, communicating environmental health risks to the public has been tagged on as the "tail end" of agencies' efforts to identify, assess and remediate environmental health hazards. However, to DSR, the inclusion of risk communication as an integral component of an environmental health investigation represents a logical step forward in our efforts to improve the way that environmental health hazards are addressed by government. Including risk communication up-front in our efforts to identify and assess environmental health risks not only allows the affected public to have a genuine "stake" in the decisions made, but it also increases the likelihood that the decisions made will be supported both by the agency and by the community.

The research investigation that provided the basis for developing this manual was one of DSR's first efforts to investigate better ways for agencies to generate productive dialogues with communities. Since undertaking this project, our efforts in this area have grown. DSR has established a three-person Risk Communication Unit which is specificially charged with conducting research to identify effective risk communication and public participation strategies. In addition, the Risk Communication Unit is involved in testing and practicing these strategies in a variety of case studies. We intend to continue our efforts in this area by undertaking even more challenging research and case studies.

We appreciate the hard work and insight of the researchers at the Rutgers University Environmental Communication Research Program (ECRP), Billie Jo Hance, Caron Chess and Peter Sandman, who undertook this research investigation and prepared this manual. Special thanks are extended to Caron Chess who initiated this research investigation while she was a staff person at NJDEP. I would like to personally thank the members of the DSR Risk Communication Unit who worked closely with the researchers to develop this manual as well as the members of the interagency advisory group that was established to consult on the direction of this research investigation. Lastly, I would like to thank DSR Assistant Director Hank Garie and DSR Manager of Policy and Administration, Marty Rosen, who provided the management support that is essential to the success of a project of this kind.

There are two companion pieces to this manual: a condensed version of the guidelines and a report discussing policy implications of incorporating risk communication into environmental risk management. If you would like additional copies of this manual or the two companion reports, please contact the DSR Risk Communication Unit at the address above or at (609) 984-6072. I hope that this manual provides you with inspiration and guidance for integrating the public into your environmental health decision-making.

Sincerely,

Robert K. Tucker

Robert K. Tucker, Ph.D.
Director

TABLE OF CONTENTS

ISSUES OF PARTICULAR INTEREST

The chapters in the manual are divided into sections that provide easy reference to important topics. These are listed in the Table of Contents. There are, however, a few key issues that cut across chapters. These are listed below, with corresponding chapter, guideline, and page numbers.

[p. iv blank]

LIST OF INTERVIEWEES

The following people are quoted and referred to throughout the manual. A description of the individual's risk communication experience is provided for those whose titles are not self-explanatory.

U.S. ENVIRONMENTAL PROTECTION AGENCY

Marc R. Alston
Chief
Public Water Supply Section
U.S. Environmental Protection Agency, Region VIII
Drinking Water Section
Denver, CO

Ann Fenn
Community Relations Coordinator
Superfund Program
U.S. Environmental Protection Agency
Washington, D.C.

Randall F. Smith
Chief
Hazardous Waste Policy Branch
U.S. Environmental Protection Agency, Region X
Seattle, WA

OTHER FEDERAL AGENCIES

Jerome Delli Priscoli
Senior Policy Analyst
U.S. Army Corps of Engineers
Institute for Water Resources
Fort Belvoir, VA

Robert O'Connor
Formerly: Manager, Intergovernmental Analysis Section
Institutional Affairs Department
Technical Support Team to the Office of Civilian Radioactive Waste Management
U.S. Department of Energy
Now: Professor of Political Science
Pennsylvania State University
University Park, PA

STATE AGENCIES

Bruce Bentley
Citizen Participation Specialist
New York State Department of Environmental Conservation
Albany, NY

Susan Boyle
Assistant Director
Hazardous Waste Facilities Siting Commission
New Jersey Department of Environmental Protection
Trenton, NJ

Thomas Burke
Formerly: Director, Division of Science & Research
New Jersey Department of Environmental Protection
Trenton, NJ
Now: Deputy Commissioner
New Jersey Department of Health
Trenton, NJ

Jacquelyn (Ruddie) Clarkson
Chief Environmental Epidemiologist
Environmental Epidemiology Program
Louisiana Department of Health and Human Resources
New Orleans, LA

Kenneth H. Cobb
Program Specialist, Cooperative Extension Service
Cornell University
Ithaca, NY
(Cobb advises communities on dealing with environmental risk issues.)

Donald A. Deieso
Assistant Commissioner for Environmental Management & Control
New Jersey Department of Environmental Protection
Trenton, NJ

Richard Dime
Bureau Chief
Bureau of Hazardous Substances Information
New Jersey Department of Environmental Protection
Trenton, NJ

Jason Gaertner
Community Relations Coordinator
Radon Monitoring Program
Pennsylvania Department of Environmental Resources
Gilbertsville, PA

Joan N. Gardner
Director
Massachusetts Hazardous Waste Facility Site Safety Council
Boston, MA

Barker Hamill
Chief
Bureau of Safe Drinking Water
New Jersey Department of Environmental Protection
Trenton, NJ

Ernest Kuhlwein
Chief
Bureau of Hazardous Waste Engineering
New Jersey Department of Environmental Protection
Trenton, NJ

Edgar Miller
Community Relations Coordinator
North Carolina Governor's Waste Management Board
Raleigh, NC

Raymond Neutra
Chief
Epidemiological Studies and Surveillance Section
California Department of Health Services
Berkeley, CA

Faith Schottenfeld
Community Relations Specialist
New York State Department of Health
Albany, NY

Grace L. Singer
Chief
Bureau of Community Relations
Division of Hazardous Site Mitigation
New Jersey Department of Environmental Protection
Trenton, NJ

Gary Sondermeyer
Acting Bureau Chief
Bureau of Solid Waste & Resource Recovery Planning
New Jersey Department of Environmental Protection
Trenton, NJ

Brian C. Strohm
Special Assistant for Health Risk Assessment
New Hampshire Division of Public Health Services
Concord, NH

INDUSTRY

Nancy E. Blethen
Vice President
Coleman and Pellet, Inc.
Union, NJ
(Blethen advises clients on communicating with the public about environmental risk.)

James D. Callaghan
Formerly: Senior Vice President
Hill and Knowlton, Inc.
New York, NY
(Now a private consultant, Callaghan spent many years advising industry on how to communicate risks to the public.)

Geraldine V. Cox
Vice President and Technical Director
Chemical Manufacturers Association
Washington, D.C.

James Hulm
Vice President
Solvents Recovery Service of New Jersey
Linden, NJ

W. Larry Petcovic
President
Advanced Communication Techniques
Columbia, MD
(Petcovic advises health physicists and other science professionals on how to communicate health risks.)

Susan Santos
Formerly: Superfund Program
U.S. Environmental Protection Agency, Region I
Boston, MA
Now: Manager, Risk Assessment Group
E.C. Jordan Company
Portland, ME

ACADEMIA

Vincent Covello
Director, Risk Assessment Program
National Science Foundation
Washington, DC

June Fessenden-Raden
Associate Professor
Institute for Comparative and Environmental Toxicology
Program on Science, Technology, and Society
Cornell University
Ithaca, NY

Baruch Fischhoff
Professor of Engineering and Public Policy and Professor of Social and Decision Sciences
Carnegie-Mellon University
Pittsburgh, PA

Allan Mazur
Professor of Sociology
Syracuse University
Syracuse, NY

CITIZEN GROUPS

Ken Brown
Director
New Jersey Environmental Federation
New Brunswick, NJ

Lois Gibbs
Executive Director
Citizen's Clearinghouse for Hazardous Wastes
Arlington, VA
(Gibbs also played a key role in organizing homeowners at Love Canal.)

Kay Jones
President
Pennsylvanians Against Radon
Boyertown, PA

John O'Connor
Director
National Campaign Against Toxic Hazards
Boston, MA

INTRODUCTION

Agency representatives who deal with environmental health issues often feel frustrated with communities that don't seem to listen and that many times appear to be frightened of the "wrong" risks. In response, agency policy-makers and staff can choose to ignore communities (and in all likelihood face increased hostility). Or they can choose to interact more effectively with them. This manual was written for those who understand that they must deal with communities, but want some help in doing so.

Effective risk communication can help agencies to:

- understand public perception and more easily predict community response to agency actions;
- increase the effectiveness of risk management decisions by involving concerned publics;
- improve dialogue and reduce unwarranted tension between communities and agencies;
- explain risks more effectively; and
- alert communities to risk in productive ways.

Risk communication must be two-way to be effective. Although talking to communities is a good start, listening to them is even more important. Improved dialogue between communities and agencies will, in the short term, permit a more productive relationship and help avoid the locking of horns that typifies many government/community encounters. In the long term, decisions made cooperatively will be both more workable and more acceptable to communities.

No matter how well done, risk communication cannot (and should not) replace effective risk management or aggressive environmental regulation. This manual will not provide techniques to make environmental problems or community concerns disappear. Although it may be possible to sell "bad" policy with "good" communication, we doubt that communities will buy the approach.

DEVELOPMENT OF THIS MANUAL

Improving Dialogue With Communities was made possible by a contract from the Division of Science and Research (as part of the Spill Research Fund), New Jersey Department of Environmental Protection. Not only did DSR fund this project, but it also contributed significant substantive input and cooperated in setting up an advisory committee with members of NJDEP and the New Jersey Department of Health.

The field of risk communication, which explores perception and communication of a variety of risks, is growing rapidly. However, the research literature lags significantly behind the wisdom of the best practitioners, who have been "experimenting" for years with a variety of approaches to communicating risk. In addition, the literature does not immediately translate to agency practice. Therefore, this manual is based largely on interviews with academic experts, industry representatives, citizen leaders, and agency staff throughout the country in policy, technical, and community relations positions.

Based on a list of risk communication issues most pressing to environmental health agencies, we developed interview protocols that elicited success stories and "horror stories" related to these issues. We spent considerable effort locating people whom their peers consider effective communicators. After conducting more than 50 interviews (including 30 of more than an hour each), we sorted the interview summaries by risk communication topic. The guidelines included in this manual, and the quotations and anecdotes used to illustrate them, reflect the consensus of those we interviewed.

At various stages throughout the research we received feedback from the DEP/DOH advisory committee. In addition, we interviewed members of the advisory committee who wished to share their experiences more thoroughly.

The draft manual received feedback from a variety of sources, including interviewees and advisory committee members. We also conducted several workshops for agency representatives in California and New England, during which we presented ideas from this manual. Many suggestions have been incorporated into this draft.

While based on extensive interviewing and a review of the research literature, this manual does not purport to be derived from quantitative analysis or entirely free of bias. Like much social science, risk communication is based, in part, on values, judgments, and intuitions. We attempted to distill those of people we interviewed in terms that would be useful to agency practitioners.

Ultimately, more careful empirical research may test—and revise—many of the guidelines in this manual. Unfortunately, agency practitioners cannot wait until all the data are in.

WHAT THIS MANUAL CAN'T DO

Risk communication does not provide quick-fix solutions. *Improving Dialogue With Communities* does not outline a new approach to explaining parts per billion so that communities will understand risks as agency scientists do. Nor does it attempt to be a "cookbook," providing step-by-step instructions to deal with the complex, highly situational problems that agencies face daily. Neither does this manual attempt to cover all subjects equally. Because agency representatives are generally far more interested in learning how to deal with communities that already are concerned about risk, this manual spends considerably less time providing guidance about how to alert communities to new risks.[1] Above all, this volume does not tell you how to limit your dealings with communities. In fact, this manual, conforming to the advice of both academic experts and practitioners, suggests very strongly that agencies often need to increase their dialogue with the public.

Although agency staff can do much to improve their risk communication performance, a theme we heard repeated again and again while interviewing for this project was the importance of consistent support from management in order to carry out effective risk communication. Practitioners and academic experts have impressed on us the need for a clear mandate from top policy-makers. To that end, we have provided

---

[1] In addition, dealing with the media is not included because (a) the subject is sufficiently broad to warrant its own manual, currently being developed by the Environmental Communication Research Program under a separate grant; and (b) this project's advisory committee suggested that most NJDEP staff had limited contact with the media.

recommendations for ways management can support and encourage effective risk communication on the staff level in a report entitled, "Encouraging Effective Risk Communication In Government: Suggestions for Agency Management."

WHAT THIS MANUAL CAN DO

The guidance in this manual may help you to:

- understand public responses to environmental risk;
- avoid unwittingly outraging the community;
- improve your dialogue with the community;
- initiate interaction with the community;
- more effectively handle routine tasks such as coordinating public meetings and making presentations;
- think more creatively when you are stymied by a communications problem; and
- supervise staff who deal with the public.

A shorter version of this manual has also been prepared. This version may be suitable for orienting new staff or assisting those who have less extensive interactions with the public. The shorter version is available from NJDEP's Division of Science and Research, 401 East State Street, CN-409, Trenton NJ, 08625.

HOW TO USE THIS MANUAL

We suggest that you set aside some time to read the entire manual; most risk communication issues are so interrelated that they are difficult to appreciate out of context. We also recommend that you pay particular attention to Chapter I, "How Communities See Risk," which lays the groundwork for much of the manual.

A section entitled "Issues of Particular Interest" appears after the Table of Contents at the start of the manual. This may be used as a reference for guidelines that apply to specific issues practitioners may find themselves dealing with frequently—for example, explaining uncertainty or dealing with community anger. This index may help you to narrow down the field when you are looking for specific guidance.

The next section, "List of Interviewees" lists the names, titles, and affiliations of the government, industry, and citizen group representatives and the academic experts quoted most extensively in the manual. (Short descriptions of people's risk communication activities are also provided when their titles are not self-explanatory.) We have avoided repeated references to titles in the manual itself. Affiliations are given only the first time each interviewee is mentioned in a chapter. If you want to know more about a person quoted in the body of the manual, please refer to the list. Additionally, we would like to acknowledge the considerable time and energy these people devoted to this project, both in interviews and in subsequent reviewing and commenting. We thank them for giving freely of their experiences and insights, without which this manual could not have been written.

Each chapter includes:

- an introduction that gives background and an overview;
- guidelines, printed in bold, followed by background explanations, quotations, and illustrative anecdotes; and
- a final section entitled "Yes, But...." to respond to the most likely objections and concerns of readers.

When you are involved in a risk communication problem, use the Table of Contents to locate the section most likely to be of help. Use the headings within chapters to locate specific guidelines pertaining to your problem.

A FINAL NOTE

Much of the guidance in this manual may seem common sense. In fact, some of the most "obvious" guidelines appear in several chapters in different forms. Unfortunately, these common-sense guidelines are routinely violated in agency practice, leading to the all-too-common battles between agencies and communities. We hope that this manual will help common sense become more common than the battles.

I. HOW COMMUNITIES SEE RISK

NJDEP Assistant Commissioner Donald Deieso pointed out in an interview for this manual: "Since the 1970s, I've watched a change. In the early days ... when we came into a public meeting, we were believed. People walked away relieved or alarmed, depending on the message, but they believed us and felt that we were competent and had the best intentions. Now the presumption is that we're incompetent, that we have a hidden agenda, that they've got to ferret out the truth for themselves, and that the agency is an obstacle in getting to the truth." Deieso's statement reflects the frustration felt by many within agencies, who feel their expertise, experience, and commitment are unappreciated by the communities they seek to serve.

Agency scientists and policy-makers are particularly confused and frustrated by public reactions to environmental risk. Tempers flare at a public meeting concerning a risk that the agency estimates might cause considerably fewer than one-in-a-million increased cancer deaths. Yet, people will smoke during the break and drive home without seat belts—risks far greater than those discussed at the public meeting. When agency scientists point out this apparent contradiction (ignoring the fact that smoking and driving without a seat belt are risks that people choose, not an environmental risk that chooses them), people become even angrier. Conversely, risks that the agency sees as serious—geological radon in homes, for example—can be met with relative indifference by the public.

Agencies sometimes respond to such community reactions by dismissing them as irrational and concluding that the public is unable to understand the scientific aspects of risk. Consequently, agencies may believe that communities are in no position to make decisions about how to deal with the risks that confront them. But when agencies make decisions that affect communities without involving those communities, they often elicit even angrier responses.

In order to break this cycle, agencies might begin by recognizing that communities are quite capable of understanding the scientific aspects of risk assessment. "The public" includes doctors, chemists, and teachers, as well as persons with less scientific background, who manage to teach themselves many of the technical intricacies of particular risk situations. In fact, while government personnel may change over the life of an environmental issue, residents of affected communities often remember studies, reports, and agency actions with an impressive amount of recall. Too often government assumes that because communities don't agree with an agency action, they don't understand it.

Because outbursts of citizen anger make agencies understandably uncomfortable, they also tend to forget that public outrage can be extremely positive. In fact, most environmental agencies and a significant number of the laws they enforce are the results of citizen campaigns, fueled by anger over environmental degradation. Funding for these laws, and consequently for agency staff, also depends in some cases on tough legislative battles fought by citizens. In addition, most agencies can admit to a number of environmental problems that wouldn't have been uncovered were it not for community action.

On the other hand, agencies particularly resent anger directed at them rather than at the environmental problem. Unfortunately, agencies tend to act (often unwittingly) in ways that provoke such anger. In order to reduce the level of hostility between agencies and the public, those who work within agencies need to understand better how communities perceive risk.

FACTORS IN COMMUNITY OUTRAGE

Admittedly, public fears are often not well-correlated with agency assessments. While agencies focus on data gathered from hazard evaluations, monitoring, and risk assessments, the public takes into account many other factors besides scientific data. Collectively, it is helpful to think of these non-technical factors as the "outrage" dimension of risk, as opposed to the "hazard" dimension more familiar to agency professionals. Because the public pays more attention to outrage than the experts do, public risk assessments are likely to be very different from agency risk assessments. Ignoring the variables that influence public perception—or worse, labeling them irrational and then discounting them—is guaranteed to raise the level of hostility between community members and agency representatives and ultimately stand in the way of a successful resolution of the problem.

Merely hammering away at the scientific information will rarely help. Most agency representatives can recall instances when explaining the science made little difference—or made people even angrier. While it may be tempting to conclude from this that laypeople cannot understand risk assessment data, research in the field of risk perception, backed by much anecdotal evidence, strongly suggests that other factors are at work. Below are some of the key variables that underlie community perception of risk—and community anger at agencies that treat these factors as irrelevant:[1]

a. *Voluntary risks are accepted more readily than those that are imposed.* When people don't have choices, they become angry. Similarly, when communities feel coerced into accepting risks, they tend to feel furious about the coercion. As a result, they focus on government's process and pay far less attention to substantive risk issues; ultimately, they come to see the risk as more risky. For example, if you dragged someone to a mountain, put boards under his feet, and shoved him downhill, your actions would be considered outrageous. Ask the same person to accompany you on a ski trip, however, and the picture changes radically.

b. *Risks under individual control are accepted more readily than those under government control.* Most people feel safer with risks under their own control. For example, most of us feel safer driving than riding as a passenger. Our feeling has nothing to do with the data—our driving record versus the driving record of others. Similarly, people tend to feel more comfortable with environmental risks they can do something about themselves, rather than having to rely on government to protect them.

c. *Risks that seem fair are more acceptable than those that seem unfair.* A coerced risk will always seem unfair. In addition, a community that feels stuck with the risk and gets little of the benefit will find the risk unfair—and thus more serious. This factor explains, in part, why communities that depend on a particular industry for jobs sometimes see pollution from that industry as less risky.

d. *Risk information that comes from trustworthy sources is more readily believed than information from untrustworthy sources.* If a mechanic with whom you have quarrelled in the past suggests he can't find a problem with a car that seems faulty to you, you will respond quite differently than if a friend delivers the same

[1] Baruch Fischhoff, Paul Slovic, and Sarah Lichtenstein conducted much of the ground-breaking research that developed an understanding of risk perception variables.

news. You are more apt to demand justification, rather than ask neutral questions, of the mechanic. Unfortunately, on-going battles with communities erode trust and make the agency message far less believable.

While the above factors are those most frequently stumbled over by government agencies, social scientists have identified a variety of others that also can play a significant role. The following are also likely to be relevant to agencies dealing with environmental health issues:

e. *Risks that seem ethically objectionable will seem more risky than those that don't.* To many people, pollution is morally wrong. As former EPA Assistant Administrator Milton Russell put it, speaking to some people about an optimal level of pollution is like talking about an acceptable number of child molesters.

f. *Natural risks seem more acceptable than artificial risks.* Natural risks provide no focus for anger; a risk caused by God is more acceptable than one caused by people. For example, consider the difference between the reactions to naturally occurring radon in homes and the reactions to high radon levels caused by uranium mill tailings or industrial sources.

g. *Exotic risks seem more risky than familiar risks.* A cabinet full of household cleansers, for example, seems much less risky than a high-tech chemical facility that makes the cleansers.

h. *Risks that are associated with other, memorable events are considered more risky.* Risks that bring to mind Bhopal or Love Canal, for example, are more likely to be feared than those that lack such associations.

i. *Risks that are "dreaded" seem less acceptable than those that carry less dread.* For example, an industrial emission that may cause cancer seems much less acceptable to many people than one that may increase the risk of emphysema, even though both diseases can kill.

j. *Risks that are undetectable create more fear than detectable risks.* As an experienced war correspondent said at Three Mile Island, "at least in a war you know you haven't been hit *yet*." Similarly, risks with effects that may take years to show up are more likely to be feared.

k. *Risks that are well understood by science are more acceptable than those that are not.* Risks that scientists can explain to communities seem more acceptable than those about which scientists have to admit a great deal of uncertainty.

The greater the number and seriousness of these factors, the greater the likelihood of public concern about the risk, regardless of the data. As government agencies have seen many times, the risks that elicit the greatest public concern may not be the same ones that scientists have identified as most significant. When officials dismiss the public's concern as misguided, moreover, the result is controversy, anger, distrust, and still greater concern. None of this is meant to suggest that people disregard scientific information and make decisions based only on outrage factors. It does suggest, however, that outrage *also* matters, and that by ignoring the outrage factors, agencies skew the balance and cause people to become still more outraged. This is the logic that leads to the guideline that follows.

Pay as much attention to outrage factors, and to the community's concerns, as to scientific variables. At the same time, don't underestimate the public's ability to understand the science.

Agencies too often focus on the data and ignore the outrage factors. They pay the price for doing so. Insistence on dealing with the "right" risks, the "right" way, may seem to many outside the agency as arrogant at best. If you fail to attend to the outrage factors and people's concerns from the outset, you will often be forced to attend to them later, after you have angered the public— a far more difficult situation.

Unfortunately, this manual is full of examples in which this has happened. Agency practitioners can recall far more horror stories than success stories because it is still unusual for agencies to attend consistently to variables other than scientific ones. There are many examples of agencies failing to realize, for example, that communities resent risks that are imposed and not under their control. As a result, communities which were not consulted during the decision-making process more readily fight agency decisions. Similarly, agency representatives have also been shouted down when trying to present data because communities have felt their concerns were not acknowledged, much less addressed.

Nonetheless, there are examples of agency successes. The New York Department of Health asked office workers their concerns and gave them opportunities for input following a fire that contaminated their office building with dioxin. Trust was built in the process. NJDEP listened to— and responded to— community concerns in Clinton where extremely high radon levels were found, leading to a community response to NJDEP that seemed far more positive than in many other instances. In Virginia a developer involved the community in the risk assessment process, building sufficient credibility that when the risk assessment showed negligible risks, the results were believed. In most of these instances of success, communities that were consulted about their concerns were also helped to understand the science, and their understanding seemed to increase.

In short, response to risk is more complex than a linear response to "the facts." This does not mean that people don't need to know— or want to know— the facts. It means rather that agencies need to take into account other factors as well.

YES, BUT....

• ***Our job is to protect public health. That means relying on data, not dealing with outrage factors.***

There are basically three responses to this point.

First, if you merely run with the data and ignore the outrage factors, you will outrage the public. As a result, risks the agency deems minimal will become battlegrounds. Agencies will have less time for serious risks. In short, one way or another agencies will have to deal with these factors.

Second, in a democracy controversial issues are not merely determined by those with technical expertise. To use an analogy, the experts in the Pentagon have great technical expertise in weaponry, but few people, regardless of their political beliefs, feel that American defense policy should be determined solely by the Pentagon.

Third, data are not always complete, and management options are rarely perfect. The public's raising other concerns can lead to better technical solutions.

• ***If it were not for advocacy groups, there would be no outrage.***

As anyone who has tried to organize a community can attest, it is hard to create outrage when none exists. Advocacy groups can focus or direct the community's anger, but rarely create it. In fact, most environmental activists count on government to create the outrage. Unfortunately, in many cases where environmental officials blame public-interest groups for blocking solutions, the blame needs to be shared by the officials themselves, who unwittingly goaded the outrage by failing from the outset to listen to community concerns. Instead of blaming citizens for not understanding risk, in short, agencies might spend more time trying to understand outrage.

II. EARNING TRUST AND CREDIBILITY

Agencies achieve trust, in large part, by being consistently competent, caring, and honest. If you communicate with honesty and fairness, your audience will often respond in kind. If you fail to do so, trust is unlikely.

Trust is rarely built through slick packaging; a veneer of honesty is easy to see through. According to James Callaghan of Hill and Knowlton, the only way to achieve credibility is to "be credible."

Trust and credibility are fundamental to many of the stories told by practitioners for this manual. The stories go two ways: interaction between the agency and the public builds mutual respect and understanding ... or degenerates into antagonism and hostility. While many of the stories have their ups and downs, those consistently marked by anger and tension tend to end with regulatory action, legal intervention, or abandonment of agency plans. In most cases the practitioner could, in retrospect, identify a point at which the ending of the story was predictable. Problems with trust and credibility were at the heart and were often linked to the agency's failure to communicate openly or to involve the public early.

Of course, even if you deal with communities honestly and involve them in the decision-making process, there is no guarantee that they will agree with the proposed action or that all concerned will walk away happy with the resolution. Also, most experts and practitioners concede that a small segment of the public will not trust you no matter how trustworthy you act.

However, if you fail to "be credible," you will virtually guarantee people's opposition. That opposition will express itself as a confusing mixture of resentment of the agency and disagreement with the science. As Baruch Fischhoff of Carnegie-Mellon University explains, "When people are mad, they'll fight on whatever issues they can fight most effectively ... and risk is the Achilles heel of technology."

The guidelines in this chapter offer a framework for the more specific recommendations that follow in the rest of the manual. While they may seem obvious, these guidelines are often overlooked or ignored.

1. Be aware of the factors that inspire trust.

Trust of an agency depends, in large part, on the answers to five questions: (a) Does the agency seem competent? (b) Does the agency seem caring? (c) Does the agency encourage meaningful public involvement? (d) Does the agency seem honorable? and (e) Is the agency taking outrage factors into account when dealing with the public? Agencies and their staff need to be asking these questions of themselves consistently. In essence, instead of pushing the public to trust them, agencies should strive towards acting consistently trustworthy.

2. Pay attention to process.

Process is (almost) everything. Everyone— academic experts, practitioners, and citizen leaders— agrees that the process by which agencies make decisions is crucial. According to Baruch Fischhoff: "People read the agencies and their actions more carefully than they read the details of the studies.... That's what we have some generalized skill at. If the process works, that's all you need to know." In most stories that involved citizen opposition to a government proposal, the opposition was not only to the action but also to the manner in which the agency proceeded towards that action.

Ann Fenn of the EPA Superfund program says that many times the obvious is overlooked: "Lots of times ... the telephone calls aren't made, or enough fact sheets aren't taken, or enough individual person-to-person briefings aren't done...."

Bruce Bentley of the New York Department of Environmental Conservation says that the controversy over what to do with the PCBs in the Hudson River has been about process more than science. From the beginning, says Bentley, the public was not fully involved in the process. A disposal site for the dredged PCBs was selected without involving the public in either the development of the site selection criteria or the actual selection of the site: "We failed to involve people in determining what the criteria for a site should be and then went ahead and selected the site and then told them, 'Here's what criteria we used and this is what the site is.' By that time, people were not willing to buy into the criteria and certainly, therefore, not willing to buy into the site."

Joan Gardner of the Massachusetts Hazardous Waste Site Safety Council says that the "developer-driven" process of selecting sites in Massachusetts shuts the community out: "The community comes to the table because the state makes them," says Gardner. It doesn't matter that the state is giving the community money to hire its own consultants, because the site has already been chosen by a developer who has been solicited by the state. By the time the community finds out about the proposed site, it is the outsider and uses its consulting money to try to find ways to fight the facility.

3. Explain agency process.

Agencies can improve relationships with the community by providing an understanding of government's internal workings, which are often a mystery to people outside the agency.

Communities need a better sense of why agencies and their representatives behave as they do, says Raymond Neutra of the California Department of Health Services. He says that because government agencies are analogous to black boxes that the public can't see inside of, it is important to open up the "box" and demystify the process. Bruce Bentley adds that it is also important to explain where the public can fit into the process.

Barker Hamill of NJDEP also stresses the need to show that government functions in a logical manner. Hamill cites a case in which private water-supply wells were contaminated. At a public meeting he and other agency representatives explained the agency's problem-solving approach and constraints as well as the technical information. "Sometimes people want to see that you've put an effort into the problem," says Hamill.

4. Be forthcoming with information and involve the public from the outset.

There are numerous examples throughout the manual, especially in Chapter III, "Deciding When to Release Information," that illustrate loss of credibility because an agency held onto information too long or failed to involve the public from the outset. In most of these situations, once credibility was lost it was difficult or impossible to regain and the situation deteriorated. Practitioners recommend being up-front with all information—good and bad—or it will come back to haunt you later.

Early involvement of the public can lead to a cooperative effort to solve a problem. Alternatively, interest can dwindle as the public finds that its major concerns have been addressed. Failure to involve the public early, on the other hand, causes the public to mistrust the agency and puts the agency on the defensive.

Thomas Burke of the New Jersey Department of Health says: "When you are faced with difficult decisions, the effectiveness of implementing those decisions has to do with the public trust in you.... An agency has to develop credibility by showing that it is responsive, that it is involving the public in the decision-making process, that it is open to suggestion, that it is a two-way street, that the decision-making is a dialogue between the affected publics and the agency. The best way to shut out credibility is to shut out that process."

5. Focus on building trust as well as generating good data.

Agency scientists are dismayed when their science seems to be overlooked by the public. As we have discussed previously, however, people's risk judgments are seldom based solely on the data, but rather on a combination of the data, their perception of the risk due to other variables, and their feelings about the agency. Agencies should monitor not only the environment but also the impression they create.

In the controversy over whether to dredge or leave PCBs in the Hudson River, Bruce Bentley says that there are basically two choices: to leave the PCBs in the sediment and water column or to remove them and place them in containers in secure landfills. Although this is by no means an easy decision, Bentley feels that the public's responses have more to do with lack of faith in government than with the scientific information: "They [communities] don't trust government, and therefore despite the fact that it would seem logical that containing them in one place is better than leaving them free in the environment ... because they don't trust us they forget what is logical. The reason they don't trust us is that we didn't involve them in the decisions."

6. Follow up.

Get back to people. Do what you say you are going to do. Check to see if what was promised actually happened. These suggestions may seem overwhelmingly obvious, but they are not easy to implement. Few officials arrange to have notes taken about the small and large commitments they may make during a public meeting. Even fewer go as far as NJDEP's Grace Singer, who has her staff follow up with memos to officials about the promises they have made. Singer's staff, whom she calls "professional nudges," also keep track of whether the commitments are carried out. Without such a system, staff at all levels of the agency would be hard-pressed to know if commitments were being kept.

Just as important, there should be a clear system for handling telephone calls from the public, to avoid their being bounced endlessly or falling through the cracks. Singer gives people her name before transferring calls and promises that if the person to whom she has referred the call is not appropriate, she will handle the matter herself. Susan Boyle of New Jersey's Hazardous Waste Facilities Siting Commission feels it has been critical for her to return telephone calls from people considering whether to buy homes near a proposed site, and then to explain the process as clearly as possible.

7. Make only promises you are sure you can keep.

Agency employees are often tempted to make unrealistic promises when pressed by the public. Or they promise something they genuinely expect to be able to deliver, only to find out later that they can't. Grace Singer says she has learned to be extremely careful about making commitments, because Superfund is so technically and administratively complex that progress can be slow. Instead she states goals, with an explanation that there could be hold-ups. Perhaps most important, her bureau gives people progress reports in the interim.

8. Provide information that meets people's needs.

Agencies should anticipate what people need to know in order to make decisions. (See Chapter V, "Explaining Risk.") Agencies should not only answer questions that come up at meetings but also prepare ahead of time for questions that they feel the public might ask. (See Chapter IV, "Interacting with the Community.") Additionally, agencies should give people the information they need even if they don't ask for it. Bruce Bentley says that often communities do not know all the questions to ask to get at the information that is important. Agencies should point that information out to communities if it is key for communities' understanding of the problem.

Citizens sometimes accuse agencies of stonewalling— that is, refusing to honor requests for information and instead providing rationalizations for the refusal. If there are reasons why you must withhold information, they should be explained.

9. Get the facts straight.

Clearly, agency representatives work hard to provide information that is accurate. Occasionally, however, wrong information gets to the public, or key information is left out that causes people to feel misled later on. Make sure that all information has been checked and double-checked for accuracy, and that it is complete and truthful. If a mistake does slip through, acknowledge it and correct it as soon as it is discovered. Don't assume that people overlooked it.

It is important that agency scientists are seen not only as competent but also as honest. While getting all the data and other information correct will not guarantee trust, inaccurate or incomplete information will almost guarantee distrust.

10. Try to coordinate with other agencies.

Practitioners say that when agencies do not coordinate their actions and their responses to the public, the result is very confusing. Ultimately, trust is eroded.

When there are honest differences of opinion among agencies, they should be acknowledged. (Of course it is difficult for agencies to deal with these differences on an ad hoc basis. In some areas of the country, regional boards consisting of the health and environmental officials from several states encourage discussion and consensus among participating agencies.)

More often, however, agencies give different responses because they have failed to coordinate sufficiently. Marc Alston of EPA Region VIII says that when the EPA Superfund program found trichloroethylene (TCE) in wells surrounding the Rocky Mountain Arsenal in South Adams County, Colorado, neither the EPA drinking water program nor the state health department had known that EPA had been sampling the wells for the contaminant. To make matters worse, different messages were given out at different times by the various agencies. Initially, people were told that the levels they were finding were not an immediate problem because the proposed standard was based on lifetime exposure and the contamination was relatively recent. Several months later, the health department advised people to drink bottled water. People found it very difficult to decide which agency they were supposed to believe, and basically felt that all the agencies were in "cahoots with the Army," which the people blamed as the source of the problem in the first place. (Subsequently, other sources were identified.)

11. Make sure to coordinate within your agency.

Lack of coordination *within* the agency creates confusion and an impression of agency ineptness. Responses to various issues should be consistent from one division to another, or the differences should be acknowledged and explained. (See Chapter IV, "Interacting with the Community.")

Richard Dime of NJDEP says that an agency increases its credibility problems "by having ten different people give ten different answers to the same question. The public gets a different viewpoint depending on who they are talking to. It gives the impression that no one knows what they are talking about." According to Dime, "If someone asks, 'Should I shower with this water?', I might say 'no.' Someone else might say 'yes.' And someone else might say 'yes, but.'" Dime says that the problem is not the difference in technical analyses so much as the internal organizational problem of how to coordinate a response. "We don't share enough internally about how to apply it [risk assessment] and how to share it with the public.... [There is] not enough internal guidance on how to deal with these issues."

12. Don't give mixed messages.

Risk issues are difficult for people to understand and deal with, and agencies frequently make the situation worse by giving the public mixed messages. For example, agency safety policy may dictate that under certain conditions field personnel must wear protective gear while collecting samples. However, says June Fessenden-Raden of Cornell University, "Don't tell [the community] there is nothing wrong and then come in and sample with moonsuits on." If you have to take an action such as this, which may seem inconsistent, explain *before* you take the action in order to reduce confusion.

Likewise, the agency's multiple objectives may at times seem conflicting to communities. An effort should be made to review agency objectives for congruence and address up-front those that may seem disparate. Agencies may not be aware of the mixed messages they give—for example, saying that a particular action or facility is low-risk and then issuing regulations or criteria that imply a higher risk to those outside the agency. As a citizen asked at a hazardous waste facility siting hearing: "If it's too dangerous to put where there are endangered species of animals and plants, isn't it too dangerous to put where my children live?"

Another example, says John O'Connor of the National Campaign Against Toxic Hazards, is the conflicting messages about Superfund. Top officials, says O'Connor, have stated that there was no need for expanded funding for Superfund because they could not possibly spend that much money. However, he says, site managers say that the agency doesn't have the resources to clean up a site as fully as the community is demanding. O'Connor says that these different messages create a situation in which no one is trusted.

13. *Listen* to what various groups are telling you. Avoid offending any group.

Some agencies have had running battles with activist groups. Officials in several states have suggested that were it not for outside "rabble-rousers" coaching local communities, the agency would encounter relatively little opposition. However, as pointed out previously, agencies overestimate the power of activist groups. These groups can't create outrage; they can only focus such feelings and direct the energy. In most cases when communities are angry, the agency precipitated the hostility and the activist organization took the opportunity to make a case.

Agencies should try to be particularly aware of seeming insensitive. Kay Jones of Pennsylvanians Against Radon tells the story of an agency spokesperson who said in a newspaper interview that the affluent communities were handling the radon problem well but the people in Jones's area were different and would cry over anything. Jones and her neighbors were deeply offended and felt that the agency thought they didn't deserve to have a voice because they weren't wealthy.

14. Enlist the help of organizations that have credibility with communities.

It may be helpful to the agency to enlist the help of trusted and respected groups to explain risks. Some agency representatives have worked with such groups as the League of Women Voters in helping to educate people about risks. Others— Brian Strohm of the New Hampshire Division of Public Health Services, for example— rely on groups that involve a range of experts, such as the Northeast Center for Environmental Health, to help them provide answers and lend them increased credibility. Still others, such as Raymond Neutra of the California Department of Health Services, have used the advisory group concept to communicate with and involve interested parties.

In some instances, practitioners have used physicians to help them communicate environmental risks to people, because doctors have a sort of "built-in" credibility with their patients. This works only when the exchange between physicians and health or environmental agencies is on-going, however, because the physicians need to be updated about epidemiology and other environmental health issues.

Agencies can also work effectively with groups that disagree with them on some issues. For example, if a group disagrees on the extent of the risk, but agrees on a recommendation, it might be helpful for the agency to acknowledge the area of disagreement while citing the recommendation: "Citizens for Clean Water have said that the risk is greater than our estimate, though they agree with us that bottled water isn't called for at this time." Of course, be sure that you are citing the group accurately; the goal is to build— not tear down— trust.

Associations such as those described may enhance credibility, but agencies cannot rely on them to replace agency forthrightness or community involvement. Ken Brown of the New Jersey Environmental Federation cautions that there is a distinction between using other organizations as a front and working in partnership with them. Further, says Brown, agencies cannot expect groups to want to work together unless the agency is addressing their concerns. Brown notes as well that agencies are often not familiar enough with the community to identify correctly the groups that have credibility.

15. Avoid secret meetings.

When trust is high and the public is actively involved in decision-making, the agency has leeway to conduct private meetings. However, when trust is low, even routine private conversations can look like evidence of untrustworthiness. This does not mean that the agency should conduct all its business publicly, rather that it should be sensitive to community concerns about secrecy.

Obviously, there are distinctions between different types of meetings. Casual meetings— the routine turning of government wheels— are generally not suspect. Private meetings— those that are closed to the public— are more suspect, and agency staff should ask whether there is truly a need for privacy. If not, open them up to the public.

Secret meetings are the ones the agency feels that it can't afford for people to know about. However, these are the very meetings that the public eventually hears of. When this happens, the agency loses trust and credibility because of the cover-up. Consequently, a private meeting that you must keep secret is rarely worth the cost in credibility. You probably should open the meeting or, at least, inform people that it is happening— and be prepared for questions about the secrecy. If you want to hold private meetings with industry or elected officials or local government agencies, it is usually wisest to schedule meetings with community groups soon after, and to tell all parties about both meetings in advance. Better yet, solicit community input about other groups you should contact. (See Chapter IV, "Interacting with the Community.")

Bruce Bentley says that some aspects of the siting of a dumpsite for the disposal of PCB-contaminated river sediment were decided at closed meetings with town boards. He attributes some of the resulting citizen opposition to this type of "private" activity and to the public's not being at the center of the decision-making.

Faith Schottenfeld of the New York State Department of Health says, "One thing we learned from Love Canal is that secret meetings are a disaster.... Even if you're not hiding anything, the damage that's done ... is so extreme that you're better off having an open meeting where nobody understands what's going on." In the case of the Binghamton Office Building fire, the department decided to make all working sessions of the technical risk assessment committee open to the public and the media. The committee, which consisted of people from the county and city, union members, and technical people not connected with the health department, held all discussions and made decisions in full view of anyone who wanted to attend. Schottenfeld says that the meetings were not "public information meetings," but that there was time allotted for questions at the end of each session. (Other meetings were designated as public information meetings.)

In addition to avoiding the suspicion that surrounds a closed-door meeting, Schottenfeld says that there were other advantages to the open meetings: "It was interesting to see that the people on the committee were struggling with the same kinds of issues the people [in the community] were. It was really helpful for people to see the kind of interchange that went on between these 'experts' when it came to making difficult decisions." From a community relations standpoint, says Schottenfeld, the open meetings gave her an opportunity to prepare background materials for people and to assist the media in their coverage of the situation.

16. If you are dealing with a situation in which trust is low, consider taking the following steps.

a. Review the outrage factors listed in Chapter I and the guidelines in this chapter, and consider which ones may have been violated.

b. Acknowledge the lack of trust: "I know you may feel I can't be trusted because the person who handled this case before me delayed in giving you information...."

c. Indicate what steps you plan to take to prevent the trust- eroding actions from happening again: "In order to make sure you get information as quickly as possible, I am going to send you biweekly updates about the status of the situation. These updates will include all new data."

d. Ask those who distrust you what *they* feel would make them more likely to trust you. To the extent possible, implement their suggestions.

e. Personalize your responses when appropriate. (See Chapter IV, "Interacting with the Community.")

f. Try to reduce the *need* for trust by sharing information and involving the public in developing solutions to the risk problem. (See Chapter IV, "Interacting with the Community.")

g. Be patient. Don't expect all the people to trust you all the time, even if you feel that you are totally trustworthy.

The practitioners interviewed who had recouped trust spent considerable energy doing so. (See, in particular, the stories related in Chapter IV.) Expect to go out of your way for people and to bend over backwards to meet their concerns.

If you are the person who aroused the distrust (as opposed to walking into a situation damaged by someone else's mistakes), try not to be defensive. Acknowledge your mistakes. Expect to work twice as hard at the above steps.

YES, BUT....

• ***It seems that no matter what we do, some people will never trust us.***

True. However, the fact that you can't earn the trust of all the people all the time does not imply that the agency should forgo making the effort to be trustworthy. It may take some time to overcome a long history of distrust. The agency should check to make sure that— despite its commitment to trustworthiness— there is not some basic violation of the principles in this manual. (The best way to find this out is to ask those people who don't trust you why they feel as they do.) The agency may also be confusing trust with agreement; people can trust each other's integrity and still disagree on fundamental issues.

III. DECIDING WHEN TO RELEASE INFORMATION

Perhaps no other aspect of agency communication of environmental risk is so closely related to the agency's credibility as its decision about when to share risk information with the public. It is also probably the toughest decision to make. Agencies fear that releasing information early may cause undue alarm or lead to disclosure of incorrect or misinterpreted data. Agencies also prefer to hold onto information while developing management options, rather than going to the public empty-handed.

Citizens view these reasons with suspicion. Although agency policy-makers believe they are acting prudently and with appropriate scientific caution, they may be overlooking two important factors: the anxiety that people feel when they are kept waiting for information that concerns the well-being of their families, and the anger that people feel when they learn later that they have been kept waiting. When health risks are involved, regardless of the level of the risks, the public often finds it difficult to believe that holding onto information is justified. What an agency views as scientific caution, the community may see as a "cover-up" or as bureaucratic intransigence.

Waiting to release information may therefore cause the risk issue to be eclipsed by the public's anger at the agency process. Trust plummets and dialogue becomes more difficult. (For further discussion about the causes of public anger, see Chapter I, "How Communities See Risk.")

Good arguments can be made both for holding onto information and for releasing it. The answer is often situational. Nonetheless, agencies tend to err on the side of delaying release too long, rarely on the side of releasing too quickly. In fact, many risk communication "horror stories" involving a battle between an embittered, untrusting public and an increasingly frustrated agency have resulted, in part, from the agency's decision to hold onto information longer than the public felt was justified.

This is not to suggest that information should always be released early, or that essential quality assurance procedures should be circumvented. It does suggest, however, that agencies should seriously examine the implications of holding onto information. The next time you contemplate whether to make information public, consider some of the reasons to release information early:

a. Early release of information sets the pace for resolution of the problem.

b. If you wait, the story may leak anyway. When it does, you are apt to lose trust and credibility.

c. You can better control the accuracy of information if you are the first to present it.

d. There is more likely to be time for meaningful public involvement in decision-making if the information is released promptly.

e. People are entitled to information that affects their lives.

f. Prompt release of information about one situation may prevent similar situations elsewhere.

g. Less work is required to release information early than to respond to inquiries, attacks, etc. that might result from delayed release. Also, your project is more likely to stay on schedule if you don't have to backtrack over steps you took without the public's knowledge.

h. You are more apt to earn public trust if you release information promptly.

i. If you wait, people may feel angry and resentful about not learning of information earlier.

j. People are more likely to overestimate the risk if you hold onto information.

DECIDING WHETHER TO RELEASE INFORMATION

1. If people are immediately at risk, do not wait to communicate—and to act on—risk information.

Everyone interviewed, practitioners and experts alike, agreed that if a hazard is putting people at immediate risk, the agency should follow its mandate to protect public health without hesitation. If strong indications—for example, unconfirmed preliminary data—are all the agency has to go on, the agency should probably release the information rather than put people at more risk by waiting for confirmation of the data.

2. If the agency is investigating a potential risk that people aren't aware of, the agency should seriously consider making known what it is doing and why.

Agencies tend not to talk too much about investigations that take place out of the public eye; they are concerned about raising undue alarm or being accused of "crying wolf." But when an agency announces findings from an investigation people have not been aware of, the agency is open to attack for not communicating its concern sooner. The agency is then forced to defend its delay in announcing the investigation and to justify the possibility that people were exposed to a risk longer than necessary. The public, in its anger over not being told, is more likely to overestimate the risk and far less likely to trust any recommendations the agency makes concerning the risk itself.

New Jersey has had many experiences with this type of situation, according to Thomas Burke of the New Jersey Department of Health: "You routinely see headlines like 'NJ discovers dioxin in Ironbound,' and people had no idea you were even in there looking ... so they're convinced that you knew all along and that there have been secret studies.... I've seen enough cases like that [to think that] when you're designing an investigation ... or a regulatory strategy, the communication should begin just as you sit down to design it if you're going to be successful and if you're going to build credibility." Even if an investigation suggests that no problem exists, when people find out about it belatedly they are apt to suspect a cover-up. As Ken Brown of the New Jersey Environmental Federation suggests, when communities are not told about an investigation at the beginning, they are less willing to believe the results of the investigation.

Bruce Bentley of the New York Department of Environmental Conservation relates a story in which early communication with the public about an investigation, he feels, made all the difference in people's reaction to the risk. Bentley says that as soon as the state and county had reason to believe that the particular county might have TCE in its private wells, the county health department began sampling, going door-to-door and explaining to people what was going on. Results were sent to each person by mail with a letter giving times of "availability sessions" the state and county had set up in the town to answer people's questions about the data. Further work was always preceded by a letter to each homeowner, naming people to contact with questions. "People were told what we were going to do and when we were going to do it and given a chance to come and discuss it with us," says Bentley. Remediation consisted of installing filters on private water supplies. Bentley says that even though the community still has concerns about whether the filters are sufficient and what risks they were exposed to before the problem was found, the discussion is centered on the risk, not on the way people were treated.

Citizen leaders agree that they want to be told even if there is only a suspicion. They feel even more strongly about being told if the agency is monitoring or testing. Ken Brown says that when an agency holds information for more than a day or two for the purpose of confirmation, the delay destroys agency credibility, leads to "widespread distrust," and has repercussions on future situations. He cites as an example the case of the Ciba-Geigy plant in Toms River. The state had information on the nature of the company's discharge for quite a while, Brown say, but failed to make that information public. When the company's ocean discharge pipe ultimately burst and people discovered that this information had been on file, DEP's credibility was seriously damaged.

3. If it seems likely that the media or someone else may release the information before you are ready, release it yourself.

Leaks of information are not uncommon in government agencies. In fact, a startling number of environmental issues have been uncovered when the media or a citizens group dug up information that an agency was sitting on—for whatever reason. In these situations, agencies lose the ability to shape the issue and are instead engaged in playing "catch-up," often at the expense of both their credibility *and* the accurate portrayal of the information.

For example, a 1986 controversy over lead in drinking water occurred after a report prepared for the EPA Office of Drinking Water in Washington, DC was leaked to the media, according to Marc Alston, Chief of the Public Water Supply Section, USEPA Region VIII in Denver. Alston says that the media used numbers in the report as the basis for misleading averages and comparisons, which his office then had to work diligently to refute.

James Callaghan of Hill and Knowlton, a consulting firm that helps industry explain risks to the public, was involved in a similar situation when a company he represented reported the presence of dioxin-containing soil on-site to the state but failed to alert the community. Eventually, the media got the story through a leak at the state agency. Callaghan feels that the company should at least have let the "official community" (i.e., the mayor and local fire and health departments) know because "that would have permitted local officials to deal with the facts rather than simply joining in the outrage when questioned by constituents and the media." Also, says Callaghan, in a leak like this the media don't always check with the company first, so the company has no chance to correct wrong information or misinterpretation.

4. If it is likely that the media will "fill in" with information concerning an on-going story while they are waiting for you to speak, speak first.

If the news on a story has already been released—either by you or by somebody else—you are often better off continuing to feed reporters information than letting them rely on less accurate sources. Once again, your releasing information can make the difference in both the accuracy of the story and the agency's credibility. When you wait to communicate about something that is already news, the press will shape the issue without you. You may then end up spending time defending your views or your credibility.

Ruddie Clarkson of the Louisiana Department of Health and Human Resources was forced to wait to communicate the health risks of a derailed train carrying "a real chemical soup" because of the need to coordinate with another state agency. "The reporters were left on their own to dig up what they would about public health, and they did.... A real campaign of fear was put out in the newspapers. What was missing from that was a lot of the technical information that would have negated that fear."

For example, a car containing tetra-ethyl lead had exploded very early in the crisis, converting the lead to its inorganic form and greatly reducing its risk off-site. Because the Department of Health and Human Resources was not able to talk to reporters about health risks, this information was not getting into the newspapers, and peoples' concerns were often misplaced. The Department began its official communication in the middle of the second week of the accident. At that time, the health department "slowly began this process of retrieving credibility and ... the proportion of risk ... but it took almost 18 months to regain." That incident, says Clarkson, forced Louisiana agencies to rethink the entire communication process. (For more information about explaining health risks, please refer to Chapter V, "Explaining Risk.")

5. If you really don't trust the data, talk to the public about your procedures but don't release your data.

If preliminary review shows some serious problems with the data (for example, if a blank is contaminated or if you have reason to believe that the sampling procedure was way off base), don't release the data. However, you need to make the distinction between (a) data that have not yet gone through confirmatory testing although you have every reason to believe they are sound, and (b) data that are truly suspect for whatever reason. In the case of suspicious data, wait. *But do talk to the public.* Be up-front and tell citizens what has happened and when they will be able to get some results that are meaningful. Explain the process rather than remaining silent. In the case of preliminary data you consider reliable, refer to Guideline 6 below.

There is one exception to withholding information you do not trust: When dealing with data that may be shaky, but that could point to immediate risks if true, you should release the information. Underline the uncertainty of the data but stress your need to err on the side of protecting public health. In this case, advise people what actions they can take until more reliable data are available, and make the new data available as soon as possible.

6. If the preliminary results do show a problem—and you are fairly confident of the results—release them and explain the tentativeness of the data.

Often agencies are more willing to release tentative good news than tentative bad news, reasoning that they want to be totally sure of the bad news to avoid needlessly alarming people. Although it is appropriate not to want to alarm people unnecessarily, if you are fairly confident of data that show a problem, then holding them for any length of time for any reason will be considered unconscionable. You will leave the agency vulnerable to charges of a cover-up later on, and to resulting community outrage (see Chapter I).

As explained above, there is a difference between data, still unconfirmed, that adhered to quality assurance procedures and data that are suspect due to deviation from standard practices. In the latter case, the data should be withheld unless the potential health risk is substantial. But in the former case, the data should probably be released to citizens, explaining that formal quality assurance procedures have yet to be done. This has several advantages: It allows citizens to take necessary action as soon as possible; it reduces the chance that people's outrage over the agency's waiting will lead them to overestimate the risk; it greatly enhances the agency's credibility by demonstrating concern not only about people's health but also about their feelings.

Citizen leaders agree that the value of going to the public early outweighs the risks, that by including people in the process you actually reduce stress. "We can deal with tests not being 100% accurate, but we can't deal with tests still going through QA six months later," says Lois Gibbs of the Citizens Clearinghouse for Hazardous Wastes.

If the agency does release preliminary data with tentative interpretation, it is important to explain the uncertainty of the data. The agency should be up-front about what the numbers indicate; how confident the agency is in the numbers; and when more certain numbers will be available. Outlining the process for approving the data can avoid people's suspicions about what you are doing with the data in the interim. Otherwise, points out Faith Schottenfeld of the New York Department of Health, people may feel the data are being manipulated. (For more information on communicating uncertainty, please refer to Chapter V, "Explaining Risk.")

Despite the feelings of citizens, there are many agency policy-makers who disagree on the value of releasing preliminary data, regardless of agency confidence in them. As NJDEP's Donald Deieso says, "When we have hard information ... that's when we reveal it.... We're being paid to offer the best number, the number with the greatest integrity.... Others may choose to run with preliminary [data], but I don't think a regulator should." However, as pointed out throughout this chapter, the risk of holding onto data is great. Scientific prudence is likely to be mistaken for callousness or worse.

7. Before deciding to wait to communicate—especially if the news is bad—consider the effect on the credibility of the agency representative dealing with the public.

An agency decision to withhold information can greatly jeopardize the credibility of agency staff members who are dealing with the public. Because credibility is often a scarce commodity that is difficult to replace, it should be an important variable in your decision.

Susan Santos, formerly with the Superfund program in EPA Region I and currently with E.C. Jordan Company, says that at one point she had to make a community wait for three months while the agency analyzed the samples and tried to determine whether the data indicated a problem or there was a problem with the data. It also took time to decide if the federal or state agency should take the lead in communicating the risk. By the time EPA released the data "no amount of communicating helped" because the people were so upset. Santos was torn between the needs of the community she was dealing with and the orders she received from her superiors. The situation was so untenable that she decided that if the same thing happened in the future, she'd have to divulge the information and risk the repercussions at work. "Agencies have to make more conscious decisions about what their responsibilities are in terms of ... when you let somebody know.... I think it's too loose.... It's an aspect of my job that I did not enjoy at all."

8. Release information while the risk management options are tentative, rather than waiting to develop solutions.

Agencies tend to wait to release information about a problem until they have defined a solution. They then announce the solution, and defend it from the onslaught of public opinion. This practice makes the agency vulnerable, once again, to charges of callousness from those who feel they should have been alerted earlier to the risk. Waiting also tends to elicit hostility from people who resent an agency's determining solutions without their input on problems that affect their lives. (See Chapter I, "How Communities See Risk.")

Practitioners we interviewed tended to disagree somewhat about the extent to which an agency should develop risk management strategies before releasing risk information. All felt that information should always be released in a context of some sort. Most felt that the agency should at least present options when releasing the data, but disagreed about the degree to which those options need to be worked out.

Thomas Burke said that it is "irresponsible not to have it all figured out as to what potential options you have ... but you also have to be open to receiving new information from the local leaders and the community." Raymond Neutra of the California Department of Health Services felt that releasing data early and saying, "Here are the data, and here are the steps and the temporary measures...." was the way to handle situations where the agency did not have definite solutions yet. Grace Singer of NJDEP felt that she would inform people as soon as possible but would "temper that with how useful the information would be in my view to the person, i.e., whether telling the person without explaining the implications about it would be helpful."

Citizen leaders assert that they want to know as soon as the agency knows for two reasons: (a) It is the citizens' right to know about situations that affect their lives; and (b) Citizens can help find the solutions and evaluate the tentative options the agency has to solve the problem. According to Ken Brown, "The sooner the information is out, the more quickly people can work on it." The academics interviewed also pointed out that giving people time to comment on tentative options gives them a greater sense of power over their lives. As a result, they are less likely to argue with the agency about process concerns. A final solution will often be arrived at more quickly using this approach than when an agency waits until it knows what final solution it prefers.

9. If you feel the information will not make sense unless released with other relevant information, and you don't have the rest of the information yet, wait to release it all at once. But explain to the public why you are waiting and get the information as soon as you can.

There are times when an agency must hold onto information until it can release it in a comprehensive fashion. Barker Hamill of NJDEP cites as an example the release of information related to the DEP's drinking water testing program. Data came in at different times and, says Hamill, "The press was on us to release it in a piecemeal fashion and said 'We want to look at all your data that's come in and we want to pick out the high [in toxics] supplies right now.' We said no.... It was a new program and ... we felt that it wouldn't be doing it justice ... to say we had gotten back one result ... until we had done all our homework on it, because clearly what the media were interested in was getting the first [few] results that were high and making a big media splash with it." In cases such as this one, it is particularly important to plan an overall communication strategy for the program and know where releases to the media fit into that strategy. Says Hamill: "You have to determine how big an impact this particular case of risk communication will have on your overall program and what it means to your overall program to have it come out early or late and how much flack you're going to have to take...."

IF YOU WAIT TO COMMUNICATE

10. If you wait until the data are quality assured to release them, use the time—and the preliminary data—to develop management options and to advise the community on interim actions, if necessary.

While the agency may choose not to release data until it is fully confident, it can still use those preliminary results internally to guide discussions about the risk and possible mitigation efforts.

Thomas Burke says, "I think that these data should be used from a policy point of view to indicate potential scenarios so that you are able to be responsive to the indications [of preliminary data]." Burke adds that he would be "cautious and protective in my guidance" to the affected community based on preliminary results, particularly if the second test or quality assurance would take a relatively long time.

11. If you are waiting to communicate data or information for some other reason, don't say that you are waiting for data to be quality assured. Use this rationale only when it is the real reason.

Agencies lose credibility when they tell half-truths or remain silent and let others fill in the information gaps—often incorrectly. If you need to delay releasing information for some reason, be forthright rather than let people conjecture. Unless you have a great deal of credibility—and most practitioners suggest that assuming that much credibility is dangerous—people are apt to suspect more serious reasons for your withholding information. People are often rightfully suspicious of the quality assurance excuse. They will ask incredulously how it can take months to confirm data.

In the example in Guideline 7 of this chapter, in which a project manager was asked not to communicate data to concerned people for three months, the agency's uncertainty about the data was only part of the problem. The other reasons for not letting people know had to do with interpretation of the data, development of risk management options, and interagency coordination. Making false excuses is likely to make the situation worse.

12. If you have decided that you can't communicate right away about the risk, talk to the public about the process you are going through to get more information. *Don't merely remain silent.*

If for whatever reason you have decided to delay the communication of a particular risk, it is crucial for the agency's credibility—especially for future communications about that risk—that you communicate *something.* Communication shouldn't be like an on/off switch—either you do it or you don't.

Practitioners agree that people get upset when they feel they don't know what is going on about something that directly affects them, and that it is easy for them to be suspicious if the agency is saying nothing. Gary Sondermeyer of NJDEP says: "We get a great deal of criticism because people don't know what we're doing.... There's always going to be delay; there's always going to be problems. But at least we can tell them what we're doing."

Some practitioners have suggestions for keeping communities informed about what is happening with a particular project. Bruce Bentley says an update letter that goes out periodically to concerned citizens is very helpful. Bentley says that ongoing news helps people feel confident that something is still happening—that their situation hasn't been forgotten. Faith Schottenfeld recommends giving communities a sequence of actions—when X is completed, Y will occur—so they can measure the progress of a particular project. She feels this is more accurate and helpful than a time frame that may prove impossible to stick to.

Larry Petcovic of Advanced Communication Techniques suggests that the process for responding to situations be laid out so that the public eventually begins to see that there is a method for agency response to hazards, that "the wheels are turning in some recognizable and effective way." He also recommends that time frames for specific action be given, but that they be flexible enough to allow for inevitable government delays. The purpose of these steps, says Petcovic, is to keep the public informed throughout the process.

YES, BUT....

• Releasing information early, while data are still preliminary and we don't have a clear game plan, leaves the agency vulnerable to criticism.

This manual is not suggesting releasing information without forethought and planning. We are suggesting, however, that you consider releasing the data if you trust them, and if you have developed some management options or a process leading to development of options. Yes, this strategy is not without risk. The agency is vulnerable to criticism. As suggested, however, in the introduction and in Guidelines 2,3,4,7, and 8, you are far *more* vulnerable when you hold onto information. Think back to your agency's horror stories involving the public. In most cases they will involve anger and hostility caused, in part, by delayed release of information.

Withholding information can also result in leaks—which can best be viewed as the agency waiting too long, not as someone else releasing too early. One of the best reasons for releasing information early is so that you can make the facts public accurately and appropriately.

• By releasing information early, we may cause undue alarm.

As pointed out in the above guidelines, you may cause greater alarm, compounded by resentment and hostility, if you hold onto information. When people are not given information, they may think that the truth is too awful to be told. We suggest that the information be released in context and with caveats, if necessary.

•We run the risk of legal liability if we release information early.

We don't pretend to be legal experts, but we do question the number of cases in which liability is a primary concern. In many cases it can be a convenient rationale. Certainly major legal battles have been fought over situations in which information was withheld or people felt their rights had been overlooked and went to court to win them back. If, in fact, there might be a liability problem, vulnerability to legal action should be weighed against the ten reasons given in the introduction for considering early release of information. Over the long term, agency attorneys can help agencies to plan overall strategy to reduce liability and to permit maximum release of information.

IV. INTERACTING WITH THE COMMUNITY

Many agency technical people come to their positions with little or no experience interacting with communities. All too frequently, their early exposure is at a public hearing full of citizens who are angry, in part because of the factors discussed in Chapter I. Agency representatives are then put in the position of defending the agency and themselves. The result is anger and frustration on both sides, and confirmation of the scientist's belief that numbers are easier to deal with than people.

Although agency practitioners often find it difficult to explain risks to communities, it is usually the quality of the interaction—not the technical information—that stands in the way of communities' understanding. Agency staff sometimes feel that technical information is lost on communities, and that no matter what they say, people's minds are made up. Communities, on the other hand, sometimes feel that agency representatives will never give them honest answers about certain issues. In fact, *both* agencies and communities can feel that what they have to say will have no impact on what the other believes.

As a result, some agency people feel the best interaction with the public is no interaction. They fervently hope that risk communication techniques will just make the public go away and leave the agency to make decisions in peace. However, as discussed at many points in this manual, shutting the public out of the process is likely to precipitate more anger. In fact, the literature and most practitioners agree that the solution to the problems described above is usually more interaction, not less.

When communication can be established between an agency and a community, the result is nearly always productive. Frustration is reduced on both sides and better decisions are made. Unfortunately, there are not many examples of successful interactions between agencies and communities. This does not mean, however, that citizen involvement doesn't work—only that there haven't been enough sincere and creative attempts.

INVOLVING THE PUBLIC

The literature and interviews point out five important reasons for agencies to encourage citizen involvement: (a) People are entitled to be involved in issues that directly affect them; (b) Involvement in the process leads to greater understanding of—and more appropriate reactions to—the particular risk; (c) The input of those who live with the risk every day and are familiar with their own needs can lead to better policy decisions and solutions; (d) Cooperation between the agency and citizens can increase agency credibility; and (e) Outrage is reduced.

1. To the extent possible, involve the community in the decision-making process.

Communities and agencies often have very different notions of what public participation looks like. Sometimes agencies essentially ask for community ratification of agency decisions rather than community input. While the agency may feel that the public participated in the process, the affected community may feel quite differently.

The "Ladder of Citizen Participation" on the following page (which is derived, in part, from the work of planner Sherry Arnstein) illustrates the distinctions among different types of citizen participation.[1] In many cases the agency errs by giving too little power to the public, essentially placing interactions with the community at lower levels on the "citizen participation ladder" than might be appropriate.

In fact, much agency communication is appropriately at the level of "Consult 1" or lower. Routine functions of government rarely demand very much interaction with the public. But increasing the level of public participation is particularly important when (a) controversy exists; (b) feelings run high; (c) the agency genuinely needs input; or (d) citizens request it.

Government agencies should attempt to err on the side of giving the public more input than the agency might think is required. Interactions with communities are more apt to be successful if the agency proposes a higher level of interaction from the outset than if it is pushed by the community to the next rung of the "citizen participation ladder."

Bruce Bentley of the New York Department of Environmental Conservation sums up what many experienced practitioners feel about involving citizens in risk decisions: "The public should be involved in all aspects of all the decisions whether they are considered highly technical or economic.... Out of that ... the risk factors and risk assessment become more understandable and more acceptable. Problems, confusions, and misunderstandings or lack of faith relative to risk assessment are a direct outgrowth of not involving the public in the development of these factors."

Some agency representatives express concern about the additional time it takes to involve communities in decision- making. While agency people might prefer to make decisions independently, failing to involve the public will run afoul of a variety of outrage factors described in Chapter I and may ultimately undermine the "efficient" agency decision. Many such efficient decisions end up in court. As a result, the agency spends more time dealing with angry people and suffers irreparable damage to its credibility. Just as important, variables may be overlooked due to the lack of local input, and thus policy-making may suffer.

---

[1] S. Arnstein, "A Ladder of Citizen Participation" in *The Politics of Technology*, pp. 240-243, (1977).

THE STATE UNIVERSITY OF NEW JERSEY
RUTGERS

Environmental Communication Research Program
A program of the Agricultural Experiment Station
Cook College • 122 Ryders Lane • New Brunswick • New Jersey 08903 • 201/932-8795

LADDER of CITIZEN PARTICIPATION

Citizen Power	**Citizens act without communicating with government**	• volunteer fire department; • citizen investigation; • citizen development and implementation of programs
Power-Sharing	**Citizens and government solve problems together**	• funding of citizen groups to hire technical consultants and/or implement projects; • citizen oversight and monitoring; • meetings called jointly by government and citizen groups
Consult 2	**Government asks citizens for meaningful input and intends to listen**	• citizen advisory committees; • informal meetings; • on-going dialogue; • some public hearings
Consult 1	**Government asks citizens for limited input and would prefer not to listen**	• most public hearings; • most requests for responses to formal proposals; • pro-forma meetings and advisory committees
Inform	**Government talks; citizens listen**	• some public meetings; • press releases and other informational strategies: newsletters, brochures, etc.
Government Power	**Government acts without communicating with citizens**	• some investigations; • legal and enforcement actions

2. Recognize that input from the community can help the agency make a better decision.

Many practitioners agree that very often a community can supply agency scientists with valuable technical information about the problem and alternative solutions.

Raymond Neutra of the California Department of Health Services (DOHS) says, "The community is the expert about possible routes of exposure and what they're most concerned about." He points out that communities have told his agency many things that the agency otherwise might not have considered. For example, the DOHS hired consultants to look at cancer rates in a community south of the BKK Landfill in southern California. When the study was released, the community to the north pointed out that, even though most of the air drainage occurred to the south, the northern community had considerable problems with odors from the landfill, and they had lived there longer, thus increasing their potential for exposure. Says Neutra: "By not having that input—we were just looking at the map and the wind [patterns]—we made a decision that ended up costing a lot more money," because the agency had to go back and do a separate study on the community north of the site.

Ken Brown of the New Jersey Environmental Federation agrees that citizens can provide invaluable information, particularly in ongoing cases. Says Brown: "With continual transition in site managers, citizens have the continuity and the shared memory that the agency doesn't have."

3. Involve the community at the earliest possible stage in the assessment of the risk. (See also Chapter III, "Deciding When to Release Information.")

Nearly everyone interviewed agreed that citizen involvement should begin early. Even in situations in which the agency feels confident about the best technical solution, a focus on technical factors alone may not lead to the best solution, particularly when there is a potential for controversy. Involving communities from the outset is the best way to deal with both the technical aspects of a problem and the value-centric concerns that will ultimately need to be a part of the risk management decision.

Vincent Covello of the National Science Foundation's Risk Assessment Program says that citizens should participate in defining the problem and determining how serious it is. "Involvement should be at the earliest possible stage ... so that people are assured that their interests are being represented.... If you allow the assessment part, which is usually the one that is done behind closed doors, to become part of the public involvement process ... then it is a lot less likely that issues will surface later and become points of contention."

Citizen leaders overwhelmingly agree. Lois Gibbs of the Citizens Clearinghouse for Hazardous Wastes believes that involving citizens in the risk assessment process overcomes trust and credibility problems that can otherwise undermine the process. Says Gibbs: "Value judgments are part of the risk assessment process, but if you are part of defining those judgments and those decisions, then the outcome of it is something you can trust." For example, in Manchester Lakes, Virginia, a developer found that subsurface water below the development was significantly contaminated with arsenic. Because he wanted to sell the houses—and avoid litigation—he was willing to pay for the citizens to bring in their own consultant to ensure that the arsenic would not pose a problem. Gibbs says that prospective homeowners or their consultant were involved in every phase of the process, including determining the assumptions on which the risk assessment was based and developing a sampling plan. When the risk assessment revealed a negligible risk, people trusted the results sufficiently to purchase the homes.

Ernest Kuhlwein of NJDEP says that if people's concerns were addressed when a facility applies for a permit—rather than waiting for the public hearing when the permit has already been drafted—the process of permitting might move more smoothly. Says Kuhlwein, "That whole process where [we] go to a public hearing with a draft permit in our hands ... is a little ludicrous. Most people on the outside feel 'They have already made their decision.'" In contrast, Kuhlwein cites a case in which the Pennwalt Company wanted to upgrade one of its old plants in West Deptford and reopen it as a new plant with an attached incinerator. The company felt that there would be much opposition from citizens and local environmental groups, so it decided to get everyone involved in the process from the start. "From the minute they started talking to us, they also started talking to the town," says Kuhlwein. Pennwalt had several meetings with town officials and citizens, and actually flew some people to a similar plant to show them how it operated.

At the point of permitting, only 20 people attended the hearing, and testimony was presented only by a local official who summed up the town's comments. Kuhlwein said that the comments there were "recommendations for additional safety and notification." Although there is a routine "official notification" procedure that is adhered to in most permit applications, it is a process that tends to go unnoticed by most local citizens. This story suggests that official notification is not a substitute for real communication with the public.

4. Be clear about the public's role from the outset.

Sometimes there is tension between agencies and the public because the public's role in the decision-making process is not clearly defined. For example, it is not uncommon for agencies to promise "public input" and, in fact, deliver what the "Ladder of Citizen Participation" dubs "Consult 1," simply announcing and defending the agency position.

Citizens need to know, or better yet to help define, their role in the decision-making process, says Larry Petcovic of Advanced Communication Techniques. If agency and citizen expectations—and agency limitations—are not expressed at the beginning, people will feel misled further down the road. Any credibility and trust developed along the way will be lost as the agency assumes a defensive position.

For example, when EPA Region X asked citizens for input regarding regulation of a smelter that emitted arsenic, the agency was careful to be clear about the role of the public. Randall Smith of Region X says that although the newspapers were framing the workshops conducted by EPA as a chance for citizens to vote for their future, the regional administrator made it very clear from the outset that the final decision rested with the agency. The agency also made it clear that the opinions and values of the public would be given considerable weight in the final decision.

5. Acknowledge situations where the agency can give the community only limited power in the decision-making.

There are situations in which the agency is bound by legislation to act in specific ways regarding permitting and other regulatory functions, and cannot consider variables other than those mandated by law. These legal constraints should be explained when they are legitimate— and they should not be used as excuses for excluding the public at other times.

Randall Smith says that in permitting RCRA facilities, for example, there is a certain set of regulations that must be met, and if the company meets the regulations, it must get the permit no matter how unpopular the decision. Smith says that it is important for the agency to be up-front early in the process about the limitations of public involvement, "to accurately convey the constraints the law puts on you as a decision-maker."

6. Find out from communities what type of involvement they would prefer.

Different communities have different needs and concerns, as well as different ways of receiving information. For meaningful involvement, you must consider the needs of each community.

Ann Fenn of the EPA says that her experience with Superfund sites suggests that the best way to involve people in the process is to ask them how they want to be involved. For example, in a farming community in Idaho, local people told the agency, "Look, you can have all the meetings you want, but we don't have the time to attend your public meetings. But if you give the information to Margaret Delavan down at the county courthouse and she posts it up on her bulletin board, we'll get it from her."

Bruce Bentley says that citizens may not want to be involved in every decision, and that it is important to find out what decisions are important to people. For example, says Bentley, some people may want to be involved in the decisions about where the wells are placed, but won't particularly care who the contract lab is. Bentley says the process of involving citizens should be "citizen-focused rather than agency-focused."

DEVELOPING APPROPRIATE FORUMS

Because of laws that mandate a public hearing process, most agencies have learned to rely on formal public meetings as a way to interact with the public. Yet most practitioners interviewed saw large public meetings as having distinct limitations. If agencies want to have meaningful dialogue, they may need to look beyond such traditional approaches.

7. When appropriate, develop alternatives to public hearings. In particular, hold smaller, more informal meetings.

Most interviewees felt that large public meetings and formal hearings did not encourage meaningful dialogue between citizens and government. Practitioners see large public meetings as opportunities for people to "grandstand for their neighbors" and "posture for the record." Citizens see such meetings as a one-way situation in which the agency delivers its message and doesn't really want to hear the concerns of the community.

In fact, large public meetings and hearings are not the appropriate forum for most problem-solving efforts. However, they do have a variety of uses, including: (a) alerting people to risks, particularly those for which individuals must take action; (b) receiving information on low-controversy issues; (c) creating a sense of closure and meeting official obligations at the end of a less formal process; and (d) allowing both the agency and the public to have their views aired on the record and for the media on high-controversy issues. Although most agencies find this last option painful, it is nonetheless legitimate, and activist groups that use hearings as a means to oppose the agency are well within their rights.

Agencies consistently make the mistake of waiting to communicate until formal hearings are necessary. By communicating as the issue develops, agencies can employ forums that are much more conducive than formal meetings to joint problem-solving. Smaller-scale and more informal work groups and subsessions are much better forums in which to share views, seek consensus, build trust, and develop compromises.

Some of the more frequently used alternatives to public meetings include drop-in hours at the local library for questions, newsletters, information booths, telephone hot lines, and advisory committees.

Often the most effective approach is small, informal meetings. June Fessenden-Raden of Cornell University emphasizes the importance of such small-group meetings. Many ideas that are nearly impossible to explain at a large meeting—for example, relative risks or the uncertainty of risk numbers—can be communicated in a small group because you can see the expressions on people's faces, can backtrack when it seems they don't understand, and can respond more easily to personal questions.

Fessenden-Raden says that one of the most effective ways to use small groups is to bring people with similar concerns together frequently enough with the same agency representatives to build trust and credibility. She adds that meetings with town officials should not be overlooked.

8. If you cannot avoid a large public meeting, the logistics should be developed so that both agency and community are treated fairly.

It is not uncommon for large public meetings to be one-sided: either called and conducted by citizen groups with the agency representatives at a severe disadvantage, or arranged by agencies with citizens feeling they have no control over the process. Just as agencies sometimes feel that they have walked into meetings and "were dead from the start," so are citizens discouraged by being kept waiting or by being treated with less respect than the experts.

To the extent possible, structure meetings so that people aren't put on the defensive. For example, develop a way of scheduling testimony so that citizens do not have to be kept waiting until the end of the hearing. For meetings involving controversy, consider the suggestion of Robert O'Connor of Pennsylvania State University to use a neutral moderator such as a member of the League of Women Voters, "someone with a local flair who won't set you up."

9. Consider breaking larger groups into smaller ones.

Another suggestion for handling a large public meeting is to break it down into smaller groups after a presentation to the larger group. Practitioners have had success with this approach because it combines a general education and informational presentation with a greater opportunity for people to ask questions.

The workshops conducted by the EPA concerning regulation of the ASARCO smelter in Tacoma, Washington are an example of informational presentations being combined with an opportunity for people to be heard by the agency. The community was very concerned about both the health effects of the smelter and the possible economic impact of regulation. The meetings started off with short technical briefings for the large group, then broke down into smaller workshops for discussing the information, asking questions of the experts who were rotating from group to group, and talking about related concerns. These smaller discussion groups were facilitated by people who did not work for EPA (a member of the League of Women Voters, a local attorney, etc.) to "let the public know that EPA was not trying to manipulate this process and was willing to turn over some measure of control," according to Randall Smith. Also present was an "official observer" (also non-EPA) who circulated among the groups and summed up the concerns at the end of the evening to give a kind of closure to the proceedings, "so people didn't go out into the night air saying, 'That was nice. What did it all mean?'"

Robert O'Connor observed similar success at a public meeting he attended in Deaf Smith County, Texas on the ranking of sites for geological repositories for radioactive waste. O'Connor says that the DOE knew the meeting would be large and wanted to "reduce the lynch mob factor." Since the purpose of the meeting was to help citizens understand the impact assessment, DOE had a short presentation about siting and the assessment. Then people were directed to tables labeled with the various parts of the assessment, for example, "Hydrology" or "Socioeconomic impact" or "Employment." The moderator told people, "At each of these tables is the person who was responsible for writing that portion of the impact statement. You can direct your questions to the appropriate person." O'Connor says that this approach had three advantages: (a) It showed people that "the DOE didn't have horns," that they were human beings with whom people could talk one-on-one; (b) There was no grandstanding because the multiple-table forum wasn't suitable for it; and (c) The professionals were less intimidated and didn't lapse into professional jargon as a defense.

This type of approach is meaningful only if the purpose of the meeting is made clear in advance and citizen concerns are addressed. If the format is used to dodge people, they will resent it.

10. Be clear about the goals of the meeting. If you cannot adequately fulfill a citizen request for a meeting, propose alternatives.

Sometimes communities want to meet with an agency, but the agency does not know the concerns citizens want addressed. Or citizens may be demanding answers to questions that the agency has not yet thought through.

A productive way to handle this type of situation is to try to find out what the community's underlying needs for a meeting are. Instead of refusing a request for a meeting or holding a meeting without being able to respond to concerns, develop some meaningful alternatives that address the community's concerns. For example, propose a meeting about the issues you are ready to discuss or meet informally to clarify the community's key questions so that you can better respond to them later. Faith Schottenfeld suggests asking a representative group of citizens for a list of their questions beforehand, so that these concerns can be addressed and worked into the agency's presentation.

11. In certain situations, one-to-one communication may be best.

Agencies often can't afford the labor-intensive practice of sending staff door-to-door to talk to people. Also, some practitioners feel that small groups are better than one-to-one communication, not only because they are more efficient but also because small groups give people the chance to hear what their neighbors think, and gain other insights about a situation. In some situations, however, one-to-one communication is advisable.

This is particularly true when technicians are doing door-to-door sampling. In such cases, it is critical that the technicians be trained to answer people's questions, or at least be able to supply informational literature and a phone number for people to call with their concerns.

Bruce Bentley says he is a "big proponent of the one-to-one communication" because it can be more personalized. (Personalizing is discussed in detail in a later section.) "You can direct the discussion to exactly the issues the person is interested in.... [The communicator] becomes much more of an individual and another human...." As an example, Bentley relates a story about the contamination of private wells with TCE from the degreasing operation of a local business. Samplers who went door-to-door were encouraged to talk to people about the situation, results were sent to people personally in the mail with a note giving a name of someone locally they could talk to about the results, and the Department of Environmental Conservation held "availability sessions" in the town to give people a chance to go talk individually to DEC staff.

Susan Santos of E.C. Jordan Company says that when she was with EPA and first took over as project officer at a Superfund site in Rhode Island, she tried to have a meeting with concerned residents to update them on the site. People essentially shouted her down, accusing her of being just another EPA employee who would not listen to them. They suggested that before she "lectured" them she should go through their files of information. Santos agreed to review the files, and during the days she spent at people's houses going through their information, people dropped by and talked to her: "You realize that people just need a forum to get those emotions and questions out.... If you can do that outside a large public meeting which is impersonal ... it can be much more effective." Santos says that later meetings were still difficult, but that people would applaud at the end and many times stay after the meeting to talk to her.

As Santos' experience suggests, a good opportunity to talk to people one-to-one is after public meetings and workshops. Many times people have individual concerns that are not necessarily appropriate to be aired at a public forum. Ruddie Clarkson says that agency representatives need to make time to stay after meetings as long as it takes to talk to people who need help. When someone stands up at a meeting and begins telling her about an individual health problem, for example, she tells the person that she needs more information on his personal health history in order to help, and that that should be discussed privately. She then stays later to talk to the person, or offers her phone number. Says Clarkson, "I'm not so sure that relieving stress isn't a role for public health personnel anyway, and relieving stress entails getting the things that are bothering them the most solved."

COMMUNICATING WITH DIFFERENT AUDIENCES

Although the term "the public" is used throughout this manual, in fact there are obviously many publics; different constituencies are affected differently by an issue. Depending on the issue, the agency may need to communicate with environmental groups, civic organizations, industry, sporting associations, health organizations, local government agencies, local elected officials, local businesses, trade organizations, and so on. If you treat everyone as if they had the same concerns, at the very least people feel that their issues have not been addressed clearly. At worst, people are offended.

12. Try to identify all the various interest groups in a situation at the beginning and meet with each of them informally.

Practitioners and experts agree that it is important to identify all the interested parties, their views of the problem, and their thoughts about possible solutions. Ruddie Clarkson says that identifying groups early is crucial because "once the situation deteriorates into a battleground where lines are drawn" it is extremely difficult to communicate. Bruce Bentley says that there was no early attempt to reach all the interests in the Hudson River PCB controversy. As a result, he says, the situation will probably go to court because people are not open to bargaining at this late date.

June Fessenden-Raden of Cornell University suggests that agencies should find out early who the different factions are for any issue and deal with each informally and separately "so you can recognize and give time to all agendas." It is important, however, not to appear as if you are going behind the backs of other interested groups, or trying to win some groups over to the agency position in order to resist other opposing groups.

Vincent Covello points out that very often there are citizens who have not coalesced into an organized group but may be interested in and affected by a particular issue. By identifying and contacting these interested parties, says Covello, the agency can address their concerns early and avoid having them form an angry opposition later on when they find they have been overlooked.

Identifying the various interests is essentially a three- step networking process: (a) Make a list of the different aspects of the issue and the types of organizations that might be concerned as a result; (b) Contact organizations and interest groups with which you are familiar; and (c) Ask these groups the names of others who might have an interest in the issue. And, says Jim Callaghan, formerly of Hill and Knowlton, "Don't overlook the obvious ones," such as local government bodies. Faith Schottenfeld adds that identifying audiences is a continuing process, that it is important to use sign-up sheets and the like to identify *new* interested parties.

13. Respond to the different needs of different audiences.

Because constituencies have different needs, concerns, and backgrounds, you must often communicate with them differently. For example, says Faith Schottenfeld, a woman of child-bearing age will be concerned about how a risk may impact her child-bearing and child-rearing. Elderly people who have their life savings invested in their homes, on the other hand, may be more concerned about real estate values than health risks. Hence, a talk geared toward the former will not meet the needs of the latter.

Similarly, all the various groups agency representatives may be called upon to speak to will have somewhat different concerns. Local civic organizations will sometimes have a different agenda than environmental organizations. Sports fishing or hunting enthusiasts will often have other interests. As explained in Chapter V in the section about presenting technical information, agency representatives who give identical presentations to all groups are probably failing to communicate with many people.

According to Susan Santos, "Knowing the audience and its needs is a crucial first step in preparing the risk communication talk, hand-out, or graphics." Once needs are identified, says Santos, the agency communicator must balance them with the agency objectives in presenting information.

14. Recognize the strengths, weaknesses, and appropriate roles of citizen advisory groups. Define the role of such a group from the outset.

Citizen advisory groups are useful as (a) sounding-boards for agency decisions; (b) intermediaries for two-way communication with their constituencies; (c) vehicles for power-sharing; and (d) sources of input on issues where the general public isn't terribly concerned but interest groups are.

Some practitioners also see advisory committees as helpful to reach out to the community, to mend fences, and to promote better understanding between communities and the agency in the future. For example, Nancy Blethen of Coleman and Pellet, Inc. helped her client, Georgia Gulf, create an advisory committee of people who had been interested in a recent court battle that the community had lost against the company. The resulting advisory committee, says Blethen, is made up of "friends and enemies" who live near the plant (and anyone else who expressed interest in being on it) and is a "communications vehicle." Meetings consist of answering people's questions about the plant, giving them a tour of the plant, etc.

However, advisory groups should not be used as a replacement for dealing with the concerned public. Neither should they be elite groups that are privy to information that other citizens can't have. According to Thomas Burke of the New Jersey Department of Health, "What you are willing to tell one group, you should be willing to tell everyone. There should be no double standard.... It makes the advisory group an extension of you in the eyes of the public."

In order to be effective, advisory groups should be truly representative of the concerned population. An advisory group was set up on the PCB-Hudson River controversy, but Bruce Bentley feels that it was a "political unit" that did not represent citizen concerns. In addition, says Bentley, the group was "never really given a charge as to what they were supposed to do.... They don't feel that they are responsible to the public or to DEC or to anybody else but themselves." Ken Brown agrees that citizen advisory groups and oversight committees frequently don't work because the wrong publics are represented, or some concerns are represented more heavily than others.

15. Deal with everyone equally and fairly.

As mentioned in the above guideline, it's important for the agency to treat everyone fairly and not to seem to be telling one group what it is unwilling to tell another. Ann Fenn of the EPA Superfund Program says that it is very important to "treat all people equally and evenly, for example, in providing information.... Nobody gets priority access to information." In the case where homeowners are directly affected, Faith Schottenfeld suggests they should have access to the information first, and that agencies should always inform homeowners and local officials before going to the press.

DEALING WITH VALUES AND FEELINGS

Jerome Delli Priscoli of the U.S. Army Corps of Engineers relates a story about a public meeting during which a woman testified in tears about her feelings regarding a proposed project. After she was finished, the presiding officer asked, "Now do we have any factual comments?" This interaction is an extreme version of what often takes place between agency representatives and the public.

Scientists, by training, tend to focus more on data than on feelings, either their own or others'. Communities, on the other hand, focus on how a particular situation affects their lives. Unfortunately, neither side listens well to the other.

Agency representatives wish the public would pay more attention to data. The public wishes scientists would consider their concerns. Instead of merely insisting that communities listen to "reason," agencies might learn to listen to values and feelings. By doing so, many practitioners feel agencies will help community people open up to more technical information.

16. Recognize that peoples' values and feelings are a legitimate aspect of environmental health issues, and that such concerns may convey valuable information.

When people convey their feelings, they let you know what is important to *them*. Feelings provide data about what people want, and thus deserve to be heard as information directly relevant to policy-making. As discussed in Chapter I, these concerns may be more important to the community than many of the technical variables scientists see as critical. As Baruch Fischhoff of Carnegie-Mellon University puts it, "Risk is frequently put in the context of perceived versus real risk.... I prefer to look at it as the perception of two communities," experts and the public.

For example, Robert O'Connor tells of a meeting with representatives of the Department of Energy (DOE) and Indians whose reservation was near a proposed site for a radioactive waste repository. Following the meeting, the Indians told O'Connor that they had tried to explain to officials "their concerns, their heritage, why certain kinds of things might be considered sacrilegious." Regardless of DOE's intentions, the Indians felt that DOE seemed impatient, as if the agency people considered the information irrelevant. Obviously, for the Indians whose lives were being disrupted, their values were *very* relevant.

The public's feelings often lead to information about the problem itself, and a good listener can find technical clues in what people are saying. For example, listening to a community's emotional response to odors from a facility may provide information about the types of emission, their pattern, etc.

Even if community values and feelings seem inappropriate to the agency, the recommendations that evolve from them may well be useful. For example, Edgar Miller of the North Carolina Governor's Waste Management Board says that agencies should encourage people to be as specific as they can be about their concerns and fears. "Look at it with sort of a utilitarian perspective.... If someone wants zero risk, that's not a very realistic feeling. However, we *can* listen to their suggestions and try to incorporate some possibilities and options into our overall program to address the problem from a comprehensive standpoint." Some of the issues other than risk that people are generally concerned about, says Joan Gardner of the Massachusetts Hazardous Waste

Facility Site Safety Council, are the value of their homes and their community's reputation. Rather than ignoring or trying to diminish concerns like these, agencies can acknowledge and deal with them.

Finally, values are central to risk management. The public's values are no less "facts" than experts' values, and should figure as prominently in deciding what to do. There is a tendency for scientific experts to see their own values as "facts" and the community's values as mere values. It is important to remember, however, that experts' opinions may have more legitimacy than laypeople's opinions only in the domain of data, *not* in the domain of values. In fact, the values of the affected community are more relevant to a risk management decision than the values of the expert risk manager.

17. *Listen* to people when they express their values and feelings.

Internal agency meetings rarely involve much emotion. In fact, as in most work settings, emotional responses are frowned upon. As a result, it can be disconcerting to respond to people who are dealing very emotionally with the same subject.

The first step is to listen to people's concerns. When people do not feel they are being heard, they feel frustrated, at best. Often, they will express their concerns more strongly or more loudly in order to be heard. This type of interaction contributes to the battles between communities and agencies that have become all too common.

If you fail to listen to people's feelings, people are unlikely to trust or listen to you when it is your turn to speak. An agency representative who appears uncaring has little credibility. In addition, when people feel their concerns are not being heard, they will have difficulty absorbing much information.

Most practitioners have experienced going to a meeting where feeling was intense and trying to open the meeting with a technical presentation. There are usually two responses: either they get "hooted down" immediately, or they give the information and ask for questions. The first question, typically, is unrelated to the technical presentation, leaving the agency official wondering: "Didn't they hear anything I had to say?" This interaction is the result of failing to pay attention to community concerns. An alternative approach might have included spending some time informally on the telephone or in small meetings listening to people's feelings and concerns. Then the formal agency presentation could acknowledge the feelings and respond to the concerns.

18. Acknowledge people's feelings about an issue.

Acknowledging people's feelings is a way of indicating that you have heard what they have said. If you believe that emotions have validity, indicating so will not be problematic, though you have to remember to do it. If you genuinely don't believe that emotions or community concerns have a legitimate place in the risk management process, your response to people's feelings will probably be wooden or condescending. People can tell the difference.

Many practitioners have found that when they say "I understand how you feel," they are attacked by citizens who say they could not possibly understand. There *are* ways to acknowledge people's feelings without seeming to assume too much. One is simply to state what you have heard: "I can see that you're angry about this proposal because...." Another response might be: "Many people would be angry in a situation like yours." A third, more personal approach is to respond "*I* would be angry in a situation like yours." While none of these is perfect and certainly none will eliminate the anger, they are still ways to show you listened. Once the feeling is acknowledged, it should be easier to deal with the issue or question that went along with the feeling.

19. Provide a forum for people to air their feelings.

A meeting agenda that allows no room for people to express their feelings will rarely result in a tame meeting. Such an approach will probably lead to greater frustration. If communities have emotional responses and heartfelt concerns, they will express those concerns sooner or later, one way or another.

Kenneth Cobb of the Cornell University Cooperative Extension Service says that it helps if the agency consciously provides an opportunity for people to talk about their concerns and to hear what others' feelings are about the issue. Ideally, this opportunity should come in a setting that is less threatening and less antagonistic than a large meeting; most practitioners recommend small-group meetings and one-to-one conversations. (See the section in this chapter on Forums.)

20. When people are speaking emotionally, respond to their emotions. Do not merely follow with data.

The following is a common exchange in meetings between citizens and agencies. Members of the affected community angrily tell agency representatives about their concerns about property values or the quality of their lives. The agency people respond with scientific information that indicates, they say, that the community should not be concerned. And the community then gets angrier. When people are concerned about values, it's generally not possible to calm them with the scientific evidence alone, and it's generally not wise to try.

Instead, acknowledge the emotion as discussed previously and repeat the concern, as you understand it: "You are angry because you believe your property values are going to drop." If such issues are outside the agency's purview, that should be acknowledged clearly. If the agency can possibly address the concerns, it should indicate how.

Many practitioners say that citizens have concerns other than those they express. For example, Jason Gaertner of the Pennsylvania Radon Monitoring Program says that people tend to confuse health concerns with concerns over real estate values. He generally tries to get behind the expressed concern to the underlying concerns that may be bothering people. Other practitioners say that you shouldn't second-guess people, that you have to deal with what they tell you.

Regardless, blaming people for their values will not be helpful. Neither will discounting people's concerns, such as property values, because they are not the "right" issues as far as your agency is concerned.

21. Be aware of your own values and feelings about the issue and the effect they have on you.

Agency representatives often care deeply about issues and about their agency's risk management approach. After investing months, if not years, in a project it would be difficult not to care about its resolution. Agency representatives have their own legitimate emotions and can feel as angry and frustrated with the community as the community feels with them. They just express these feelings differently, or not at all.

However, agency representatives should recognize when their feelings influence their actions. For example, anger may lead staff to resist "giving in to community demands." More usually, the investment of months of effort in a project will lead to a staff person's resistance to the project's modification.

Randall Smith says that the more government employees can think about and articulate their own values, which, he says, are "similar [to] values of a lot of the people that are coming to talk to you," the better off they will be. However, he says, thinking about their own values is something that "government officials don't do enough. They hide it or, even worse, don't think about it themselves and keep it buried deep within them...." Smith thinks this is one reason Ernesta Barnes, Regional Administrator of Region X, was so successful in leading the workshops the EPA conducted in Tacoma, Washington concerning arsenic emissions from an ASARCO smelter. "She had been in EPA ... three weeks when ASARCO hit, so she had zero background on all this. But what she did have was a great feel for what her own values as a public official were and how she thought decisions should be made, and she had a great ability to articulate that. People understood right away that she wasn't pretending to be an expert, but they understood what her notion of her job was and how she was going to make decisions...."

22. Show respect by developing a system to respond promptly to telephone calls from community residents.

A number of practitioners, including many members of the DEP/DOH advisory committee, stressed the need to respond quickly to telephone calls from community residents. People failing to receive responses to their calls develop a picture of an uncaring agency, even if the real causes are misplaced messages or a backlog of calls. Because community concerns often do not fit neatly into any staff person's area of expertise, they are often avoided or bounced about the agency, reducing credibility and causing tension.

Grace Singer of NJDEP asks her staff members to give the caller their name before they transfer a call. In this way if a person is bounced, he or she has a point of reference. Singer adds that she tells people, "If you do not get the information you want, call me and I will deal with it directly."

23. Recognize and be honest about the values incorporated into agency decisions.

Agencies very seldom acknowledge that risk management decisions are not based purely on scientific data, that the agency has political and economic constraints that go into decision-making. Ken Brown says that it is important for agency people to be up-front about the values incorporated into technical information and agency decisions, rather than to create a false dichotomy between the agency's science and the peoples' values: "There is an attempt to portray technical information as pure and totally unbiased and certain, but that's not necessarily the case." Communities sense when there is more going on than simply science, and the agency loses credibility unless it acknowledges those issues.

RESPONDING PERSONALLY

Inevitably, community residents are concerned about how a situation affects them and their families. As explained by Harold Sharlin in his 1985 study of EDB (ethylene dibromide) for EPA, the agency spoke in policy terms about the "macro-risk" to public health from EDB, when people were more concerned with the "micro-risk": "Can I eat the bread?" According to Sharlin, EPA's failure to anticipate and respond to these concerns accounted for much of the confusion about the issue.

Practitioners and academics agree that questions about individual risk give the agency an opportunity to put risk in perspective. Often an audience will demand such a response. For example, nearly every practitioner interviewed has been asked: "Would *you* drink the water?" Responding to such concerns offers agency representatives an invaluable opportunity to relate to the community more personally.

24. When you speak at a public meeting or similar event, tell people who you are, what your background is, and why you are there.

It is helpful for agency communicators' credibility if they give information about themselves first, before they simply deliver a presentation or answer questions. Richard Dime of NJDEP says that "a lot of times people get up in front of a group and don't tell how they fit into a program and what their background and experience is.... [For example,] when Terry Shehata comes in from the Health Department, I think people feel more comfortable because he explains who he is. I know I feel more comfortable...."

25. Let people see that you are human.

It is relatively easy to tear apart a bureaucrat. In fact, unyielding, "faceless" representatives who mouth agency policy are perfect targets. Agency representatives who let their "real selves" show are much less vulnerable and rightfully earn greater respect by virtue of their honesty.

According to Larry Petcovic, when agency communicators confront an audience, they can be in any of four social roles: the organizational role ("my agency believes..."); the professional role ("as a chemist for thirty years, I believe..."); the political role ("I believe this is the best decision for the greatest number of people"); and the human role ("as a person with a small child at home, I would do this..."). When someone gets up and tells you about his or her child, that citizen is inviting you to make the transition into the human role, which may be far more helpful for giving people perspective than any amount of data. Agency people can and do wear several different hats, including the personal one. It is important to keep track of which hat you are wearing at the moment, and it is particularly important to be clear with the community which hat you are wearing.

Susan Santos says that speaking personally is very important in her communication of risk, and agrees that agency people need to show that they are human beings, too. "As professionals," says Santos, "we put on this professional air that seems to take the person out of us.... As a public official you go out there and, because no one wants to be on the firing line, you try to come up with too many answers that in fact aren't good legitimate answers."

Faith Schottenfeld relates a story about calling a citizen leader to introduce herself when she was assigned to the Binghamton Office Building case. (The office building had burned three years before, spreading dioxin throughout.) Schottenfeld says the woman attacked her professionally and personally, refused to listen to her, and classified her as a do-nothing state employee. In a subsequent conversation, the woman began to react the same way again, and Schottenfeld said, "You know, the last time we talked ... you made me cry. I honestly came in here just trying to help.... You don't even know me.... If, in a few months, I turn out to be just like everybody else, then you can call me those names...." The woman's attitude toward Schottenfeld changed significantly, and she admitted that she, too, had been upset after their previous conversation. Schottenfeld says that she subsequently worked very hard to include the citizen leader in everything that happened regarding the office building, but that the initial honesty went a long way in opening doors to communication.

26. Prepare responses to personal questions about risk.

Clearly, agencies need to address individual concerns. Vincent Covello says that "it's important not to duck the issue," and that agency people should prepare in advance to answer personal questions. Barker Hamill of the NJDEP says that you must prepare sufficiently so that you don't hesitate, because if you hesitate, you lose people's trust. Thomas Burke agrees that preparation is important and says that in weekly meetings among upper-level staff they try to anticipate questions and think about answers that are consistent with agency policy. However, as most agency communicators will agree, people know the difference between an honest answer and a well-rehearsed, slick response designed to calm people down.

It is critical to give people guidance even when there is not yet a clear-cut scientific answer or an "action number." If agencies can't make policy statements for whatever reasons, agency representatives should consider making personal statements. For example, Jason Gaertner says that he tends to personalize in the "fuzzy area," that is, radon levels that are close to the standard, telling people what he would do if the radon levels in his home were the same as theirs. He feels that this gives people a better frame of reference than just the standard, even though they may not necessarily take the same action.

Grace Singer says she sometimes tells people, "Look, if I were in your position and were worried the way you obviously are, I would get bottled water. You will feel better about it." While making this suggestion, Singer is also honest with people about the potential problems with bottled water due to lack of regulation and advises that they check out the source of the water. Despite the caveat, says Singer, "people really appreciate it.... It gives them an avenue when there is no official avenue."

27. When speaking personally, put your views into the context of your own values, and urge your audience to do the same.

By speaking in personal terms, agency representatives are not telling people what to do so much as giving them a context that helps them to decide. Therefore, it is important when you personalize to let people know *your* framework of values and attitudes. For example, when Raymond Neutra is asked a personal question, he puts his answer in terms of his "personal value system" and contrasts that against other value systems. For example, he once replied, "I would drink [the water], but my wife wouldn't," and went on to explain that his wife is much more sensitive about particular risks than he is, and that some people are much less willing to take risks from certain sources than others.

Other practitioners agree with this approach. Many give information about their diet, whether they smoke or not, whether they exercise, how careful they are to avoid certain types of risks, etc. Practitioners who have actually had to deal with an environmental risk near their homes find that relating this information and talking about how they dealt with it is very helpful for putting the issue into context. (See also Chapter V, "Explaining Risk," especially the section on explaining the numbers.)

28. If personalizing makes you uncomfortable, work on it until it gets easier. If you just don't think it's appropriate, don't do it.

Not all agency people feel comfortable speaking personally. According to Vincent Covello of the National Science Foundation, "To answer personal questions you must be very personable. I would not put people in the position to answer those kinds of questions unless they have attractive, amiable personalities. People have to identify with people as human beings.... Rapport is the key."

If you are not comfortable being as personal as these guidelines suggest, there are several things you can do: (a) Use concrete information and anecdotes from your own experience that will help people see the risk in context. You need not tell them what you would do if you were in their position, but perhaps you had a similar experience that relates to the situation; (b) Bring along a colleague who is willing to be more personal to help give that perspective; and (c) Try it. It may get easier to do the more you do it. But if you really feel speaking personally isn't appropriate, don't do it.

29. If your personal position does not agree with agency policy, avoid misleading the community.

There are times for every practitioner when his or her personal feelings do not agree with the agency's official position. Academic experts and practitioners have different opinions about how to handle this difficult situation. Vincent Covello suggests that an agency representative compare his or her personal response to the agency position; if it does not conform, Covello says, then that person should not represent the agency. This is a very untenable choice for most practitioners, however; many feel that their job is to represent the agency and not refuse to handle an assigned task.

However, misrepresenting your personal views undermines your and the agency's credibility and should be avoided. Potential options for avoiding acting as spokesperson for views which you oppose include trying to modify the agency position and recommending that someone else be assigned to the task. Another option might be to indicate to your supervisor that to avoid lying you might have to take an approach such as the following: "The agency was faced with two options. There were good reasons for each, and it was decided to go with this option for the following reasons. I personally did not support this option. But it was a close decision and I understand why the agency chose as it did."

When faced with this dilemma, some practitioners deliver the agency position but make it clear through their actions that they do not necessarily agree. Kay Jones of

Pennsylvanians Against Radon says that some agency representatives made after-hours calls and visits to give people advice about what to do about extremely high radon levels when the state failed to offer any official recommendations.

Of course, disagreeing with agency policy isn't the same thing as having personal views that go beyond official policy. Both agency credibility and personal credibility are helped by an answer that combines the official recommendation and a well-thought out personal recommendation.

DECIDING WHO SHOULD COMMUNICATE

Agency representatives can be responsible for people's impression of the entire agency. If an agency person seems understanding and responsive, the impression created can be one of an understanding and responsive agency. If the person speaking for the agency seems cold, unsympathetic, or defensive, this will also reflect on the agency. Therefore, agencies should choose carefully the people who will represent them in public, train these people appropriately, and support their communication activities fully. All too often, however, agencies send out staff with no training in dealing with people but a great deal of technical expertise.

Conversely, they may send staff who do not have sufficient understanding of the technical aspects of the situation or who have little or no authority to speak for the agency. This approach can create an impression that the agency isn't doing its homework. At worst, the agency looks incompetent or scheming.[2]

Despite the importance of effective communication, the skill is often not valued highly enough within agencies. June Fessenden-Raden asserts that rather than being a task that people get stuck with, it should be a career goal to which people aspire. Ideally, says Fessenden-Raden, an agency communicator should be a highly placed, highly paid blend of scientist, listener, and spokesperson—because that person's performance may very well decide the fate of a particular management option.

30. Technically qualified people should have a major role in communicating with the public about risk.

Communities usually want to talk to those who are directly involved with the technical aspects of a problem. While community relations people can advise agencies about process, identify community concerns, set up meetings, act as liaisons with the community, deal with day-to-day issues, etc., much direct communication with communities about the risk itself should be done by the technical people and decision-makers.

Ann Fenn says that the project officers of some Superfund sites don't really feel that they can handle the communications aspect of the situation. However, says Fenn, the Superfund community relations staff have been urging upper management to "hire project managers who do have communications skills and do understand the innate interweaving of scientific and political decision-making, so that they don't see their job as being a purely scientific one— they see it as also being a political one and a humanistic one."

Randall Smith agrees that training site managers to communicate is important, because citizens have good instincts about the difference between someone who has been sent out to be a spokesperson and someone who is really involved with the site. He adds that credibility goes up when the person with whom citizens are dealing is the person wrestling with the problems. Smith says scientists in his office develop communications skills through teaming up with a community relations expert and a press person in an informal apprenticeship. They are taught and encouraged until they feel confident to assume the communication function independently.

[2] The issue of agency staffing of communications positions is discussed in a separate report, "Encouraging Effective Risk Communication in Government: Suggestions for Agency Management."

31. Use community relations people to amplify community concerns within the agency.

Sometimes community relations staff are used as buffers between the agency and the public; community relations people are considered to be effective if they keep the community off the agency's back. Instead, community relations people should act as amplifiers, bringing community needs and concerns back to others in the agency. In this way community concerns can be heard *before* people feel they must shout to have any impact.

In the example cited previously of the fire at the Binghamton office building, Faith Schottenfeld spent a great deal of time listening to community concerns and bringing them back for agency consideration. Her use of a hot-line and suggestion boxes increased the ability of people to be heard easily.

32. Regardless of their technical knowledge, people who are unable to cope with communication tasks should not be required to do so. Train those who can be trained, and keep the others away from public contact.

Although there are undeniably some people who are "born communicators," most people need help, at least initially, to communicate more effectively. Many practitioners got their experience by jumping in with both feet, but most felt that prior development of some basic communications skills would have been desirable. As Nancy Blethen of Coleman and Pellet, Inc. puts it, "You can't fly by the seat of your pants. You must know communications techniques to allay fears and handle crowds." Faith Schottenfeld adds that in unusual situations when only one person can be sent on the spur of the moment, it is best to send the "born communicator" or the community relations person who has experience "flying by the seat of the pants."

Inexperienced people need to be helped by more experienced people, and untrained people should be trained. Those who after training and some experience prove to be poor communicators or who are miserably unhappy interacting with the public should be given jobs that don't require such skills.

33. Make sure that the people sent out to meetings are appropriate for the situation.

Many times agencies send out a public information officer when a scientist would be more appropriate, or a scientist when an administrator should be sent. Ken Brown says that community relations people make excellent facilitators and information-gatherers. However, in many situations, says Brown, people like to talk with decision-makers. And when people have questions about the technical aspects of a project, they want to talk with scientists who can discuss the science clearly.

It may be advisable to send out more than one scientist, says Barker Hamill, if there are specialized areas of expertise that need to be covered. For example, he cites a meeting about drinking water contamination that included sufficient agency representatives so that each person could speak to the specific questions in his or her area of expertise.

People may also have questions about a situation that are best answered by other agencies. In the aftermath of a Livingston, Louisiana train derailment in which 27 cars carrying hazardous materials ruptured and leaked, Ruddie Clarkson says there were four agencies involved in the cleanup. To avoid confusion and unnecessarily speculative answers, Clarkson traveled to meetings in a group that included a representative from each agency. When a question was asked, it was funneled to the appropriate person, who had both the knowledge and the authority to answer it. Admittedly, this took considerable coordination, but Clarkson feels the effort was well worth it.

Practitioners advise that when it is necessary to bring several people to a meeting to answer questions adequately, care must be taken not to look too imposing and intimidating. One practitioner suggests that the experts sit in the front row at the meeting and stand up when they address a question, rather than assembling in front of the room or on stage. Always make sure all experts are introduced and their roles clearly stated.

34. The agency representative should be consistent throughout the life of the project or situation, if possible.

Trust and credibility need time to build. People are naturally suspicious of agency representatives who come and go. They feel betrayed when someone they have trusted is taken off the case, and they resent the enormous effort it takes to bring new representatives up to speed. A constant changing of the guard makes the agency response seem disjointed. People are less likely to trust subsequent representatives in an ongoing situation if there has been a lot of turnover. Just as important, it is difficult for the agency representative to get to know people and fully understand the situation.

According to Ann Fenn, at the BKK landfill, a Superfund site in California, the same person had contact with all the families around the site for the duration of the project. She developed relationships with the people, knew their children and their particular concerns, and her name was on every fact sheet and every piece of correspondence regarding the site. Fenn says that this worked very well, that otherwise it is "very confusing for people" when the participants are constantly changing.

35. In some situations, a non-agency communicator may be more useful than someone from within the agency.

According to Allan Mazur of Syracuse University, "If you lose the credibility, then you should switch the communication function to someone else." This "someone else" can be from within the agency, but in some cases the communication function might be better handled by outsiders who are considered more credible. (The replacement must be an excellent communicator, however, because as several practitioners related, going in after a situation is in progress is extremely difficult, particularly if the original communicator(s) did a poor job.)

Credibility need not necessarily be shattered in order to try using a non-agency person as communicator. Thomas Burke has often called upon scientists within universities to explain technical aspects of problems. Ann Fenn says the Superfund program used a local person (who was hired by EPA's contractor) as the community relations person for a site in Montana. Fenn says that it worked well for the Montana site, that people trusted the communicator because they felt that she would give them straight answers and that she would ultimately be living with the same levels of contaminants as they would. However, says Fenn, such a situation can be tricky because such a person would have institutional responsibilities to EPA and at the same time feel very pulled toward the community. This might raise problems, for example, if the agency asked him or her to hold onto some information for a day.

YES, BUT....

• ***As an agency, we are supposed to protect health—not deal with feelings.***

As explained in Chapter I, protecting health will be quite difficult if you do not take into account community concerns. Ignoring such concerns will not only lead to stress on the part of the community, but will ultimately undermine the agency's ability to implement risk management decisions. As explained in the section on "Dealing with Values and Feelings," people's emotions can also provide very valuable insights into the situation. Also, when you deal with people's feelings, they are more likely to trust you and take appropriate action when you recommend it.

• ***Communities worry about the "wrong" risks. Involving them in decision-making will lead to poor policy.***

"Right" and "wrong" risks are not merely a function of the numbers, but also involve other considerations, explained in Chapter I, such as equity and control. In addition, in many cases risk management decisions are based on values, not merely technical factors. Agencies' values are no more legitimate than communities'. As stressed throughout this manual, in many cases if you do not involve the public, the subsequent outrage may lead to even less logical policy decisions. Finally, communities often provide valuable insight into problems and creative approaches to solutions.

• ***We don't have the time or resources to do the type of outreach recommended in this manual.***

Some changes suggested in this manual do not take more time and money—merely a shift in attitude. For example, it takes no more time to listen to people's feelings than to argue with them. Although involving the public in decision-making can be labor- intensive, in most cases it is far more efficient than dealing with subsequent lawsuits. Finally, the quality of projects can increase as a result of a diversity of input, thus reducing the likelihood of having to rectify oversights.

V. EXPLAINING RISK

Agency representatives are frequently frustrated in their attempts to explain risks in ways laypeople can understand. Talking about one in a million increased cancer deaths or comparing one part per billion to one second of time in 32 years can lead to blank stares or even anger on the part of the community. Scientists struggle to convey complex, technical information, believing that if they could only find a way to explain the data more clearly communities would understand the risks the way that scientists do. As a result, they hope, communities would accept the risks scientists define as minimal and take seriously the risks scientists see as serious.

However, simply finding ways to explain the data more clearly is not the panacea practitioners might hope for. While searching for the magic formula that will help people calm down about the small risks and wake up about the big ones, agencies tend to overlook key variables that influence public perception of risk, such as those explained in Chapter I, "How Communities See Risk." Because of the other variables that significantly affect how communities view risk, agencies must, in addition to explaining the risk in clear terms, place a greater priority on: (a) understanding the community's concerns and values; (b) involving people in risk decisions that affect their lives; (c) developing a meaningful process for explaining the risk; and (d) developing sufficient trust and credibility. These and other factors are at least as important—and in many instances more important—than how agencies talk about the science. In fact, according to the practitioners interviewed, most of the cases of successful communication with the public—that is, dialogue with mutual respect and understanding—did not rely on innovative methods to explain the data, but instead focused on improving the interaction with the public.

Nonetheless, it is crucial for agency representatives to try to explain risk information to the public as completely and as clearly as possible. Communities not only want to know risk information, but they are also far more capable of understanding complicated technical material than agencies generally assume they are. According to Ken Brown of the New Jersey Environmental Federation, "As people walk through the process, if they are given ownership, they understand the complexity."

AVOIDING OUTRAGE WHEN EXPLAINING RISK

Although some of the factors that contribute to people's outrage over environmental risks (see Chapter I) are beyond the control of the agency—for example, whether the risk is a dreaded one like cancer or whether the effect of the risk is delayed—there are other variables that the agency can affect. For example, the extent to which a community perceives a risk as fair often has a lot to do with the extent to which citizens have been consulted. As explained more fully in Chapter IV, "Interacting with the Community," the more input people have in decisions about risk, the less likely they are to respond inappropriately to them.

The following guidelines discuss what agencies should be thinking about in addition to explaining the technical information about risk.

1. Consider the outrage factors when explaining risk.

In order to avoid upsetting people, you must first understand what upsets them. We suggest you thoroughly grasp the concepts in Chapter I, "How Communities See Risk," before you attempt to explain any risk.

Larry Petcovic of Advanced Communication Techniques says that communities are more likely to base decisions about risk on agency process than on the technical aspects of the risk. If the agency is forthright in its communications and involves the public in risk decisions, public perception of the risk is more likely to be on target. If, on the other hand, the agency fails to acknowledge people's values and feelings, or fails to involve them early and often in the decision-making process, the public will mistrust the agency. There will be greater resistance to the agency's message, no matter how clearly that message is expressed.

There are many examples of people refusing to listen to risk information when the "outrage factors" are violated. NJDEP's Donald Deieso tells the story of trying to explain the additional risk of a resource recovery facility in the Ironbound section of Newark, a facility for which DEP had already granted a permit with little opportunity for input by the community most affected. At the public hearing, Deieso attempted to explain the minimal risk of one in one million increased cancer deaths that would result from the facility. Instead of responding to the information, members of the audience (reacting, in part, to their distrust of the agency and their anger about not being consulted), jeered, "We hope you're the one." Although scientists felt that the increased risk was negligible, the agency's process spoke louder than the risk numbers.

2. Be prepared to give people's concerns as much emphasis as the numbers.

According to Larry Petcovic only half the population bases its decisions on information, while the other half decides on equity and feelings. "For those who go this way," says Petcovic, "numbers will never do."

This is not to say that communities do not want to be told the numbers, but rather that their values and feelings need to be addressed *first*. Vincent Covello of the National Science Foundation says, "Health matters raise very strong fears, concerns, and emotions among people. To treat it as a technical analysis and not to recognize the extent to which people feel strongly, and not to acknowledge their concerns and fears and to attempt to deal with them, are fatal mistakes in dealing with many of these kinds of problems."

Stressing feelings as much as data is difficult but not impossible, according to Susan Santos of E.C. Jordan Company. When she was with the Superfund program at EPA, she was assigned as project officer for a site in Maine that had a history of unsatisfactory interaction between EPA and the community. Santos says she "got very involved in finding out what their concerns and fears were—whether they were real or not—and initially not worrying about trying to confirm or sway their fears, but just letting them know that someone was out there to listen to what their concerns were...." Santos' obvious caring helped to turn the situation around so some meaningful dialogue could occur between her and the citizens. Obviously, this kind of involvement and listening takes a good deal of time. However, failing to understand people's concerns at the outset can cost the agency more time in the long run. (See Chapter IV, "Interacting with the Community," for further discussion of values and feelings.)

3. Be forthcoming with information about the situation from the outset.

Once the agency has lost credibility because the community suspects you withheld information, people are unlikely to be open to agency interpretations of the data. (See Chapter II, "Earning Trust and Credibility," and Chapter III, "Deciding When to Release Information.")

There are many examples of problems resulting from violation of this guideline, including the following story related in Chapter II. In the early 1980s, EPA found volatiles and other organic pollutants in wells around the Rocky Mountain Arsenal in South Adams County, Colorado, but did not notify the health department or the citizens. When the information was finally released, the agency found it very difficult to get past the community's distrust in order to explain the risk. At the time, the proposed standard for TCE was 5 parts per billion; the agency was finding levels around 10 ppb. Marc Alston of EPA Region VIII tried to explain that the risk was relatively low because the standard was based on lifetime exposure, whereas the problem hadn't been there very long. According to Alston, citizens found that "tough to swallow.... People kept saying 'Why should we trust you?... You know more than you tell us.'"

4. Be sensitive to related issues that may be more important to people than the risk itself. Expect different people to see the risk differently.

Often, the risk that practitioners are trying so hard to explain is secondary to other concerns of the community or of various groups within the community. These concerns must be identified and addressed up-front.

Ken Cobb of the Cornell University Cooperative Extension Service says that when an upstate New York community found nitrates in the public well, the community had three distinct perspectives on the problem: (a) Local officials were interested in the remedies and the cost of remediating; (b) Farmers were interested in possible lawsuits, as well as what would happen to their crops if they decreased the amounts of nitrate they used; and (c) Citizens were concerned about the health effects of drinking nitrates.

In another situation, Faith Schottenfeld of the New York State Department of Health relates that concerns and questions were solicited of state employees about their move back into a Binghamton office building that had previously been contaminated with dioxin from a fire. Schottenfeld felt people would have to deal with many emotional and psychological issues before they felt comfortable about going back into the remediated building. People were urged by their unions to drop off lists of their concerns and questions at certain checkpoints in several state office buildings, and a committee reviewed and classified the concerns. The committee dealt with the easiest ones first, thereby earning trust for those they had trouble answering. They answered specific concerns by individual letter if a person had requested that. Many people, it turned out, were worried about parking. When the committee addressed the parking issue, some of the tension felt by those people was alleviated. As a result, when the more complex issues took longer to solve, people weren't already upset because of parking problems. They were more receptive because there was a track record of responsiveness to their concerns. According to Schottenfeld, "Any stress we can reduce is to our advantage."

5. Be careful comparing environmental risks with other risks.

Inappropriate risk comparisons can greatly undermine your explanations of risk. See "Comparing Risks" in this chapter.

EXPLAINING THE NUMBERS

Although agencies may overemphasize the importance of explaining the data, it is nonetheless an important variable in conveying risk information. In fact, explaining your data clearly may be as vital to the agency's credibility as the quality of the data.

6. Find out what risk information people want and in what form.

There may be vast differences between the risk information scientists and regulators think communities should have and the information communities actually want. Informational needs vary dramatically from situation to situation. Before you spend a lot of time preparing a risk presentation, therefore, it is best to meet with citizens in the community and find out what they want and need to know, or talk with key community leaders who you know have their fingers on the pulse of the community and ask them. At a minimum, develop a checklist of the likely concerns and questions of the community, based on the concerns people have had in similar situations in which the agency has been involved.

According to Ken Cobb, "A lot of it [putting risk into context] evolves as you work with a community.... People are at different stages on that continuum of understanding." Different people "don't read the same types of materials ... or listen to the same radio stations...." Ann Fenn of EPA says that the information needs she has heard from people range from "just tell us: safe or not safe?" to "don't tell us what you think we should know or talk around the problem, tell us the whole problem—we're big boys and girls now."

Risk information should also be in a form that is accessible to people. Interviewees have several suggestions for giving risk information to communities in a form they can use. Ann Fenn has had success in the Superfund program with materials developed by the community itself: "The writing style and content of material ... differs [according to] who produces the material.... The trust level is a lot higher in material produced in the community for the community...."

Ken Cobb suggests that in situations where "neighbors teach neighbors," risk information is more easily understood. "Maybe the question won't be answered in as technical a manner, but it will be answered so that it speaks to the concerns" of the person asking the question. Larry Petcovic agrees that using peer groups to explain risk to one another is effective. He also suggests using different ways of conveying information so people can choose the explanation that feels most comfortable.

7. Anticipate and respond to people's concerns about their personal risk. Consider responding personally.

As explained more completely in Chapter IV, "Interacting with the Community" (particularly in the section on "Responding Personally"), agencies are usually concerned with public policy issues while people are more interested in their own risk and that of their families. When agencies don't clearly respond to questions about their own personal risk, people are often confused and frustrated.

Agency representatives should prepare to respond to questions about personal risk, or better yet, to incorporate answers to such concerns in presentations and informational materials before they are raised as questions. Dealing with people's concerns about their individual risk gives agency representatives an opportunity to put the risk in perspective in terms that people can understand.

Some experts and practitioners also think agency representatives should consider responding to such concerns personally, in relationship to their own lives. Agency representatives who take this approach, however, make clear distinctions between their personal values and agency policy. Discussing such issues personally gives communities an additional perspective on how individuals can respond to risk problems. It also allows communities to see agency representatives as human beings rather than as just bureaucrats. As discussed in Chapter IV, replying personally is not appropriate for all situations or all agency representatives.

Some examples from practitioners and experts:

Vincent Covello agrees that, in certain situations, personalizing can help people put risks into their own context. He says that it is important for the agency representative to indicate that different people have different degrees of risk aversiveness ("some people have three locks on their doors instead of one"), which may or may not be related to different degrees of risk. Covello also feels that it is useful, to offer specific anecdotes about yourself— for example, if you have lived near a waste site or the particular risks you do or do not take— so people can understand your perspective.

Ruddie Clarkson of the Louisiana Department of Health and Human Resources describes a meeting with the affected community just before residents were about to be moved back into their homes following the derailment of a train carrying toxic materials. After the presentation, which included charts, graphs, and reports, there was a five-hour question-and-answer period. Although the agency had been communicating with people throughout the situation, the questions that people wanted answers to during that meeting were very basic: "Do I have to burn all my clothes?" "What about all the furniture in my house?" "What about my garden?" Most citizens have similar questions; answering these questions is crucial to help them put the risk into an individual context.

Jason Gaertner of the Pennsylvania Radon Monitoring Program says that personalizing the risk in the "fuzzy" area around a standard is very helpful. He tells people what he would do and, even though they may decide to do something else, he feels they have a better frame of reference than just the statistics can convey.

8. If you are explaining numbers that are derived from a risk assessment, explain the risk assessment process before you present the numbers.

Many of the practitioners interviewed agreed that people need to understand how risk numbers are developed before they can begin to understand and have faith in the numbers themselves. Richard Dime of NJDEP summarizes what most practitioners feel: "People have to understand how we assess risk.... You have to give some background. You can't say, 'The risk associated with a chemical is X.' You have to say, 'Here is the process and here is the information that comes out of it.'"

Susan Santos conducted a workshop on the risk assessment process before the data were available. She felt that the workshop gave people the background to understand the data better when they were available. It also provided a less charged setting for people to grasp the basics than while they were first confronting their test results.

9. Explain the routes of exposure and, if possible, show them in clear and simple graphics.

Frequently, the issue is not whether a dangerous substance exists in relatively high quantities in a particular location but whether the routes of exposure put people at risk. In cases where there is minimal likelihood of such exposure, the agency may put a lower priority on cleaning up a particular site. Explaining exposure in these cases is crucial to helping the public understand that, whatever their other objections may be to the site, it is not posing them a significant health risk. Similarly, if the exposure is significant—for example, exposure to radon in homes over long periods of time—explaining the exposure routes may help people understand the seriousness of the risk.

In meetings with the community about a Superfund site, Susan Santos used the analogy of a bottle of poison carefully labeled and locked in a safe. If a child came into the room, there would be almost no chance of exposure and, consequently, little risk. However, if she were to take the poison out of the safe, put it in a brightly colored dish on a table and let the child into the room, the likelihood of exposure would increase the risk dramatically. According to Santos, this analogy worked well because "at least they got the idea of risk—whether or not that meant public acceptability.... That doesn't mean that you don't still want it out of there; it doesn't mean you like it. But let's at least agree that it may not be posing you a risk." She also carefully explained the groundwater movement at the site: "I did a lot of transport and fate work and hydrogeology to educate them about where the groundwater was flowing."

10. Avoid dichotomizing risk. Put the data in perspective.

Practitioners often claim that communities create risk dichotomies—that they tend to demand absolute safety and are unable to see any gray area between safe and dangerous. In fact, very often the decisions people face *are* dichotomizing ones: Should we evacuate or not? Should we drink the water or not? Nonetheless, agencies should avoid feeding this tendency. As Baruch Fischhoff of Carnegie-Mellon University points out, people sometimes create risk dichotomies in response to messages from both agencies and the media about safety. Among other factors, standards tend to lead to dichotomizing. If the standard is 5 parts per billion, for example, people may tend to deduce that 4 ppb is quite safe, and 6 ppb very dangerous.

In order to avoid dichotomizing, risk numbers of various types should be expressed in relative rather than absolute terms. For example, avoid making a standard into a watershed figure with everything above the standard "dangerous" and everything below the standard "safe." Instead, express risk numbers in ranges such as 1-10 parts per billion as low risk, 15-25 as moderate risk, etc.

You can also put the data in perspective by showing how they relate to other similar data. For example, when explaining drinking water contamination, you might show one community's contamination level within a spectrum that includes the action level and the levels found in other communities in the state. EPA and the New Jersey Department of Health have used both these approaches to explain ranges of radon risk, indicating how different levels of radon suggest the need for different actions. (See also the following section in this chapter on using risk comparisons.)

11. Express risks in several different ways, making sure not to evade the risk question.

Research indicates that people whose minds are not already made up are very sensitive to how data are presented. For example, one study showed that physicians would prescribe a procedure with significantly different frequency depending on whether the outcome of the procedure was described to them in terms of survival rates or death rates. In fact, research suggests that no presentation of risk numbers is entirely "objective." Every way of expressing the risk "frames" it in a manner that affects how the audience is likely to respond.

When agency communicators wish to reassure a community that is overly alarmed by a small risk, they typically express the risk in ways that minimize it. Conversely, when communicators try to arouse concern about a serious risk in an apathetic community, they look for expressions that seem more alarming. This is inevitable, since no risk expression is really neutral. But leaning too far in either direction (especially in the reassuring direction) can cost credibility and open an agency up to charges of manipulation. Expressing the risk in several different ways— some more alarming and some more reassuring— is the fairest, most thorough way to help the audience understand the risk.

For example, the tobacco industry can cite statistics indicating that the decrease in life expectancy from smoking one cigarette is extremely low. While such estimates may be technically accurate, they are misleading without citations of figures such as the increased likelihood of contracting lung cancer over a lifetime of smoking. Describing the effect of any risk exposure for a brief period such as a week or a year will always sound less ominous than the same data expressed in terms of lifetime exposure. The best strategy is to offer several risk estimates based on different exposure periods.

According to a workshop on risk comparisons held by the Chemical Manufacturers Association in Alexandria, Virginia in September 1987, there are several elements of risk that can be used to describe it to communities. For example:

a. Quantities - how much effluent was released, how much soil was contaminated, etc.
b. Concentrations - parts per million, picocuries per liter, etc.
c. Exposures - how much is likely to be absorbed, inhaled, etc.
d. Probabilities - how likely is it to happen.
e. Risk levels - expected mortalities per year, per decade, per lifetime, etc.

All of these elements describe different aspects of a risk, but a mistake practitioners tend to make is to confuse aspects when putting risks into context. For example, to say that a risk is like a drop of water in an olympic-sized pool is using concentration to explain the risk. This may well be misleading— a small concentration of a very hazardous chemical can be associated with a substantial risk. Even where it is not misleading, it doesn't tell the public what it needs to know to make a decision about the risk. Whether or not you include additional information about quantities, concentrations, and other factors, be sure to respond to risk questions with *risk* answers.

12. Explain the agency's cautious approach to risk assessment and standard-setting. Substitute "cautious" for the term "conservative" in order to avoid confusion.

People generally are not aware that the numbers used to set standards are quite cautious and that, in many cases, state standards or guidelines are more stringent than federal ones. In addition, they often do not know the types of buffers built into risk assessments to ensure that they err on the side of caution.

In explaining this cautious approach, agencies have often used the word "conservative" to mean cautious. This is misunderstood by people who think that a "conservative" estimate is a low estimate, and that a "conservative" risk assessment procedure thus means that the agency is not regulating strictly enough. Therefore, substitute the word "cautious" or "protective" for the word "conservative."

COMPARING ENVIRONMENTAL RISKS TO OTHER RISKS

Risk comparisons can be useful. Unlike scientists who are used to dealing with quantitative data and therefore have a frame of reference for numbers, most citizens do not have a context for the data. But as many agency representatives have found, comparing risks can be extremely risky. The public will consider inappropriate comparisons at best, irrelevant, and at worst, extremely offensive.

13. Avoid comparisons that ignore the "outrage factors."

Probably the least useful and most inflammatory comparisons agencies can use to explain a risk, according to nearly everyone we interviewed, are those that cut across the "outrage factors" discussed in Chapter I. For example, you may cause anger by comparing an imposed risk to a risk that people take every day of their own accord. This accounts for why people resist most comparisons to smoking. The nuclear power industry's comparison of bicycling to living near a nuclear power plant falls flat for the same reason.

Vincent Covello stresses that the reason such comparisons do not work is that they do not acknowledge the legitimacy of the outrage people are feeling: "It has been shown in the literature many times that risk comparisons to daily life that have no direct relationship to the risk in question tend to backfire because they show a lack of understanding and concern about people's own concerns.... There is no relationship for most people between driving or sunbathing and a hazardous waste dump."

Randall Smith of EPA Region X discusses the reactions to such comparisons at information workshops in Tacoma, Washington, to help the agency determine what to do about ASARCO smelter emissions. One of the presentations included a slide that compared the cancer risk of the smelter with the cancer risk of drinking diet soft drinks. "It provoked a lot of negative reaction at the workshop," says Smith. "People said, 'I can choose to drink or not drink diet coke, but I can't choose not to breathe,' or 'I don't drink diet coke, so that is cold comfort.'" Before the next presentation, they pulled the slide from the presentation. Says Smith: "Nobody is going to make a decision on a smelter based on how the risk stacks up against the ingestion risk from saccharin in diet coke...."

It should be pointed out that these comparisons tend to backfire most often when the purpose is to reassure people. Risk comparisons can be used much more freely when you are trying to alert people to a risk than when you are trying to calm them down about a risk.

14. Avoid comparisons that seem to minimize or trivialize the risk.

People are rightfully suspicious of comparisons they feel are used to soothe them or to minimize the risk, rather than to put it into context for them.

For example, Ken Brown relates the story of a person standing up in a hearing and reading federal agency guidelines which stated that there was no acceptable exposure to a carcinogen. The agency representative in turn pointed out, "You can get cancer from peanut butter." A comparison such as this not only trivializes the risk, it also fails to acknowledge the very real concerns people have about environmental health risks. Almost any comparison to a little-known "homey" hazard such as peanut butter or bicycling will strike the community as an effort to trivialize the risk, no matter how solid the data.

Lois Gibbs of the Citizens Clearinghouse for Hazardous Wastes expresses similar frustration with the analogies agency representatives sometimes use for parts per billion. She stresses that a relatively low concentration of a substance does not necessarily mean that the risk is small. A discussion of chemical risks that compares one part per billion of the chemical to one sheet in a roll of toilet paper stretching from New York to England, for example, makes two errors: (a) It assumes that low concentration means low risk, and (b) It trivializes the risk and seems contemptuous of citizen concerns.

15. Develop comparisons of similar situations or substances.

If you use comparisons— and they must be used very judiciously— compare similar things. Vincent Covello suggests looking at a list of the various dimensions of a situation and checking off the outrage factors that are most relevant, then trying to find a more familiar risk for your comparison that is similar in its outrage-provoking potential.

In trying to develop comparisons that won't backfire, the key is to compare risks that will seem *similar* to the audience. The following guidance from the Chemical Manufacturers Association workshop on risk comparisons may be helpful:

a. Use comparisons of the same risk at two different times. For example: "The risk from X is 40% less than it was before the latest discharge permit." Or: "We plan to institute new standards next year that will reduce the risk by 10%."

b. Compare with a standard. "The emissions are 10% of what is permitted under the old EPA standard, and slightly under the level established by the new EPA standard."

c. Compare different estimates of the same risk. For example, compare the most cautious "worst case" estimate with the most likely estimate. Or compare the agency's estimate using one methodology with its estimate using another methodology. Or compare the agency's estimate with industry's or an environmental group's estimate.

d. As explained in Guideline 10, compare with similar data found elsewhere. For example, compare one community's drinking water data with levels found in other communities in the state.

The following are some suggestions for putting data into context from practitioners and citizens:

Jason Gaertner uses comparisons within the scope of the radon problem rather than comparisons to other risks. He explains the range of readings in different situations, in different parts of the house, using different tests, etc. rather than comparing to other risks.

Kay Jones of Pennsylvanians Against Radon (PAR) says that at the time she and other families received their radon results, they wanted to know the radon levels in the homes that were being evacuated. "We weren't being nosy," says Jones. They also wanted information on levels in homes in other areas of the country (homes that were built on mill tailings, for example) to put their readings into perspective.

Thomas Burke of the New Jersey Department of Health says that he tries to put specific risks into context with "the baseline kind of risk ... the big picture." For example, if you know that the benzene in your air is only slightly higher than the level in the national forests, says Burke, "That's something that's helpful. You're not going to understand whether it's going to cause leukemia in you, but certainly your risks are no higher than anyone else's in the country."

Edgar Miller of the North Carolina Governor's Waste Management Board addresses relative risks "from a multi-media perspective ... the hierarchy of waste management strategies," in explaining the risk of hazardous waste treatment technologies, and talks about the risks of treatment technology options versus other management options. "We try to be careful about comparing apples and oranges," says Miller, "and try not to use comparisons outside the sphere of waste management." The Board does talk about types of industrial manufacturing and service industries that use hazardous materials, explaining that these are highly regulated and pose about the same degree of risk that waste management facilities do if they are properly managed and monitored. (However, cautions Ken Brown, don't limit discussion of options to the agency's favored ones, "the ones that are politically expedient or cheapest or whatever," because people will see through this. For example, Brown cites the ocean incineration controversy, where he says in the early days the government framed the issue as if there were only two options, "polluting your own backyard or burning it 250 miles out to sea where there are no people."

According to Martha Bean of CH2M Hill, an environmental consulting firm, people often ask "how much?" when they mean "what does it mean to me?" Bean says answering only the "how much?" question may cause fear and confusion. In the following progression of progressively more complete answers, Bean demonstrates how practitioners can incorporate the answer to "how much?" in a context that is truly meaningful to people:

a. "The excess lifetime cancer risk will be 10^{-6} at this site after cleanup."

b. "The excess lifetime cancer risk will be 10^{-6} at this site after cleanup, meaning that the average incidence of cancer is increased by 1 per million people exposed over a lifetime."

c. "At this site, we would expect that among one million people drinking 2 liters (about 8 glasses) of water per day for their entire lives, one person may get cancer caused by contaminants in the water. This person may not die of it."

d. "Let me try to explain what we call a 10^{-6} risk of cancer in personal terms. First, let's assume that you know 200 people in this city. Of these 200 people, 50 will probably contract cancer, regardless of where they live or what water they drink. If all 200 people you know drink the water from your well all of their lives, there is a 1 in 5,000 chance that one more of the 200 people you know will contract cancer."[1]

[1] From "Effective Risk Communication: Foundation for Making Difficult Choices," by Martha Bean, CH2M Hill, Reston VA, p. 6.

DEALING WITH UNCERTAINTY

Although scientists are used to dealing with uncertainties in the decision-making process, they find it very difficult to acknowledge and explain these uncertainties to the public. There are at least four types of uncertainty that agency scientists typically deal with the public about: (a) the uncertainty of science in general—that is, that science is *never* 100% certain; (b) the inexactness of the risk assessment process; (c) the incompleteness of the information the agency has gathered so far; and (d) differences of opinion as to the implications of the information and the optimum risk management option.

Agency people are reluctant to acknowledge any of these kinds of uncertainty. There is a tendency for both laypeople and experts to sound more certain than they feel and to become more certain as they continue arguing their case. These are inevitable human characteristics. Admittedly, there is also special pressure on agency people to sound certain, particularly when they are emotionally caught up in a conflict with citizens.

However, most of the practitioners and experts interviewed strongly suggest that agencies should acknowledge and explain uncertainty. According to James Hulm of Solvents Recovery Service, Inc., "Not knowing is simply a point in a continuum.... The next step is finding out." Probably the worst approach to dealing with uncertainty is defensiveness, which implies that you have something to be defensive about.

16. Acknowledge uncertainty.

Learning to say "I don't know" may be one of the most difficult risk communication lessons. But a number of practitioners have suggested that it is also one of the most important.

If someone asks a question that an agency representative cannot answer, admitting uncertainty is difficult for several reasons. Many practitioners point out that there is a natural tendency to be defensive when they don't have all the answers. It is human nature to feel that doing a good job means having all the answers. Agencies also correctly perceive that the uncertainties in risk assessments do not inspire public confidence. In addition, agencies are put in an uncomfortable position by disagreements among experts about the interpretation of data and the resulting implications for risk management strategies.

Trying to cover up these uncertainties can make you extremely vulnerable. You are better off to "lead" with uncertainty. That is, explain the uncertainties before being confronted with them. If you wait until being confronted with the uncertainties, you are more likely to be attacked for them.

Vincent Covello says, "The literature suggests that admitting your uncertainty ... is a much better strategy than claiming to know more than you do.... In some cases it enhances your credibility because people will recognize your honesty and forthrightness." Most practitioners agree that it makes more sense in the long run to be honest about the uncertainties than to try to hide them or not to talk about them. Ken Brown notes that when an agency person says he or she is uncertain, the community may be pleased that "finally they are being honest."

NJDEP's Richard Dime sums up the general feeling about talking about uncertainties: "People are not pleased that you can't give them an answer to the question. But they are pleased that you are not going to sit there ... and say there are no problems to their health."

17. Give people background about scientific uncertainties.

Citizens need to be given enough background so they do not automatically assume something is amiss when the agency says it doesn't know; they need to understand that uncertainty is part of a process. Particularly in the case of the uncertainty of risk assessment, the process has to be explained to people so they can understand the thinking behind the conclusions.

Richard Dime says he gives as much information as possible; he not only says that he can't predict but also says why: "At certain times you may have to add additional information to round out the question or put the question into proper context." It also helps to use comparisons to other decisions—for example, "We are as certain as we were last year when we did thus and so...."

Ruddie Clarkson explains the uncertainty inherent in science in general and then goes into the uncertainty of the specific situation: "I educate them to the uncertainties of science up-front ... then ... go into the chemicals and the data that's available for their specific incident. Then go back to general education about ... the fact of public health ... that you have to make the best recommendation for the majority of the people, taking into mind target populations.... It's an education of 'We have never been able to give you an absolute; you're laboring under a wrong assumption that public health has always given you an absolute. We never have....'" Clarkson goes on to point out the uncertainties in things people may mistakenly take for granted as being guaranteed—for example, doctors prescribing medicine, vaccines, etc.

18. Be specific about what you are doing to find the answers.

When you say you don't know, you don't want people to think that you are hiding something or are incompetent. To avoid this, explain the process you are using to find the information. According to Nancy Blethen of Coleman and Pellet, Inc., "You have to give an explanation of how research is being conducted, why it takes time, and therefore why it can be relied upon. You have to tell them what you're doing to get the information that you want and that they want."

Ann Fenn says that she advises Superfund project officers to say they don't know, but also to say what is being done to find out. Fenn says that you can't just say "I don't know" and stop there: "You have to detail the process, where you've been and where you're going, so that if people don't understand the conclusion or like the conclusion, at least they understand the process behind the conclusion and the reasoning behind the conclusion."

Explaining the process is also important to building trust. According to Baruch Fischhoff, it's important to say "I don't know" in a way that doesn't sound like "I don't care."

19. Consider involving the public in resolving the uncertainty.

It is easier for people to accept uncertainty if they can play a role in its resolution. Involving the public in dealing with uncertainty not only is likely to be perceived as fairer but also may lead to better solutions.

Ken Brown says that involving the public takes some of the burden for the decision off the agency. "If people feel they are part of the process ... they will have more empathy and understanding for the people who are making the tough decisions."

Randall Smith says that this was the key advantage of the technical workshops EPA held with Tacoma citizens about regulating a copper smelter: "We succeeded in communicating that life's not perfect in the way government makes decisions ... that there are pressures to decide, inadequate information and uncertainty ... but what we are doing at a minimum is sharing the entire problem we face with the public...."

Also, says Brown, the public should be able to contribute to the decision of whether the current level of uncertainty is acceptable or whether there is something the government should be doing to make the number more certain.

20. Give people as much individual control as possible over an uncertain situation.

As explained in Chapter I, people are apt to feel more comfortable with risks over which they have individual control. Involving the community in resolving the uncertainty, as suggested in the above guideline, is helpful. But actually giving people some individual control is even more useful.

For example, Grace Singer of NJDEP offers people the option of drinking bottled water (while cautioning that the lack of regulations for bottled water makes it an unknown quantity as well). While this may seem a contradiction to agency policy, it need not be. It is, rather, a personal recommendation that gives people some control over the uncertainty. She adds that she gives people a DEP number to call if they haven't heard from the agency within two weeks about test results. As Singer puts it, "Let the person know that they have their own resources ... that they don't just have to sit back and wait for a phone call."

21. Stress the caution built into standard-setting and risk assessment.

Frequently citizens are concerned about uncertainty because they feel it leads to their being at increased risk when, in fact, agencies build into risk assessments and standards wide margins of safety to account for the uncertainty and protect the public. Grace Singer says that she explains to people that because the national experts are not always in agreement, standards are set to err on the side of health protection. Even though people don't necessarily like the idea that the agency isn't sure, they may be reassured to know that you are taking a protective approach in response to the uncertainty.

22. If people are demanding absolute certainty, pay attention to values and other concerns, not just the science.

When people demand certainty, what lies behind the demand is often a question of values and process, not science. The demand for absolute certainty can result, for example, from people being frustrated because agency representatives did not involve them in the decision-making process, or because the agency did not listen to their concerns.

Agency people sometimes act as though their science were being attacked when the real disagreement is over values—how people are being treated, the equity of decisions, etc. Also, communities sense that they make more headway with agencies when they talk about science than when they talk about values, so they sometimes focus on science when they are really upset about judgment calls. Thus, agencies and communities talk at cross-purposes to the increasing frustration of both sides.

People often demand certainty because they feel that the agency isn't protecting them adequately. For example, if the agency recommends no action because a risk is low, the community might demand certainty that the risk is low. Rather than debate why uncertainty is inevitable, the agency could stress appropriate protective actions that are available if people are worried.

When confronted by a demand for certainty, back up and listen to the concerns behind the demand. Address those concerns, which are usually more to the point than the uncertainty issue itself. Realize that you will probably need to involve people in developing solutions that meet their concerns.

23. Acknowledge the policy disagreements that arise from uncertainty.

Disagreement on risk issues is inevitable. Agencies, experts, and publics within communities will disagree among themselves and with each other. Often this disagreement increases the community's feelings of uncertainty about the situation. The key is to understand what the disagreement is about (for example, whether it is over science or values), and to deal with the roots of the disagreement.

Opposing recommendations from within the agency are often a result of lack of coordination rather than disagreement. Agencies should make an effort to "get the story straight" so that communities are not further confused. When there is genuine disagreement, on the other hand, it may be more useful to explain the range of views that exists within the agency, and what the majority view is and why, than to try to hide a professional disagreement. (For more on this, see Chapter II, "Earning Trust and Credibility.")

When experts outside the agency disagree with the agency's position—indeed, they may be from another agency—it is best to acknowledge the range of opinion from the outset rather than being attacked later when the disagreements become apparent.

According to Ann Fenn, when agencies disagree on how to handle the same situation (for example, when the state wants to move faster and the EPA has reasons for waiting to clean up a Superfund site), "It's advantageous to have scientists explain that there are differences of opinion rather than have a bureaucrat explaining that there are differences.... There's a higher level of credibility." Of course, if the difference of opinion is about issues other than science, having scientists explain may not help much.

Citizens are sometimes supported in disagreements with the agency by independent experts who adopt advocacy positions on particular issues. Barry Commoner was mentioned as an example by a number of practitioners for his work with citizens against siting incinerators. Agencies sometimes react by trying to highlight the limitations of the expertise or credentials of such experts, framing the disagreement as a battle between objective science and unscientific advocacy.

These battles may reduce the agency's credibility rather than enhance it. In such situations, agency scientists should by all means state their own credentials, argue the merits of their position, and articulate why they think the position of the opposing expert is inappropriate. But it should also be made very clear when the differences of opinion are about values (how much protection is appropriate, for example) rather than data. Suggesting that opposing experts are not sincere—for example, that they are "carpetbaggers" or "paid advocates"—is extremely likely to backfire. If the conflict is over science, discuss science. If it is over values, discuss values. It is seldom over character or integrity, and personal charges and countercharges are unlikely to help resolve the uncertainty.

DEALING WITH RISK ACCEPTABILITY

One of the major stumbling blocks between agencies and the public is the notion of "acceptable risk." Agencies realize that even with unlimited funds they could not reduce most risks to zero. However, when their family's health is at stake, many people demand just that. This type of situation is difficult, at best, but agencies must realize that "acceptable" is a relative term. The more agencies try to impose a definition of "acceptable risk" on communities, the more communities will resist that definition. In fact, in some cases, part of a community's fight for zero risk is the feeling that if they don't fight for zero risk, they will get levels they consider unacceptable.

It is important to realize that a community's notion of "acceptable risk" is closely tied to the outrage factors described in Chapter I. For example, siting a new risk in the community, such as an incinerator, will often feel very different to residents than coping with an existing risk, such as a local industry. The incinerator is a new rather than a familiar risk; the risk may seem unfair (assuming other people's waste for negligible benefits); and it is imposed. Facility siting is an extremely complex issue, and some aspects are beyond the scope of this manual. However, below is some basic guidance for dealing with the notion of acceptable risk.

24. Don't confuse people's understanding of the risk with their acceptance of it.

It is important to remember that understanding and acceptance are two very different issues. Even if you succeed in helping people understand a risk, they will not necessarily reward your success by saying, "Now that we understand what a part per billion is, we will accept 2 ppb of TCE in our water." In fact, your expectation that understanding will lead automatically to acceptance can actually prevent understanding; the community may feel it is easier not to understand than to understand and disagree. However, you obviously cannot gain acceptance without some understanding. The best you can do is to help people to understand the risk, as described elsewhere in this chapter, and leave acceptability up to them.

You cannot force acceptance. To understand this better, imagine taking the NIMBY ("Not In My Backyard") syndrome and the notion of acceptable risk literally. You come home from a hard day's work at the office, and as you turn into your driveway you see a group of strangers picnicking on your back lawn. They didn't ask your permission; they didn't even tell you they were coming. They're not inviting you to share their picnic. They don't even want to tell you what they're eating, because the information is proprietary and they doubt you would understand it anyway. When you ask what they are doing in your backyard, they reply that you are being concerned unnecessarily. In fact, they say, the probability of damage to your backyard is extremely low, and careful research has shown that your backyard is the very best place to have their picnic.

Your understanding that the picnic is probably not very harmful to your lawn is unlikely to eliminate your anger at the uninvited picnickers. Similarly, in some situations communities may, in fact, understand that a risk is relatively low. That fact may not make the risk "acceptable."

According to Susan Santos, "Somehow being able to separate acceptability from being able to say whether a risk is significant is a leap that has to be made or we're not communicating." Santos says she tries to help people separate the two issues for their own understanding. She says of the outcome of one project: "That didn't mean that in the end there wasn't fighting and screaming, but at least we knew what the issues were.... There was a real good relationship established...."

25. Remember that communities must determine what is acceptable to them, not the agency.

The more an agency pushes the notion of acceptable risk, the less acceptable the risk is apt to become. Imagine the hypothetical picnickers in the previous example badgering you to accept the picnic by calling in additional experts on the relative risk of damage to lawns due to picnicking.

Randall Smith illustrates the notion of acceptable risk with a story related to EPA's decision to get input from citizens concerning the regulation of a local smelter. EPA had announced its intention to get citizen input on the decision, and the issue had been framed in the newspapers as one where the people of Tacoma were going to be asked to choose between jobs and health. At some point in the process, after informational workshops and sessions that encouraged dialogue among citizens, government, and experts, citizens began wearing buttons that said "BOTH" [jobs and health]. A visiting economist remarked to Smith that the expectation was unrealistic, that there had to be a choice. Smith told him, "That's how an economist thinks, but it's not the way people think...." By wearing those buttons, Smith explains, people were saying, "I am not prepared to pick either jobs or my health.... I want to do a damn good job in trying to do both." Smith felt people realized that life would not be perfect around the smelter, but they focused on what they could do to minimize the risk, and felt that their suggestions and input were relevant to decision-makers.

In this case, people were given the opportunity to look at all the options and to discuss how each would affect their lives compared to the others. Even though the final decision was the agency's, there was a sense that all the information was out in the open, and that the people themselves had the chance to impress on EPA which options they favored. Ken Brown says that when the public digs in its heels and refuses to accept any risk, this is often a result of the fact that the agency has presented only the options that the agency favors.

26. Recognize that people are unlikely to accept a risk without a benefit.

Lois Gibbs says it is "unfair" for the government to tell people to take risks without offering them any benefits. Baruch Fischhoff agrees: "People don't accept risk without some compensation. It makes no sense to talk about acceptable levels of risk without talking about the things that go along with it."

The benefits have to be real benefits, moreover, not ones conceived by the agency to make the public feel better about a risk. Allan Mazur of Syracuse University says that it doesn't help credibility to suggest that there are benefits when there are clearly not.

27. Try to emphasize the positive aspects of alternatives rather than being defensive about them.

Thomas Burke says that agencies tend to be defensive because they know that accidents can happen, that they cannot guarantee absolute safety. "What New Jersey's pretty bad at ... we play defense when we talk about siting a new hazardous waste facility.... Right away people are talking about explosions, leachate.... But we really haven't been able to adequately describe the benefits of our environmental decision-making and the risk-reduction that accompanies appropriate control.... I try to stress the positive as well...."

Industry tends to express the more positive side of alternatives. Geraldine Cox of the Chemical Manufacturers Association says that rather than communicate risk, "I feel we need to communicate safety," and the other risks people will be exposed to if they do not accept the one in question. Nancy Blethen says that she stressed the benefits of phenol in day-to-day life to people concerned about the reopening of her client's phenol plant. Of course, too much stress on the positive can easily backfire if it seems to be ignoring or trivializing real community concerns.

28. Be careful about attempting to use monetary benefits to compensate for an imposed risk.

Nancy Blethen says that people do not want to hear about the economic benefits of a risk—that is, jobs, rateables, etc. "We have this concept," says Blethen, "that it's un-American to equate health and dollars.... The unspoken comment is ... this may be acceptable in other countries where they don't value human life as highly, but here it is much more important and therefore I don't even want to consider these trade-offs."

Joan Gardner of the Massachusetts Hazardous Waste Facility Site Safety Council agrees that, particularly with siting, offers of monetary compensation don't work because they imply that there is something seriously wrong with the facility: "People see other big facilities locate in communities without compensation ... so they are particularly suspicious when they are offered money for this facility."

In a negotiation in which the community has the right to say no to a particular risk, it may feel freer to discuss the price it might charge to accept that risk. However, this has to come from the community and cannot be presented by the government or industry as compensation for being forced to take a risk.

29. To the extent possible, build in ways for people to have control over a risk.

As explained in Chapter I, people feel more comfortable with risks over which they have control. Rather than expecting communities to accept the relative safety of a situation, some practitioners advocate giving communities more control over the risk.

Gary Sondermeyer of NJDEP says that recent modeling has shown that all landfills will leak eventually. Rather than tell people not to worry about leaks, DEP now stresses that landfill design includes systems for leak detection and mitigation. This emphasis on the control system seems to be more credible to people than talking about how reliable landfills are, but Sondermeyer stresses that getting people involved at the earliest possible point in the process really makes the difference, avoiding objections "that we get killed on all the time which are mainly procedural."

Optimally, agencies not only would build in systems to control leaks, but also would build in citizen oversight of those systems. Jerome Balter of the Public Interest Law Center of Philadelphia strongly supports the idea of giving communities the ability to monitor facilities. For example, as part of the terms of settlement of a lawsuit, a company, in addition to being required to take steps to reduce emissions, was required to submit monthly testing results to the community. As a result, the community knew whether the company was making progress toward reducing pollution. In another instance, residents were furious that a company was warehousing barrels of PCBs in their neighborhood without their prior knowledge. The community was particularly concerned about risks due to fire and break-ins. A compromise was reached in negotiations between the community and the company that allowed the company to store the barrels temporarily if it hired an around-the-clock guard and allowed the community access on a once-a-month basis to check security measures.

30. Acknowledge that there are other aspects of decision-making besides risk, and be prepared to listen and address people's concerns.

People sometimes argue about risk when they are just as concerned about issues such as property values, because risk provides a much better basis than other issues for legal, political, and publicity activities. Agencies should realize that concerns about property values and the like are also legitimate; by accepting these issues as appropriate for discussion, the agency can avoid "forcing" the community to overstress risk. However, even people who start out concerned over other issues may become concerned about health risks as they learn more about the situation. Thus, while it is important to acknowledge people's other concerns, it is rarely useful to accuse them of not really being worried about risk.

"Part of the solution," says Vincent Covello, "is to know what people are concerned about at a particular facility and not to assume that you know what the answer is.... If the community is concerned about monitoring ... then you have to provide resources ... or some other management strategy that addresses that concern, including handing control over monitoring to that specific community. If the main concern is property values, then you have to deal with that issue ... so that the specific concern is addressed in the trade-off equation." For example, by stressing the confidentiality of test results to homeowners in Clinton, a community in which high levels of radon were found, NJDEP was acknowledging and dealing with people's concern that their radon-contaminated homes might be devalued in the real estate market even after they were remediated.

31. Help people to help their neighbors decide what is acceptable to them.

Ken Cobb says that in situations where people are expressing their feelings that no risk is acceptable to them, he turns to the rest of the audience and asks a peer if he or she feels that way. Sometimes the person says yes, but often the second person is a bit less extreme in his or her thinking than the first, and can help that person get some perspective. Says Cobb, "You have to provide a forum for people to adjust [their feelings] to be more in the mainstream with others...." This technique is obviously more effective in small groups than in large, potentially hostile meetings (see the section on forums in Chapter IV).

PRESENTING TECHNICAL INFORMATION

Despite the complexity of risk information, most environmental health data can be understood by laypeople. As anyone who has worked extensively with citizen groups can attest, community residents with little scientific background have managed to teach themselves about many aspects of an issue and can often cite the latest studies in the field. Concerned citizens may view the risk issues very differently from the agency, but as discussed in previous sections, it is important not to suppose that lack of community acceptance necessarily means lack of community understanding.

Even though the public can usually understand what it needs to understand, agency representatives rightly sense that some simplification of information is appropriate to present it to the lay public. Unfortunately, what very often happens when information is simplified is that key pieces get left out, so people can grasp distinct parts of the whole picture but never seem to understand the situation fully enough to make informed judgments.

Although the distinction is difficult to make, it is helpful to distinguish between simplifying the language and simplifying the content. The former is always appropriate; plain English instead of technical jargon goes a long way in helping citizens to understand technical information. Greater care must be taken when simplifying the content.

Many of the strategies for presenting technical information are the same as those for presenting any kind of information. The following guidelines are those most frequently mentioned by practitioners. Some are quite obvious, but as with many of the risk communication guidelines in this manual, they are often overlooked.

32. Know your audience and gear your presentation to its level.

Before you give a presentation, do some thinking about: (a) what the audience already knows; (b) what the audience wants to know; and (c) what you want the audience to know. Obviously, audiences differ a great deal, but if you have had contact with the people involved in the situation before, you can get a fairly good sense of what they want to know and what level of understanding they might have. Regardless of the audience's level of knowledge, avoid being condescending. When explaining technical information to a relatively uninformed audience, it can help to imagine that you are talking to an intelligent but uninformed friend. As explained in the section about explaining the numbers, be sure to anticipate your audience's concerns. (See also the section on communicating with different audiences in Chapter IV.)

Thomas Burke suggests that it is important to provide an "interpretive, simple overview." At the same time, Burke says, you should also make the more technical information available to those who have a higher level of technical sophistication and want to know more.

33. Prepare as thoroughly as you can.

Practitioners and experts alike agree that giving a good presentation requires a lot of preparation. Gary Sondermeyer says that success in conveying technical material is "50% preparation and 50% presentation techniques," and that if either of these components is lacking the presentation will not be up to par.

Ann Fenn maintains lists of questions asked by citizens at technical briefings. The Superfund staff goes over the lists to prepare for future meetings. Many times the same questions come up from site to site.

Other practitioners practice their presentations and do role-playing. Prior to a series of workshops held in Tacoma considering the regulation of a smelter that produced arsenic, EPA employees sought out colleagues who were residents of Vashon Island—the area most opposed to the smelter—and asked them to listen to their presentations and ask questions. These people really felt the concerns, says Randall Smith, "and could flush out the pat answers." Another aspect of role-playing, says Smith, is that you can "identify people who can't cope with the anger" and pull them off the assignment.

Several people have found it helpful to videotape practice presentations.

34. Consider which information is most important to convey.

Many citizens will say they want to know everything. Others simply want to know the bottom line: safe or not safe. It is the job of agency scientists to present information in such a way that people get what they want. In practice this is often a middle ground which includes: (a) the facts the agency wants people to know about the situation; (b) the background information they need in order to understand the facts; (c) the additional background they need in order to avoid misimpressions, particularly information that seems to contradict the basic facts and that would cost the agency credibility if discovered later; and (d) the answers to the public's questions and responses to its concerns.

The facts should not stand alone, but rather should support the main points. Identify for yourself three or four main points that are the most important to convey and make sure that your presentation and informational materials highlight those points. People get particularly confused by presentations that seem like a tangle of facts rather than main ideas backed by details. Try stating each main idea first, then give the facts that support the idea, and finally sum up once again with the main idea.

Providing so much information that people are overwhelmed is as unfair as providing so little information that they can't adequately judge the situation. People should not have to wade through pages of documentation to answer basic questions about their concerns. Providing masses of technical detail without addressing the tough questions to which people want answers will strike the public as an effort to conceal, not to inform.

It may sometimes be appropriate to leave information out. According to Richard Dime, "It's so easy to get caught in dose-response curves, and the next thing you know you are getting caught in ten cancer models.... We should never be arguing in a public forum what cancer model is the best to use. This stuff is just too superfluous for John Q. Public." Dime says that in order to determine what information is important to public understanding of a concept, you have to look at how the concept applies to the situation you are explaining. "You have to really gear your argument to the issue at hand after you lay the basic foundation." Of course, audiences that want the technical details, even the cancer models, should be helped too—but not at a general public meeting.

35. Be sure to give people sufficient background. Don't assume that condensing information is the same as making it clearer.

Simplifying technical information does not necessarily mean making it shorter. On the contrary, jargon and acronyms are shortcuts we use with people who know what we're talking about. It takes *more* words to explain the same concepts without the shortcuts.

Edgar Miller says that when you try to present information succinctly, you lose a lot of background material, including what other people might be saying about the issue. "You leave a lot up to the imagination when you leave stuff out ... and people who know about the issue and are concerned about the issue ... see you making a broad, sweeping statement.... That upsets a lot of people. It may distort the perception that some people get as to what you are trying to do as a government agency if they think you are trying to gloss over the problems ... by oversimplifying."

James Callaghan agrees that you need to watch the tendency to take shortcuts: "I don't have a great belief in the one-liner in dealing with these things.... I don't think you can develop slogans or wordsmithing kinds of efforts that will make the situation any different. You have to expect that the people who are hearing you are going to have to work a little bit, are going to have to listen to something more than just a simple phrase or two.... You've got to explain what you did ... what other people have found ... and how it relates to the exposure of human beings. It can be done. It's just hard work and tedious...."

Ruddie Clarkson used this approach to communicate the risk of exposure of school children to heptachlor and chlordane after the chemicals had inadvertently gotten into the school's heating ducts: "I communicated precisely what that risk is in layman's terms.... If the chemical has the term 'carcinogen'... [we] explain to the public what constitutes a background rate in a species ... whether or not it was found in more than one species.... We communicated to them very specifically about the chemicals involved, that the chemicals were not found to be carcinogenic in dog and rat studies but heptachlor was carcinogenic in mice ... that that's what it means when we say suspected or possible carcinogen...." Clarkson then went on to explain the human epidemiological and toxicological data in very simple terms. She feels this approach gives people everything they need to know to interpret the data and make decisions. It also prevents, says Clarkson, a situation in which people are confused by data.

Richard Dime says that if he is asked a question, he "likes to put some meat around it. I find that works." Dime says that he "starts with generalities" and then gets more specific: "I've taken the time to give them a basic foundation so that they can listen to me and hear what I'm saying...."

36. Use as down-to-earth language as possible.

Every field has a language all its own that tends to exclude people on the outside. Environmental agencies may have this problem more than most. First, there is the scientific information. Then, there are government acronyms: EPA, DEP, RI/FS, etc. Finally, to make matters worse, the chemicals involved either have long, threatening names or have acronyms that are frequently confused, such as PBB and PCB or TCE and TCDD.

According to James Callaghan, "Almost everything that is in a scientific paper can be said in simpler English." All interviewees agreed that there were two rules that could immediately increase the understanding of any scientific presentation: ***(a) no acronyms, and (b) no jargon.*** Once again, use language you would use to explain the subject to an intelligent but uninformed friend.

37. Beware of the tendency to oversimplify and to give only data that support your point.

People know when you are marshalling ammunition for your argument as opposed to presenting information. The cost in credibility is high.

Ken Brown says that there is a tendency for government to oversimplify. "They hang their hat on one statistic ... like one-in-one-million increased cancer risk." Furthermore, says Brown, government tends to "come up with the number that justifies the solution [it has chosen]."

38. Choose supporting graphics that illustrate your message clearly and simply.

Most interviewees agreed that graphics can be helpful in conveying technical information. They also agreed that, if not prepared thoughtfully and carefully, graphics can be counterproductive. For example, a hastily prepared overhead that confuses the audience is worse than none at all. Graphics that are appropriate for technical presentations are often not appropriate for a lay public, which has little experience reading charts and graphs.

Maps and overlays can be helpful to show people where samples have been taken and what chemicals have been found where, says Ann Fenn. These are especially important, says Ruddie Clarkson, if you are trying to explain exposure routes. Barker Hamill of NJDEP says that he used maps to explain the groundwater and streamflow when levels of TCE were found in private and public wells in Vineland.

Gary Sondermeyer has experimented with several types of visual presentations, but thinks the use of slides is the most effective. Sondermeyer has used two projectors to make information easier to grasp. On one, for example, he can show a schematic of a resource recovery facility, and on the other, a real-life shot of garbage trucks backing up. The latter is more real and brings meaning to the former, which alone wouldn't have the impact. Sondermeyer says that he has tried very complicated "canned" presentations that have not worked because they appeared contrived.

James Callaghan cautions that graphics alone should not be relied on to convey technical information, but rather should be used to illustrate what you are properly explaining in simple terms. "Prose tells a lot more," says Callaghan. He says that he occasionally uses very simple graphs and charts but adds that "a lot of these things are so complex" that the graphics can get messy and confusing.

39. Be aware of body language and other indications people in your audience give you that they're lost. Slow down, back up, or ask questions.

Geraldine Cox says, "If I'm dealing with a live audience [as opposed to a television or radio appearance], I always watch the body language and I can tell when I'm reaching them and when I'm not." If she feels she's losing them (glazed eyes, shifting in seats, misdirected questions, etc.), "I go back and explain the same thing in different terms, use examples, anecdotal information ... to bring them back...."

40. Have background material available at meetings.

After a presentation on a subject that affects their lives, people are often looking for additional information. If you provide background information that they can pick up and take home, you are offering another way to help them understand the data. Other advantages, says Faith Schottenfeld, are that you can include a mechanism for people to follow up if they want to, and you can use the same materials to help the media in their coverage of the technical information. In addition, people can read printed information at their leisure and pass it on to those who could not attend the meeting.

41. Always have question-and-answer periods after presentations.

Question-and-answer sessions are important because: (a) You can find out what people really need to know to make their decisions; (b) You can find out what they do not understand so you can spend more time on it and clear up any misunderstandings or misconceptions; and (c) People feel more participation and control. If there is hostility or tension in the room, a question-and-answer period is even more essential.

43. Critique your presentation afterward so you can learn from the things you did right as well as those you did wrong.

June Fessenden-Raden of Cornell University recommends taking someone with you who can take notes on your presentation and the reaction of the audience so you can go over them later. She says that once an observer told her after a meeting that she had used the word "volatile" and no one had understood. Fessenden-Raden had been unaware of this and in the future she referred to "evaporation" instead. She says that scientists have to watch constantly for "jargon creeping in." Other interviewees suggest videotaping a session, if possible, and reviewing it later on.

YES, BUT....

• ***We still don't have clear ways to explain very complex information. If we did, it's likely the public would understand better.***

It is true that further research is needed about how to explain environmental health risks. EPA and DEP's Division of Science and Research are both funding projects in this area. However, regardless of our sophistication in explaining risk, people's perception of the risk will be influenced by far more than the data. If you continue to stress explaining data and fail to attend to these other variables, you will probably make less progress than you could.

• ***It is extremely difficult to help people put environmental health risks in perspective if we can't compare these risks to other risks in their lives.***

We are not suggesting that comparisons can't be used. We are suggesting, however, that comparing voluntary to involuntary risks and other comparisons that ignore the "outrage factors" are apt to make people angry. The section on comparing risks in this chapter gives examples of some useful comparisons. Further research is being done to develop and test others.

• ***It is difficult to see why an agency should admit uncertainty when people will use such admissions against us.***

This chapter suggests that people are already alert to uncertainty. Failing to disclose uncertainty is likely to undermine trust in the agency. As suggested in this chapter, agency representatives should not merely admit uncertainty and then drop the subject. The uncertainty should be put in context in several ways.

APPENDIX I

Additional Contacts in Development of Manual

The following people were contacted during the development of the manual:

U.S. ENVIRONMENTAL PROTECTION AGENCY

Frederick W. Allen
Associate Director
Office of Policy Analysis
USEPA
Washington, DC

Robert Cibulskis
Environmental Response Team
USEPA
Edison, NJ

Sally Edwards
Supervisor for Risk Assessment
USEPA Region I
Boston, MA

Margot Hunt
Director
Center for Environmental Learning
USEPA Region III
Philadelphia, PA

Arnold M. Kuzmack
Director
Office of Program Development and Evaluation
USEPA
Washington, DC

Moira LaTaille
Chemist
USEPA Region I
Boston, MA

John Perrecone
Superfund Community Relations Coordinator
USEPA Region V
Chicago, IL

Debra Prybyla
Public Affairs
USEPA Region I
Boston, MA

Greg Vanderlaan
Section Chief
Remedial Programs
USEPA Region V
Chicago, IL

STATE AGENCIES

Mary Bensman
Public Information Officer
Minnesota Waste Management Board
Crystal, MN

Elinor Blake
Associate Health Planning Analyst
Hazard Evaluation System and Information Service
California Department of Health Services
Berkeley, CA

Peter Galbraith
Chief, Bureau of Health Promotion
Connecticut Department of Health Services
Hartford, CT

Lynn Goldman
Chief, Environmental Epidemiological Unit
Epidemiological Studies and Surveillance Section
California Department of Health Services
Berkeley, CA

Tim Hartman
Administrator, Radon Monitoring Program
Pennsylvania Department of Environmental Resources
Gilbertsville, PA

Donald Lyman
Chief, Preventative Medical Services Division
California Department of Health Services
Sacramento, CA

Kate Quigley Lynch
Connecticut Hazardous Waste Management Service
Hartford, CT

Ellen Jones Mangione
Medical Consultant
Office of Health Assessment
Colorado Department of Health

Colleen Schwalbe
Division of Risk Assessment
New Hampshire Department of Public Health
Concord, NH

Michael Stetkiewicz
Massachusetts Hazardous Waste Facility Siting Council
Boston, MA

INDUSTRY

Sharon McCarthy
E.C. Jordan Company
Wakefield, MA

ACADEMIA

Edward Calabrese
Director
Northeast Regional Environmental Public Health Center
Amherst, MA

Noreen Dowling
Director
Public Service Research and Dissemination Program
Toxic Risk Information Center
University of California at Davis
Davis, CA

Nicholas Freudenberg
Associate Professor
Director, Community Health Program
Hunter College
New York, NY

Roger Kasperson
Center for Technology, Environment, and Development
Clark University
Worcester, MA

Frances Lynn
Institute for Environmental Studies
University of North Carolina
Chapel Hill, NC

William Schulze
Department of Economics
University of Colorado
Boulder, CO

Neil Weinstein
Associate Professor
Human Ecology and Social Sciences
Cook College, Rutgers University
New Brunswick, NJ

CITIZEN GROUPS

Jerome Balter
Public Interest Law Center of Philadelphia
Philadelphia, PA

Susan Sherry
Environmental Health Director
Golden Empire Health Planning Center
Sacramento, CA

APPENDIX II

New Jersey DEP/DOH Advisory Committee

**NEW JERSEY DEPARTMENT OF ENVIRONMENTAL PROTECTION
NEW JERSEY DEPARTMENT OF HEALTH
RISK COMMUNICATION MANUAL ADVISORY GROUP**

NAME	*AGENCY/DIV.*
Martin Rosen	DEP/DSR
Jeanne Herb	DEP/DSR
Thomas Belton	DEP/DSR
Richard Dime	DEP/Environmental Quality
Elaine Makatura	DEP/Environmental Quality
Larissa Kane	DEP/Environmental Quality
Joann Held	DEP/Environmental Quality
Barker Hamill	DEP/Water Resources
Judy Morgan	DEP/Water Resources
Susan Boyle	Haz. Waste Facilities Siting Comm.
Grace Singer	DEP/Haz. Site Mitigation
Russell Riggs	DEP/Haz. Waste Management
Kurt Whitford	DEP/Haz. Waste Management
Ernest Kuhlwein	DEP/Haz. Waste Management
Gary Sondermeyer	DEP/Solid Waste Management
Haydar Erdogan	DEP/Solid Waste Management
Frank W. Servis	DEP/Personnel
George Klenk	DEP/Press Office
Howard Wolf	DEP/Off. of Commun. and Public Ed.
Susan Klucharich	DOH/Occupational and Env. Health
Judith Klotz	DOH/Occupational and Env. Health
Martha Stanbury	DOH/Occupational and Env. Health

APPENDIX III

Bibliography

The following sources are likely to be useful to practitioners interested in reading more information about the practical aspects of risk communication:

- Martha C. Bean, "Effective Risk Communication: Foundation for Making Difficult Choices," presented to the American Society of Public Administrators, Boston, MA, March 1987. (Bean can be reached at CH2M Hill, Inc., P.O. Box 4400, Reston, VA 22090.)

- June Fessenden-Raden, C.A. Bisogni, and K.S. Porter, "Enhancing Risk Management by Focusing on the Local Level," in Lester Lave (ed.), *Enhancing Risk Management* (New York: Plenum, 1988).

- Baruch Fischhoff, "Managing Risk Perceptions," *Issues in Science and Technology*, Fall 1985, pp. 83-96.

- Peter M. Sandman, "Explaining Environmental Risk," TSCA Assistance Office, U.S. Environmental Protection Agency, November 1986.

- Harold I. Sharlin, "EDB: A Case Study in the Communication of Health Risk," Office of Policy Analysis, U.S. Environmental Protection Agency, January 1985.

- Paul Slovic, "Perception of Risk," *Science*, April 17, 1987, pp. 280-285.

The social science research literature on risk perception and risk communication is substantial and growing. For a guide to this literature, see Vincent T. Covello, Paul Slovic, and Detlof von Winterfeldt, "Risk Communication: A Review of the Literature," unpublished draft, July 1987. (Covello can be reached at the National Science Foundation in Washington, DC.)

Dealing with the mass media about environmental risk is a topic not covered in this manual. Sandman's "Explaining Environmental Risk" (see above) offers a brief overview of this topic. For a more detailed analysis, see Peter M. Sandman, David B. Sachsman, and Michael R. Greenberg, "The Environmental News Source: Informing the Media During an Environmental Crisis," Project on Risk Communication for Environmental News Sources, Industry/University Cooperative Center for Research in Hazardous and Toxic Substances, New Jersey Institute of Technology, March 1987. (This document is available from the Department of Journalism and Mass Media, Rutgers University, New Brunswick, NJ 08904.)

Practitioners wanting references to additional sources on particular aspects of risk communication are welcome to write or call the Environmental Communication Research Program, 122 Ryders Lane, Rutgers University, New Brunswick, NJ 08904; (201) 932-8795.

APPENDIX IV

About the Authors

THE STATE UNIVERSITY OF NEW JERSEY
RUTGERS

Environmental Communication Research Program
A program of the Agricultural Experiment Station
Cook College • 122 Ryders Lane • New Brunswick • New Jersey 08903 • 201/932-8795

The Environmental Communication Research Program, based at Rutgers University, conducts research, provides consulting services, and holds training workshops concerning how to communicate effectively with the public about environmental health issues. The following staff developed *Improving Dialogue With Communities:*

BILLIE JO HANCE is a research associate at the Environmental Communication Research Program. Formerly an environmental scientist with the U.S. Environmental Protection Agency, she has both technical and communication experience. Previous to her work at Rutgers, she was a freelance technical writer and editor, specializing in the environment. Her clients included government, industry, and non-profit environmental groups. Since coming to Rutgers in 1986, Ms. Hance has written and edited a variety of major reports for a research project that is exploring how the media cover environmental risk, as well as playing a key role in the design of research programs and training workshops.

CARON CHESS is Associate Director of the Environmental Communication Research Program. Before moving to academia, Ms. Chess coordinated programs for both advocacy organizations and government. She played a central leadership role in the campaign for the country's first Right to Know law, giving the public access to information about toxic hazards, and has written a book and many articles about the development of Right to Know laws. She was founding Executive Director of the Delaware Valley Toxics Coalition, linking environmental and labor constituencies. As Right to Know Coordinator for the New Jersey Department of Environmental Protection, Ms. Chess took a lead role in implementing the state's new Right to Know law. She also laid the groundwork for New Jersey's innovative Risk Communication Unit.

PETER M. SANDMAN is Director of the Environmental Communication Research Program and Professor of Environmental Journalism at Rutgers University. A specialist in the design of non-profit information and education campaigns, Dr. Sandman has worked on communication aspects of a wide range of environmental issues, from geological radon to hazardous waste facility siting, from nuclear power to lead in drinking water. His clients have encompassed an equally wide range, including among others the Environmental Defense Fund, the Chemical Manufacturers Association, and the U.S. Environmental Protection Agency. He is the author of eighteen books and dozens of articles in both professional journals and popular magazines.

C

Risk Communication, Risk Statistics, and Risk Comparisons

A Manual for Plant Managers

Vincent T. Covello, Peter M. Sandman, and Paul Slovic

Vincent T. Covello • Center for Risk Communication, Division of Environmental Sciences, School of Public Health, Columbia University, New York, New York 10032. *Peter M. Sandman* • Environmental Communication Research Program, New Jersey Agricultural Experiment Station, Cook College, Rutgers University, New Brunswick, New Jersey 08903. *Paul Slovic* • Decision Research, Inc., Eugene, Oregon 97401.

ACKNOWLEDGEMENTS

This manual is based in part on material developed during an intensive two-day workshop co-chaired by the authors and sponsored by the Chemical Manufacturers Association. The following persons attended the workshop and collaborated in the writing of the manual. We would like to thank them for their substantive contributions and for their comments on earlier drafts:

David Baird, Exxon Chemical Americas
Richard N. Knowles, E. I. du Pont de Nemours & Co.
Brent McGinnis, Ashland Chemical Co.
Timothy O'Leary, Chemical Manufacturers Association
John E. Slavick, Chemical Manufacturers Association
Richard Symuleski, Amoco Chemical Co.
Ben Woodhouse, Dow Chemical U.S.A.

We would also like to express special thanks to John Slavick, Robin Higgins, and the Chemical Manufacturers Association for organizing the workshop, for their assistance, and for supporting the production and publication of this manual.

Parts of the manual are also based on several papers and reports that we co-authored.

Hance, B., C. Chess and P. Sandman (1987), *Improving Dialogue with Communities: A Risk Communication Manual for Government.* Trenton, New Jersey, Office of Science and Research, New Jersey Department of Environmental Protection, December 1987.

Covello, V. and F. Allen (1988), *Seven Cardinal Rules of Risk Communication*, Washington, D.C.: U.S. Environmental Protection Agency, Office of Policy Analysis.

Covello, V., D. von Winterfeldt and P. Slovic (1987), "Communicating Risk Information to the Public," *in Risk Communication,* edited by J.C. Davies, V. Covello and F. Allen, Washington, D.C.: The Conservation Foundation.

We would like to thank the co-authors of these papers and reports for allowing us to use material from these works.

CONTENTS

RISK COMMUNICATION, RISK STATISTICS, AND RISK COMPARISONS: A MANUAL FOR PLANT MANAGERS

by

Vincent T. Covello, Peter M. Sandman, and Paul Slovic

INTRODUCTION

The Emergency Planning and Community Right-to-Know Act (Title III of Superfund) and many state and local laws are imposing much more openness on the chemical industry. During the next few years, plant managers will increasingly be called upon to provide and explain information about chemical risks to employees, customers, and communities near chemical plants.

Plant managers can use this manual for practical guidance on providing and explaining information about chemical risks. A basic assumption of the manual is that risk communication, when done properly, is always better than stonewalling. In the long run, more effective risk communication will be better for plant managers, communities, and the chemical industry as a whole.

The manual consists of five substantive parts: (I) effectively communicating risk information; (II) guidelines for providing and explaining risk-related numbers and statistics; (III) guidelines for providing and explaining risk comparisons; (IV) concrete examples of risk comparisons; and (V) anticipating objections to explanations of chemical risks. The manual also includes a set of appendices containing tables of risk statistics and warning notes about the usefulness and reliability of the statistics.

Although this manual will not try to cover all aspects of risk communication, neither will it be confined to such narrow topics as risk comparisons. To be useful, the manual must also address closely related topics, such as how best to explain information on emission levels and concentrations of chemicals in air and water. A short bibliography is provided at the end of the manual for those interested in pursuing these topics in greater depth.

Most of the material in the manual focuses on providing and explaining data on health risks, especially long-term data. The emphasis is not on providing and explaining information about the risks of accidents. In some cases, accidents raise similar communication issues—especially when most of the expected adverse health effects are long-term rather than acute. However, in dealing with risks of accidents, it is generally both more relevant and more reliable to focus on preventive measures, emergency response procedures, containment and remediation procedures, and the extent of the possible damage.

I EFFECTIVELY COMMUNICATING RISK INFORMATION

Guidelines and Rules for Effective Risk Communication

There are no easy prescriptions for effective risk communication. There are no magic bullets, no "cookbook" approaches. However, those who have studied and debated risk generally agree on seven cardinal rules (see Covello and Allen, 1988). Although many of the rules may seem obvious, they are continually and consistently violated in practice. As a plant manager, you can build a successful risk communication program on these rules.

RULE 1. ACCEPT AND INVOLVE THE PUBLIC AS A LEGITIMATE PARTNER.

Two basic tenets of risk communication in a democracy are generally understood and accepted. First, people and communities have a right to participate in decisions that affect their lives, their property, and the things they value. Second, the goal of risk communication should not be to diffuse public concerns or avoid action. The goal should be to produce an informed public that is involved, interested, reasonable, thoughtful, solution-oriented, and collaborative.

> **Guidelines:** Demonstrate your respect for the public and your sincerity by involving the community early, before important decisions are made. Make it clear that you understand the appropriateness of basing decisions about risks on factors other than the magnitude of the risk. Involve all parties that have an interest or a stake in the particular risk in question.

RULE 2. PLAN CAREFULLY AND EVALUATE PERFORMANCE.

Different goals, audiences and media require different risk communication strategies. Risk communication will be successful only if carefully planned.

> **Guidelines:** Begin with clear, explicit objectives—such as providing information to the public, motivating individuals to act, stimulating emergency response, or contributing to conflict resolution. Classify the different subgroups among your audience. Aim your communications at specific subgroups. Recruit spokespersons who are good at presentation and interaction. Train your staff—including technical staff—in communication skills; reward outstanding performance. Whenever possible, pretest your messages. Carefully evaluate your efforts and learn from your mistakes.

RULE 3. LISTEN TO YOUR AUDIENCE.

People in the community are often more concerned about issues such as trust, credibility, control, competence, voluntariness, fairness, caring, and compassion than about mortality statistics and the details of quantitative risk assessment. If you do not listen to people, you cannot expect them to listen to you. Communication is a two-way activity.

Guidelines: Do not make assumptions about what people know, think, or want done about risks. Take the time to find out what people are thinking: use techniques such as interviews, focus groups, and surveys. Let all parties that have an interest or a stake in the issue be heard. Recognize people's emotions. Let people know that you understand what they said, addressing their concerns as well as yours. Recognize the "hidden agendas," symbolic meanings, and broader economic or political considerations that often underlie and complicate the task of risk communication.

RULE 4. BE HONEST, FRANK AND OPEN.

In communicating risk information, trust and credibility are your most precious assets. Trust and credibility are difficult to obtain. Once lost they are almost impossible to regain.

Guidelines: State your credentials; but do not ask or expect to be trusted by the public. If you do not know an answer or are uncertain, say so. Get back to people with answers. Admit mistakes. Disclose risk information as soon as possible (emphasizing any appropriate reservations about reliability). If in doubt, lean toward sharing more information, not less—or people may think you are hiding something. Discuss data uncertainties, strengths and weaknesses—including the ones identified by other credible sources. Identify worst-case estimates as such, and cite ranges of risk estimates when appropriate.

RULE 5. COORDINATE AND COLLABORATE WITH OTHER CREDIBLE SOURCES.

Allies can help you communicate risk information effectively. Few things make risk communication more difficult than conflicts or public disagreements with other credible sources.

Guidelines: Closely coordinate all inter- and intra-organizational communications. Devote effort and resources to the slow, hard work of building bridges with other organizations. Use credible intermediaries. Try to issue communications jointly with other trustworthy sources such as credible university scientists, physicians, trusted local officials, and opinion leaders.

RULE 6. MEET THE NEEDS OF THE MEDIA.

The media are prime transmitters of information on risks. They play a critical role in setting agendas and in determining outcomes. The media are generally more interested in politics than in risk; more interested in simplicity than in complexity; and more interested in danger than in safety.

Guidelines: Be open with and accessible to reporters. Respect their deadlines. Provide information tailored to the needs of each type of media, such as graphics and other visual aids for television. Provide background material for the media on complex risk issues. Follow up on stories with praise or criticism, as warranted. Try to establish long-term relationships of trust with editors and reporters.

RULE 7. SPEAK CLEARLY AND WITH COMPASSION.

Technical language and jargon are useful as professional shorthand. But they are barriers to successful communication with the public.

> **Guidelines:** Use simple, non-technical language. Use vivid, concrete images that communicate on a personal level. Use examples and anecdotes that make technical risk data come alive. Avoid distant, abstract, unfeeling language about deaths, injuries, and illnesses. Acknowledge and respond (both in words and with actions) to emotions that people express—anxiety, fear, anger, outrage, helplessness. Acknowledge and respond to the distinctions that the public views as important in evaluating risks. Use risk comparisons to help put risks in perspective; but avoid comparisons that ignore distinctions that people consider important. Always try to include a discussion of actions that are under way or can be taken. Tell people what you cannot do. Promise only what you can do, and be sure to do what you promise. Never let your efforts to inform people about risks prevent you from acknowledging—and saying—that any illness, injury, or death is a tragedy.

Although these rules and guidelines can be helpful, they are no substitute for your own judgment. Much of the work needed to make research on risk communication relevant to plant managers has not been done. (For details, see Covello, von Winterfeldt, and Slovic, 1987.) Therefore, you will need to rely heavily on a combination of intuition and experience. Only you can know whether a particular piece of advice is valid and applies to your situation. Risk communication can never be made risk-free.

Actions versus Words

Virtually all communications about risks should include a discussion of what control measures and precautionary actions are being taken. In most risk situations, actions speak louder than words. Often, actions are what people most want to know about. People want to know what you are doing to prevent an accident or how you are preparing for the possibility, not how likely you think one is. People want to know what you are doing to reduce emissions, not just how much is being emitted and how many deaths or illnesses may result. People often care about the competence and conscientiousness of the plant manager more than about the risk itself. Many people perceive mismanagement, incompetence, and lack of conscientiousness as the central issues in risk assessment. Explaining what you have done, are doing, and plan to do to reduce and manage the risk is at least as important as explaining how small you think it is. Bear in mind that people may be much more willing to listen to what you have to say about how small you think the risk is *after* you have explained what you are doing to make it still smaller. At the same time, present information about plant safety records, drills, and other efforts to protect people and the environment—for example, programs to reduce or eliminate chemical odors.

Besides outlining measures you can take, be sure to tell people what you cannot do. Promises, when they are not kept, can destroy credibility. If you cannot take certain measures—for example, because they are too expensive, because they are against the law, because the technology or data are not available, or because the home office has not given approval—you are better off saying so.

Giving the impression that you will take an action that you cannot take or have no intention of taking can be disastrous.

The Role of Risk Comparisons

Because risk comparisons help put risks into perspective (see Part III), they are a powerful tool in risk communication. Still, they cannot take the place of long-term, sensitive interaction with the local community. Risk comparisons are useful only in the context of a continuing, sound community relations program. Almost any accurate risk comparison will work if you, the plant manager, have established trust and credibility with the people in the community. But if you have low credibility, inspire no trust or have no relationship with people in the community, even the best risk comparison will fail. (For more detail on establishing trust, see Hance, Chess and Sandman, 1987.)

Risk comparisons, although only a part of the answer, should be a fundamental component of any risk-communication program. In the next few years, you will be called upon constantly to explain chemical risks and to put them into perspective. Moreover, as Title III of Superfund goes into effect (not to mention various state laws and referenda, such as California's Proposition 65), the demand for information about risk will increase sharply. Many plant managers are looking for better ways to explain risk information both accurately and in a way that will make sense to people with no technical training. Finding better ways to compare risks is thus an important part of improving risk communication.

Public Perceptions of the Chemical Industry

There are limits to what one chemical plant manager—no matter how skilled—can accomplish through risk communication. The chemical industry worldwide faces the problem of explaining risk to a public that is sometimes fearful, often hostile, and almost always skeptical.

Plant managers are understandably concerned about the public's distrust of the chemical industry. However, it is important for you not to dismiss that distrust as irrational. Public distrust of the chemical industry is grounded in the belief that chemical companies have been remiss in many ways—insensitive to plant neighbors, unwilling to acknowledge problems, opposed to regulation, closed to dialogue, unwilling to disclose risk-related information, and negligent in fulfilling their responsibilities for health, safety, and the environment. Having determined (with some justification) that chemical companies are not always to be trusted, many people have been slow to notice that the industry is changing, that chemical companies are working harder to gain the public's trust and attain credibility. One of the costs of this heritage of mistrust is the public's willingness—and sometimes eagerness—to believe that chemical plants represent one of the greatest risks posed by modern technology. When people appear to be ignoring evidence that chemical risks are small, they may well be responding to evidence that the chemical industry has failed to act responsibly in the past.

Fortunately for you as a plant manager, the prospects for overcoming distrust are much better locally than globally. People stereotype less and scapegoat less when they are dealing with someone they know. Therefore, part of the solution to the global problem is local. When many plant managers have built up a track record of dealing openly, fairly, and safely with their employees, customers, and neighboring communities, the general distrust of the chemical industry may be reduced. In the meantime, anticipate initial distrust. Many people in the community—especially those who have had no direct experience with a chemical plant or have had a negative experience—

are likely to view your plant as a microcosm of an industry that they believe has been arrogant and careless; that has killed children; that has destroyed the environment for profit. Building bridges locally, and explaining risk credibly, may be difficult. But that work is essential because of the initial mistrust that faces you.

Factors Affecting Risk Acceptability

Understanding the distinction between risk and risk acceptability is critical to overcoming mistrust and communicating effectively. Even though the level of risk is related to risk acceptability, it is not a perfect correlation. Two factors affect the way people assess risk and evaluate acceptability; these factors modify the correlation.

(a) *The level of risk is only one among several variables that determines acceptability.*

Among the other variables that matter—*and should matter*—are fairness, benefits, alternatives, control, and voluntariness (see Slovic, 1987). Specifically, in deciding the acceptability of a risk, individuals will ask themselves:

- Does everyone share the risk fairly?
- How will I (or others in the community) benefit from the process that entails this risk?
- Can the risk be avoided?
- Have I chosen the risk, or is it being imposed on me without asking me beforehand?
- How much control do I (or others in the community) have over the risk?

In general, a fairly distributed risk is more acceptable than an unfairly distributed one. A risk entailing significant benefits to the parties at risk is more acceptable than a risk with no such benefits. A risk for which there are no alternatives is more acceptable than a risk that could be eliminated by using an alternative technology. A risk that the parties at risk have some control over is more acceptable than a risk that is beyond their control. A risk that the parties at risk assess and *decide* to accept is more acceptable than a risk that is imposed on them. These statements are true in exactly the same sense in which it is true that a small risk is more acceptable than a large risk. Risk is multidimensional; size is only one of the relevant dimensions.

If one grants the vailidity of these points, then a whole range of risk-management approaches will become possible and appropriate. For example, if factors such as fairness, familiarity, and voluntariness are indeed as relevant as size in judging the acceptability of a risk, then any efforts by a plant manager to make a risk more fair, more familiar, and more voluntary are as appropriate as efforts to make the risk smaller. Similarly, if control is indeed important in determining the acceptability of a risk, then any efforts by a plant manager to share power, such as setting up a community advisory board, is a good way to make a risk more acceptable.

(b) *Deciding what level of risk ought to be acceptable is not a technical question but a value question.*

People vary in how they assess risk acceptability. They weigh the various factors according to their own values, sense of risk, and stake in the outcome. Since acceptability is a matter of values and opinions, and since values and opinions differ, debates about risk are often really debates about accountability and control. The real issue is: Whose values and opinions will decide the outcome? Although the standpoint of the company is still crucial, in today's world the views of regulators, elected officials, fire and police officials, and the general public count for a great deal. That is one of the reasons why plant managers are being asked to explain risks in the first place: Public values and opinions about acceptability do matter.

When you explain and compare the risks associated with a particular chemical emission, you are providing information that you think people want to have for deciding whether the risk is acceptable. But data on risk levels are only one of many kinds of information on which people base decisions about risk acceptability. Risk comparisons cannot preempt those decisions. *No risk comparison will be successful if it appears to be trying to settle the question of whether a risk is acceptable.* To illustrate, it is often tempting to use the following argument when you meet with community groups or members of the public. However, you should always avoid it. The argument goes as follows:

> The risk of *a* (emissions from the plant) is lower than the risk of *b* (driving to the meeting or smoking during breaks). Since you (the audience) find *b* acceptable, you are obliged to find *a* acceptable.

This argument has a basic flaw in logic. Trying to use the argument can severely damage your level of trust and credibility. Some of your listeners will analyze your argument this way:

> "I do not have to accept the (small) added risk of living near your plant just because I accept the (perhaps larger, but voluntary and personally beneficial) risk of smoking or driving my car. In deciding about the acceptability of risks, I consider many factors, only one of them being the size of the risk—and I prefer to do my own evaluation. Your job as a plant manager is not to tell me about what I should accept but to tell me about the size of the risk your operation entails."

Closely tied to the issue of risk acceptability is the question of what the goal of risk communication should be. The goal of risk communication should *not* be to avoid responsible action or simply to pacify local citizens. Instead, risk communication should produce an involved, informed, interested, and fair-minded public, so that public opinions and concerns will be (or remain) reasonable, thoughtful, calm, solution-oriented, and collaborative.

Disclosing and Providing Risk-Related Information

Given the public's increasing demands to participate in decisions about risk acceptability, and given the increasing number of community right-to-know laws, industry spokespeople cannot afford to hold back relevant data about risks. But making relevant information available is not the same thing as packing it all into one incomprehensible speech, pamphlet, or news release. It is better to provide and explain two or three numbers, carefully selected, than to inundate your audience with meaningless facts. Your job is to pick a few numbers and present them well—not to use all of them. In the risk comparison examples presented in Part IV, it is not by accident that only a few numbers are used.

In providing and explaining risk-related numbers, keep in mind that such numbers are not the whole story. Generally, the community is more interested in issues such as your trustworthiness and credibility than in risk data and the details of quantitative risk assessment. Furthermore, people want you, the plant manager, to acknowledge, respect, and share those concerns. By focusing too much on "the data," you can easily fall into the trap of reinforcing the stereotype of the chemical industry as uncaring. To you, risk may mean risk statistics. But to your audience, risk means illness, suffering, and (possibly) death—not just for them, but for their families and children. Language (including numbers) that distances you from that reality defeats its purpose.

Spokespersons

In providing and explaining risk-related information, you need to decide a critical question: Who should speak? The public wants to hear from people who know what they are doing and people who have the power to make changes—that is, experts and managers. Certainly it helps to have top management support, but the outsider from the home office is probably not as good a spokesperson as a plant manager. Clearly you need to have experts on call, including health, safety, and environmental experts at the plant; but experts alone are not enough. Nor can community relations and public relations people at your plant do the job alone—they are too often seen as insulators trying to keep the public out of the manager's hair. Lawyers are also seen as insulators.

To be effective, spokespeople must have good presentation skills. They must be able to speak well in public, to recognize and avoid jargon, and to clarify technical concepts. Spokespeople also need good interactive skills. They must be able to deal well with people, to *listen,* to give feedback, and to respond to emotions. Regardless of your aptitudes, you can learn both sets of skills. This fact underlines the importance of training and experience in communicating.

Communication Channels and Media

A spokesperson can use a wide range of appropriate channels and media to communicate: public meetings; formal hearings; informal meetings, both large and small; negotiation sessions; one-on-one conversations; speeches to local groups; open-houses at the plant; pamphlets; brochures; radio and television interviews; news releases. The choice of medium should dictate the nature of the risk communication: how complex and long it can be (the two are *not* the same), how emotional it can be, and other aspects. Making good decisions about such issues is basic to planning effective risk communications programs.

Audiences

The public is not a single, undifferentiated mass. To create a good risk communication program, you should segment the audience. Some audiences you should pay attention to are:

- Employees, retirees and their families, and other plant-related people
- Environmental activists
- Health professionals
- Senior citizens, ill people, and other especially vulnerable population groups
- Emergency response people
- Plant neighbors

Audiences can be segmented even further according to demographic, educational, and vocational characteristics. Women, for example, often show a greater interest in problems of chemical risks than men do. A person's education and attitude toward technology are also determining factors in what they care to hear about. Knowledge about audience characteristics can help you formulate your communications and presentation. Knowledge about audience characteristics can also help you avoid talking down or up to people. *Always aim your risk communications at the concerns and information needs of a specific target audience.*

Each risk situation will require several formats of different lengths, different levels of complexity, and different levels of generalization. Each format should be designed for specific media and specific audiences. Information for a particular chemical might include everything from a one-paragraph risk description to be inserted in a news release to an entire slide show on the particular risk in question. You should test and evaluate public understanding of your communications before presenting them to your audience. You might first try presenting the communication to small, representative groups of local people and asking for criticism. Or try out the communication informally on non-experts. Keep records of which approaches and methods worked and which ones backfired. No matter how formal or informal an evaluation you do, it is better than reinventing the wheel with each new communication.

II GUIDELINES FOR PRESENTING AND EXPLAINING RISK-RELATED NUMBERS AND STATISTICS

Types of Risk-Related Numbers and Statistics

Levels of risk are only one among several numbers and statistics that need to be conveyed in communicating to the public. Other numbers and statistics include the following:

(a) Concentrations—such as parts per million or billion.

(b) Probabilities—The likelihood of the event.

(c) Quantities—such as how many tons of air toxic *X* were emitted into the air near the plant, how much effluent was released into the water, how much soil was contaminated.

This list is neither complete nor precise. The point to remember is that plant managers often think they are providing information about "risk" when they actually are providing risk-related numbers and statistics. There is nothing wrong with the latter. Since the most difficult number to conceptualize, present, and explain is risk itself, at times it makes sense to talk about one of the other numbers or statistics. Indeed, providing risk-related numbers and statistics often contributes to a clearer understanding of how risk is calculated. For example:

> "The plant releases *z* pounds of air toxic *X* per month (quantity) into the air, causing *y* ppb of air toxic *X* in the air at the plant gate (concentration) on a bad day. A population exposed to that dose of air toxic *X* for 70 years would experience a *w* percent increase in the rate of lung cancer (risk)."

Using Comparisons for Explaining Risk-Related Numbers and Statistics

Risk-related numbers and statistics can be presented as part of a comparison. However, comparisons often create their own problems. For example, "concentration" comparisons ("a drop of vermouth in a million-gallon martini"), though common (see Appendix A), are seldom helpful. Most concentration comparisons have the same drawbacks as the worst risk comparisons. They seem to minimize and trivialize the problem and also to prejudge its acceptability. Therefore concentration comparisons—usually designed to convince the audience to stop worrying—are likely to fail. Furthermore, concentration comparisons can also be misleading, since chemicals vary widely in potency (one drop of chemical *x* in a swimming pool might kill everyone, while one drop of chemical *y* will have no effect whatsoever). In view of these reservations and others, it is best to use concentration comparisons sparingly, and with sensitivity.

Like "concentration" comparisons, "probability" comparisons can be misleading. For example, some analysts suggest that instead of comparing the *probability* of one unlikely (chemically hazardous) event to the *probability* of another unlikely but *negative* event, such as getting hit by lightning, you would do better to compare it to an unlikely *positive* event, such as winning the Irish Sweepstakes.

"Quantity" comparisons, on the other hand, tend to be more useful. For example, it can be quite informative to translate tons of ash into Astrodomes-ful or swimming pools-ful. Quantity comparisons usually help the audience visualize how much is there.

Alternative Ways to Express Risk-Related Numbers and Statistics

Due to recent changes in the law, one of the things you will have to do is offer the public a variety of numbers and statistics related to plant inventories and emissions. There are many ways to express such data. To communicate clearly, you should not simply pass the data on to the public in the form in which you received them. Instead, you should select the best way(s) to present and explain the data. As noted below, the *terms* in which you couch the data are all-important.

(a) Often when you provide the public with a reassuring risk-related number or statistic, you will find yourself attacked by critics for "lying with statistics." The main point to remember is that in arguments about risks, *no* number can be "the right number." Each way of expressing a risk "frames" the risk a little differently and thus has a different impact. Doctors, for example, are much more likely to prescribe a medication that saves the lives of 60 percent of seriously ill patients than a medication that loses 40 percent of the patients—even though the results are exactly the same.

(b) Risk is usually presented as the expected number of deaths per unit of something per years exposed. The various ways of expressing this number, however, are not equivalent. For example, consider the issue of how many people will die annually as a result of emissions of air toxic *X*. Look at some of the ways this risk information can be expressed:

- Deaths per million people in the population
- Deaths per million people within *n* miles of the facility
- Deaths per unit of concentration (LD-50, for example, or any toxicity measure)
- Deaths per facility
- Deaths per ton of air toxic *X* released
- Deaths per ton of air toxic *X* absorbed by people
- Deaths per ton of chemical produced
- Deaths per million dollars of product produced, etc.

Depending on the circumstances, these different expressions will strike an audience as being more, or less, appropriate; more, or less, frightening; more, or less, comprehensible; and more, or less, credible. Consider and compare the first two for a minute. People living or working near a facility are obviously at much greater risk from emissions of air toxic *X* than people farther away. Therefore, dividing the expected number of deaths from air toxic *X*, virtually all of them near the plant, by the U.S. population, yields a reassuringly low risk figure—but a grossly misleading one. This approach is like including nonsmokers in a calculation of the risk of smoking.

(c) Transformations of scale are also important in presenting risk-related numbers and statistics. Should you describe the amount of effluent in pounds or tons (or barrels or truckloads)? Six parts per billion sounds like a good deal more than 0.006 parts per million.

(d) Risk data can be expressed in alternative ways by looking at different levels of exposure. One possibility, for example, is the period of exposure that is equal to some unit risk: *n* years at the plant gate, for example, equals a one-in-a-million chance of cancer. Or *n* years within 10 miles of the plant (a less alarming number). Or n years at the highest exposure so far detected (a more alarming number).

(e) One alternative unit for expressing risk data is lost life expectancy (on the basis of a conservative presumed normal life expectancy of 70 years). This measure gives more weight to early deaths and less to deaths in old age. Risk can also be expressed in terms of lost work days. This measure cannot be used, however, for estimating risks to children, non-working parents, and retired people.

(f) If data are available—which is seldom the case—risk can be calculated for health consequences other than death. These include such consequences as cancers, birth defects, genetic damage, immune-system damage, neurological damage, fertility problems, behavioral disorders, liver disorders, kidney disorders, blood problems, and cardiovascular problems. All are adverse chronic health consequences. Adverse acute health consequences include trauma, burns, rashes, and eye problems. One alternative way to express such acute consequences is to count hospital days or medical costs. Risks can also be calculated for adverse consequences on wildlife, endangered species, resources, plants, agriculture, air quality, water quality, habitat, aesthetics, climate, and so on.

(g) Having chosen a unit and calculated a number, one can choose among a variety of ways of expressing it. Suppose emissions of the air toxic is expected to kill 1.4 people in 1,000 over a lifetime. Which of the following would you want to tell people?

- The lifetime risk is 0.0014.
- The lifetime risk is 0.14 percent.
- The lifetime risk is one in 710.
- In a community of a thousand people, we could expect 1.4 to die as a result of exposure.

Although these alternatives are equivalent, their meaning to, and effect on audiences are not. Some terms may make the risk seem small, while others may make the risk seem larger. Given this fact, you should choose your terms of expression consciously and responsibly.

(h) When you present and explain risk-related numbers and statistics, be aware that (1) most risk numbers are estimates, and (2) these estimates are often based on data from animals exposed to very high doses and on modeling of one sort or another. We know how many people die each year from auto accidents and from being struck by lightning. We can measure these rates. But we can only calculate and estimate—not measure—how many people die each year from chronic exposure to trace quantities of chemicals. Given this context, you, as the plant manager, have several options. You can offer your best estimate of the risk. You can (as some federal agencies do) offer an upper-bound or "worst case" estimate. In such an estimate, each step in the calculation moves toward greater risk, thus attempting to assess the maximum risk that could reasonably be expected. Or you can offer the most likely estimate, along with the highest and lowest estimates. This last option is recommended whenever possible, since people want to be given complete information and may resent your choosing for them.

Guidelines for Providing and Explaining Risk-Related Numbers and Statistics

With this background, what then can be said about *how* best to provide and explain risk-related numbers and statistics?

(1) Do not just take the risk-related numbers and statistics as you find them. The first step in selecting numbers and statistics wisely is realizing that you need to select.

(2) Pick a risk number for which the data are good. Some of the data manipulations that have been discussed are just simple transformations of the same number. However, some transformations (for example, lost-life-expectancy data) require additional information. Similarly, if you have data about deaths and illnesses but not environmental data, discuss deaths and illnesses. If, however, you expect that people will be concerned about environmental effects such as odors or haze, be prepared to talk about the partial data that are available and what you are going to do to check into environmental effects.

(3) Use whole numbers and simple fractions whenever possible, such as 6 parts per billion instead of 0.006 parts per million. However, if you are presenting a table with several values, it is best to express all of them with the same denominator, even if it means violating the above rule. For example:

Substance	Risk per million persons exposed
Air toxic *X*	3.0
Air toxic *Y*	0.6
Air toxic *Z*	4000.0

(4) Pick a number that you think will be easy for your audience to understand. Avoid unfamiliar units or overly complex concepts. Embed the number in words that help clarify its meaning. For example, "a risk of 0.047" is comprehensible only to a select number of educated people—but everyone can understand that roughly five people in an auditorium of 100 would be affected. Similarly, "a cancer risk of 4.7×10^{-6}" is hard going even for an expert. An alternative way of expressing this number is as follows:

> "Imagine 10 cities of 100,000 people each, all exposed to *n* amount of air toxic *X*. In five of these 10 cities, probably no one would be affected. In each of the other five cities, on average there will be one additional cancer."

(5) Use graphs, charts, and other visual aids to help present and clarify the number (see the appendices for examples).

(6) Pick a number that *you*, both as the plant manager and as a member of the community, consider fair and relevant. "Fair" means that the number does not give a misleading impression of the risk—that is, the number makes serious risks look serious and modest risks look modest. "Relevant" means that the number speaks to the issue at hand. For example, if you are talking to

an audience of nearby residents, it is more relevant to discuss risk at the plant gate than average risk to the larger community.

(7) Pick a number that *your audience* will also consider fair and relevant. If you are not sure about which health or environmental consequences your audience cares about, find out. You can use various methods to obtain this information, including interviews, surveys, and focus groups. Explaining cancer risks to an audience concerned about miscarriages or property values or diminished elk hunting is pointless. Similarly, if an audience is angry or distrustful (a not uncommon state of affairs), bend over backwards to frame the risk in a way that audience will not resent—even if in doing so you must give an impression of greater risk than you think the data justify. It is pointless to offer a risk estimate that you know in advance your audience will reject as not being credible.

(8) Strive for comprehensibility and clarity, but do not oversimplify. Most people, if sufficiently motivated, are capable of understanding quite complex quantitative information. For example, people who have not been trained in probability and statistics can still understand mortgage rates and the complex odds at poker games and at race tracks. If people do not or cannot seem to understand what you are telling them about risk, you may be overloading them with technical jargon and details, or they may simply not trust you enough to want to understand what you are saying.

(9) Pay close attention to the numbers others are using. While you are not obliged to use someone else's risk numbers (especially if you think the numbers are not fair), confusion will result if everyone is using a different measure of the same risk. If you think you must change terms to an altogether different measure, explain what you are doing. This tactic can be risky, however. Many of the other participants in debates about risk have more credibility with the public than you do as a company spokesperson. All the more reason to use their measures if you can, and explain why if you cannot.

(10) If you have sufficient opportunity, consider offering several different estimates of the same risk. For example:

> "Our best estimate is *a*. Our cautious, worst-case estimate is *b*. The highest estimate we have heard, from the Environmental Defense Fund and the Sierra Club, is *c*."

If someone else has a higher calculated estimate of the risk than you do, *you* should be the first to say so.

Personalizing Risk-Related Numbers and Statistics

Technical experts see risk as a statistical number. But laypeople view risk in much more emotional terms—bound up with prospects of individual suffering and death. For many people, the term "low expected mortality" is fraught with emotional meaning—it could mean the death of the baby of the woman in the third row.

These different views are not just a matter of rational versus emotional. They also involve a matter of "macro" versus "micro." Risk calculations are on the macro level: What will happen to the community as a whole. But citizens' concerns are micro: What might happen to me and those I love.

One solution to this dilemma is to personalize the risk information—especially the quantitative risk information, which most needs personalizing. Several approaches are available:

- Use examples and anecdotes—hypothetical if necessary, real if possible—to make the risk data come alive.
- Talk about yourself—what risks you personally find unacceptable or frightening, how you and others close to you feel about the risk under discussion, or even how you feel about the emotional distress or the hostility you may be encountering at that moment.
- Use concrete images to give substance to abstract risk data.
- Avoid distant, abstract, unfeeling language about death, injury, and illness.
- Listen to people when they express their concerns. Reflect back to them your understanding of the content of their comments *and* the emotions they are expressing.

III GUIDELINES FOR PROVIDING AND EXPLAINING RISK COMPARISONS

Purposes for Providing Risk Comparisons

Assume that as part of your risk communication strategy, you have decided to explain a particular risk number. And assume that as part of that explanation, you want to compare the number to some other number. The first step is to be clear about *why* you want to make such a comparison.

Risk comparisons help put risks into perspective. Both research and experience show that people are typically less familiar with quantitative risk data than they are, for example, with quantitative length data. Most people have a solid grasp of how long 3 feet is. But they do not have a solid grasp of how risky a lifetime risk of 0.047 is. The job of risk comparisons is to make the original risk number more meaningful by comparing it to other risks.

Most risk comparisons provided by company spokespeople are intended to be reassuring. The typical risk comparison involves a risk that the company believes is small—often so small that it believes no action to reduce it further is appropriate. The purpose of the risk comparison is to help people understand why the company believes that the risk is small, so that people can make informed decisions about whether they want to accept the risk.

Less typical, but equally important, are cases involving risks that the company believes are large. The purpose of the risk comparison is to help people understand why the company believes that the risk is large. When faced with a serious risk the company should acknowledge that the risk is serious, offer comparisons that show it is serious, and focus on what is being done to reduce it.

Problems

Problems arise in presenting risk comparisons because people in the community often have good reasons to distrust industry's efforts to minimize the risk. For example, most people recognize the company's interest in minimizing public perceptions of chemical risks in general and of specific chemical risks in particular. Comparisons aimed at minimizing risk irritate the public because they are seen and resented as an effort to persuade people that the risk is smaller than they thought.

Guidelines

With this as a background, what then can be said about how *best* to provide and explain minimizing risk comparisons.

(a) Acknowledge and state the company's stake in the issue and why you are presenting comparisons. Since you hope to convince people in the community that the risk is tolerably small, you should be as explicit as possible about acknowledging this.

(b) You should not ask, or expect, to be trusted. Instead, you should point out why people need *not* put all of their trust in you. You can cite various institutions and procedural mechanisms—including government regulations, government inspections, union safety committees, community oversight committees (including the new ones established under Title III), risk assessments by independent experts (even the assessments of opponents)—to make the point that the community is not, in fact, "at the mercy of the company." As the plant manager, you should urge the community to seek out various sources of information with differing biases. *The less the community feels it has to trust you, the more the community will feel it can trust you.*

(c) The key to whether a "minimizing" risk comparison will be seen as useful or as misleading is whether you seem to be prejudging the acceptability of the risk to your audience. (See the earlier discussion on risk acceptability.) People will be more willing to learn from your risk comparison—even a minimizing risk comparison—if they are confident on two counts: (1) that you accept the community's right to participate fully in decisions that affect their lives, their property, and the things they value; and (2) that you understand the appropriateness of basing decisions about the acceptability of a risk on factors other than the size of the risk.

A Categorization and Ranking System for Risk Comparison

Experience suggests that some kinds of risk comparisons are more likely than others to be perceived as an effort to preempt judgments about the acceptability of a risk. On the basis of this experience, it is possible to rank different kinds of risk comparisons in terms of their acceptability to people in the community. The highest-ranking comparisons are those that put the east strain on the trust relationship between a plant manager and the public. These comparisons tend to strike even skeptical listeners as relevant, appropriate, and helpful information. The lowest-ranking comparisons, on the other hand, are those that have no intuitively obvious claim to relevance, appropriateness, or helpfulness. Such comparisons are more likely to be seen as manipulative or misleading—that is, as efforts to preempt judgments about the acceptability of a risk. Thus, the lowest-ranking comparisons will be much more difficult to present and will require much more effort to communicate effectively. That difficulty, though, does not mean that you should never, under any circumstances, use one of the low-ranking risk comparisons. Sometimes the only way to make a point is to use one of the less credible sorts of comparisons.

The general rule of thumb is: *Select from the highest-ranking risk comparisons whenever possible. When you have no choice but to use a low-ranking risk comparison, do so cautiously, being aware that the risk comparison could well backfire.*

FIRST-RANK RISK COMPARISONS (first choice—most acceptable)

a. Comparisons of the same risk at two different times.

Examples:

- The risk from air toxic *X* is 40 percent less than it was before we installed the scrubbers last October.
- With our new procedures, by this time next year the risk will be cut in half.

b. Comparisons with a standard.

Examples:

- Exposure of plant workers to air toxic *X* is well below the level that the Occupational Safety and Health Administration considers safe.
- Plant emissions of air toxic *X* are 10 percent of what is permitted under the old EPA standard, and slightly under the level established by the new, stricter EPA standard.

c. Comparisons with different estimates of the same risk.

Examples:

- Our best estimate of the risk is *x*, although you should be aware that EPA has calculated an upper-bound or worst-case risk estimate of *y*.
- Our best estimate of risk is *x* on the basis of methodology Alpha and *y* on the basis of methodology Beta.
- Our best estimate of the risk is *x*, whereas the government's is *y* and the Sierra Club's is *z*.

SECOND-RANK RISK COMPARISONS (second choice—less desirable)

a. Comparisons of the risk of doing something versus not doing it.

Example:

- If we buy the newest and most advanced emission control equipment, the risk will be *x*, whereas if we don't buy it, the risk will be *y*.

b. Comparisons of alternative solutions to the same problem.

Example:

- The risk associated with incinerating our waste is *x*. The risk associated with using a landfill is *y*.

  Note: In using this type of comparison, be careful not to omit alternatives with lower risks than the one you are advocating.)

c. Comparisons with the same risk as experienced in other places.

Example:

- The most serious air toxic *X* problems have been encountered in the Denver area; our air toxic *X* problem is only one-fifth as serious as Denver's.

THIRD-RANK RISK COMPARISONS (**third choice—even less desirable**)

a. Comparisons of average risk with peak risk at a particular time or location.

Examples:

- The risk posed by emissions of air toxic *X* on an average day is one-thousandth as great as the risk last Wednesday, when a valve malfunctioned.
- The risk posed by emissions of air toxic *X* to the nearest home is 90 percent less than the risk at the plant gate, and the risk two miles from the plant gate is 90 percent less than the risk at the nearest home.
- The risk posed by emissions of air toxic *X* to the average community resident is 90 percent less than the risk to plant workers.

b. Comparisons of the risk from one source of a particular adverse effect with the risk from all sources of that same adverse effect.

Examples:

- The risk of lung cancer posed by emissions of air toxic *X* is roughly three-hundredths of 1 percent of our total lung cancer risk.
- The risk of lung cancer posed by emissions of air toxic *X* would increase the total number of cases of lung cancer expected in a community our size in a typical year from 500 to 500.15.

FOURTH RANK RISK COMPARISONS (fourth choice—marginally acceptable)

a. Comparisons of risk with cost, or of one cost/risk ratio with another cost/risk ratio.

Examples:

- To reduce the risk posed by air toxic *X* by half would cost *y* dollars.
- Saving one life by controlling emissions of air toxic *X* would cost *y* dollars, whereas saving a life by improving particulate control would cost only *z* dollars.

b. Comparisons of risk with benefit.

Example:

- The chemical product whose waste by-product is air toxic *X* is used by hospitals to sterilize surgical instruments and thus contributes to the saving of many lives.

  Note: Risk/benefit comparisons tend to be more acceptable when the benefits accrue to the same people. However, even that type of comparison may strike people as bribery (the community will receive *x* amount of tax revenue from the facility) or blackmail (the community will lose *x* number of jobs if you shut down our facility). The general rule of thumb is: Explain the benefits of the chemical product separately from its risks; people generally prefer to make their own risk-benefit comparisons.

c. Comparisons of occupational risks with environmental risks.

Example:

- The community is exposed to far less air toxic *X* than our plant workers, and medical tests at the plant show no evidence of adverse health effects.

d. Comparisons with other risks from the same source.

Example:

- Our problem with air toxic *X* is no more serious than our problem with air toxic *Y* (which the community has long found acceptable).

e. Comparisons with other specific causes of the same disease, illness, or injury.

Example:

- Air toxic *X* produces far less lung cancer than exposure to natural background levels of geological radon.

Note: This last example violates at least one of the distinctions that the public considers important in evaluating risks: man-made versus natural. For that reason and others, such comparisons fall into the fourth rank.

FIFTH-RANK COMPARISONS (last choice—rarely acceptable—use with extreme caution!)

All of the types of comparisons listed above have some claim to relevance and legitimacy—a strong claim in the top ranks, a much weaker claim in the bottom ranks. In the fifth rank are all risk comparisons that have little or no claim to relevance or legitimacy. Central among these are comparisons of two or more completely unrelated risks.

Even in the fifth rank, however, distinctions can be made. For example, the more a risk comparison disregards factors that people consider important in evaluating risks, the more likely it is to be ineffective. (For a list of such factors, see Table C.1 in Appendix C.) The most important concerns people have are: (1) catastrophic potential, (2) dread, (3) voluntariness, (4) newness, (5) familiarity, and (6) controllability.

The classic example of a comparison that violates these distinctions is to tell people at a public meeting that their risk from air toxic *X* is lower than the risk they took when they drove their cars to the meeting or when they enjoyed a cigarette during a break. Unless there is already a high level of trust between the speaker and the audience, this sort of comparison is almost guaranteed to provoke outrage because it seems to make the following claim:

> "Since the risk of emissions of air toxic *X* is less than that of driving or smoking, two conclusions follow: (a) the risk of emissions of air toxic *X* must logically be more acceptable, and (b) people who drive or smoke have surrendered their right to object to the plant's emission of air toxic *X*."

This is a false argument, based on a flawed premise. To seem to be advancing such a claim is to invite resentment from your audience.

Comparing the risk from air toxic *X* to such things as the risk of food additives is also far from ideal. There is no special reason to believe that the risks of food additives are relevant to risks of air toxic *X*. But at least the comparison does not appear to do major violence to any of the most important risk distinctions. By contrast, comparing the risk of air toxic *X* to the risk from driving without a seatbelt violates most of the major risk distinctions. The latter risk is voluntary, familiar, and controlled by the individual. Comparing this risk to that of emissions of air toxic *X*—which is likely to be perceived as involuntary, unfamiliar, and beyond the citizen's control—is bound to infuriate the audience.

A comparison that is just as bad (if not worse) is to relate the risk of air toxic *X* to an unfamiliar risk from a familiar activity, such as the risk from ingesting the aflatoxin in peanut butter. At least people recognize that driving without a seatbelt is genuinely risky, though they see little analogy between that and plant emissions. People do not widely recognize eating peanut butter as risky, and they see even less analogy with plant emissions. A plant manager who tells an audience of mothers that air toxic *X* is less dangerous than the peanut butter they feed their children is likely to be seen as patronizing and not believable.

The conclusion to draw from this discussion of risk comparisons is not that risk comparisons are impossible or useless. It is just that you must take responsibility for the risk comparison, just as you must take responsibility for the plant risk data.

Warning. Throughout this discussion, it has been implied that you can count on the quality of the comparison data. Unfortunately, that is not so. A list of some of the most important data problems is provided in the appendices.

IV CONCRETE EXAMPLES OF RISK COMPARISONS

The risk comparison examples provided below are based on the following scenario:

> Imagine that you are the manager of an ethylene oxide plant in Evanston, a small town in the midwestern United States. The results of a recent risk assessment show that the risk of emissions of ethylene oxide from your plant is 0.007 additional cancers per 3,500 people per year. Your job is to present this information to the community by using various risk comparison techniques.

The purpose of the examples is to illustrate points made in the text. The examples have been organized according to the rank of the comparison.

FIRST RANK RISK COMPARISONS (first choice—most acceptable)

a. Comparisons of the same risk at two different times.

"Health risks from emissions of ethylene oxide at our plant are 40 percent less than a year ago, when we installed exhaust scrubbers. With more equipment coming in, we expect to reduce the risk another 40 percent by the end of next year."

"Despite the extremely low health risks to the community from emissions of ethylene oxide at our plant, we are still looking for ways to lower these levels further. These are some of the plans we have under way to accomplish this: [provide specifics]. As we implement these steps, we will keep you and the community informed of our progress. We will also continue to monitor our workers and keep track of health statistics within the community to ensure that the risks posed by our plant to our workers and to the community remain in the future as low as, if not lower than, they are today. Since some of you may have further questions about these and other matters concerning our plant operations, as plant manager, I am providing my work and home phone numbers so you can call me. I will do my best to supply you with answers to your questions as quickly as possible."

b. Comparisons with a standard.

"Emissions of ethylene oxide from our plant are half the levels permitted by the U.S. Environmental Protection Agency and by our state's Department of Environmental Protection."

"Emissions of ethylene oxide from our plant are five times lower than the U.S. Environmental Protection Agency's safety standard."

"Plant emissions of ethylene oxide are five times below what was permitted under the old EPA standard, and two times below the level established by the new, stricter EPA standard."

c. Comparisons with different estimates of the same risk.

"Laboratory studies on rats and mice suggest that current exposure to ethylene oxide may cause seven cancers in 1,000 generations of residents in this city. This estimate is the maximum that would occur under worst-case conditions. Actual health effects from exposure to ethylene oxide are likely to be lower."

"Let me try to put this number into the context of other numbers. We've said that our worst case prediction is seven-thousandths of one extra cancer within the next 70 years from our plant's emissions of ethylene oxide. Now, no one ever gets seven-thousandths of a cancer. A better way to see the effect is that if 130 different communities the same size as Evanston had a plant just like this one, 129 of those towns would see no effect on their cancer rate. One of the 130 Evanstons might have a single extra cancer."

"Our best estimate of the risk is 0.001 cancers per 3,500 persons using what we believe are realistic assumptions. This estimate is based on work done by our own scientists and by researchers at Evanston University. However, you should be aware that the state Department of Environmental Protection (DEP) has calculated a worst-case risk estimate of 0.007 cancers per 3,500 persons. DEP made the assumption that all individuals living in Evanston would be exposed to emissions of ethylene oxide 24 hours a day for 70 years. This formula gave DEP a human-lifetime dose. DEP then took the best available laboratory information for ethylene oxide—data obtained from studies on the laboratory mice most likely to develop cancer in response to ethylene oxide—and calculated first the lowest dose that caused adverse health effects in mice and then the equivalent dose in humans. On the basis of these and other pieces of information, DEP concluded that the maximum cancer risk to people in the community is 0.007 cancers per 3,500 persons over 70 years."

> Note: In the example provided above and in several examples provided below, decimals and fractions are used. Since decimals and fractions can sometimes be difficult to understand, consider converting these decimals and fractions to whole numbers, such as seven potential cancer cases per 3,500,000 people, or two cancer cases per million people.

"Our worst-case estimate of the risk is seven-thousandths of a cancer per 3,500 persons over the next 70 years. How sure are we that the risk is really this low? The bad news is that we're not as sure as we'd like to be. Risk assessment is a pretty new science, based on models and assumptions rather than hard data. The good news is that we're almost certain the risk is actually smaller than our estimate–we've instructed our scientists to make every assumption on the cautious side, to provide an extra margin of safety. And here's a piece of hard information. We've been manufacturing ethylene oxide in Evanston for 35 years now. We have continually monitored our employees for signs of adverse health effects associated with exposure to ethylene oxide. In all that time, as far as we know, not a single worker or retiree has had the sort of cancer normally associated with ethylene oxide. Please keep in mind that these workers are exposed to consistently higher levels of emissions than the surrounding population is. Therefore, on the basis of our workers' experience so far, the risk is zero. There are also people who think our risk estimate is too low. The Evanston chapter of the Sierra Club estimates seven-hundredths of a cancer per 3,500 persons over the next 70 years. That's 10 times higher than our estimate—but even if they're right, it's still an extremely small potential increase in the cancer rate. And we haven't found anyone with a higher estimate than theirs."

SECOND RANK RISK COMPARISONS (second choice—less desirable)

a. Comparisons of the risk of doing and not doing something.

"If we buy and install the newest and most advanced emission-control equipment available, the worst-case situation is that the maximum total risk will be 0.005 additional cancers per 3,500 persons, a very low number. If we don't buy new equipment and keep operating the plant with our current pollution-control system, the worst-case situation is that the maximum total risk will be 0.007 additional cancers per 3,500 persons—also a very low number. Please keep in mind that both of these risk estimates are worst-case estimates."

b. Comparisons of alternative solutions to the same problem.

"The maximum health risk from our plant's emissions of ethylene oxide is 0.007 additional cancers per 3,500 persons. We could switch to producing the only known chemical substitute for ethylene oxide. However, the maximum health risk of emissions of that chemical is 50 times higher."

c. Comparisons with the same risk as experienced in other places.

"We have installed in our plant the most advanced emission control system in the country. Compared with those of older plants, such as the one in Middletown, our emissions are 10 times less."

> Note: As with any risk comparison, comparisons of "the same risk as experienced in other places" must be handled fairly and carefully. For example, it would clearly be inappropriate to say that the air in Evanston is only 10 percent as polluted as downtown Mexico City.

THIRD-RANK RISK COMPARISONS (third choice—even less desirable)

a. Comparisons of average risk with peak risk at a particular time or location.

"The risk posed by emissions of ethylene oxide is extremely low, no matter where you live or work in Evanston. However, the risk posed by emissions of ethylene oxide for people living two miles from the plant is 90 percent less than for people living in the nearest home; and the risk for people living in the nearest home is 90 percent less than for people working within the plant gates. And our workers haven't had a single case of the type of cancer normally thought to be linked to ethylene oxide."

> Note: It is generally easier to make this type of comparison for exposure data. In many cases, a plant manager can confidently say that one exposure is 90 percent less than another. However, saying the same thing is more difficult in the case of risks, given the multiplicity of factors involved in estimating risks.

b. Comparisons of the risk from one source of a particular adverse effect with the risk from all sources of that same adverse effect.

"Let me see whether these numbers will help. Roughly a quarter of all of us get cancer—a disease caused by smoking, diet, heredity, radon in the soil, pollution, and many other factors. Out of 3,500 people, medical data show that one-quarter—or about 875—are going to get cancer sometime in a lifetime. So here's the predicted effect of ethylene oxide emissions from our plant on the overall cancer rate. In 129 of 130 hypothetical Evanstons, no effect—that is, no expected increase in cancer rates at all. In the 130th, cancer rates would rise from 875 to 876. Although this is only a tiny increased risk, it is still an increase. If we can find a way to make it even smaller, we should and we will. The most important thing is for all of us in Evanston to work together to find ways to bring down the *total* cancer rate, that unfortunate 875 out of 3,500. But we at our plant have a special responsibility to be safe neighbors. Much higher risks due to other factors are no reason to ignore a small risk in our facility. Here's what we're doing to make sure we keep the risk from our plant as low as it can possibly get... [Provide details]."

FOURTH RANK RISK COMPARISONS **(fourth choice—marginally acceptable)**

a. Comparisons of risk with cost, or of cost/risk ratio with cost/risk ratio.

"During the next year, our plant will spend more than $2 million to reduce our already small emissions even further. This new investment will hurt us economically but will reduce the risk of cancer in the community by more than 25 percent when fully operational."

b. Comparisons of risk with benefit.

"If we stopped producing ethylene oxide today, many more people here and throughout the United States might die than could possibly be affected by emissions from our Evanston plant. Ethylene oxide is the best sterilizing agent used by hospitals today. No equivalent substitute for ethylene oxide is available. Continued production of this product will contribute to saving many lives and will ensure that the surgical instruments that doctors and hospitals use are free from infectious agents."

c. Comparisons of occupational with environmental risks.

"One way to look at the data is to compare the risks of emissions of ethylene oxide to plant neighbors with the risks to plant employees. We have been operating this plant for 35 years, with an average employment of 400 people. We therefore have about 10,000 person-years of worker exposure to ethylene oxide at this plant. Health monitoring at our plant indicates that the average workplace concentration of ethylene oxide is 0.5 ppm, a dose 200 times higher than that in the community. The primary health concern about ethylene oxide is its potential for causing certain types of brain cancer. We have not had a single case of brain cancer in our work force. Moreover, the overall incidence of cancer in our employees is lower than that of the U.S. population as a whole. Nor has Evanston's health department documented any brain cancers among our workers. On the basis of this information, I believe that the health risk posed by the plant to the community is insignificant."

d. Comparisons with other risks from the same source, such as the same facility or the same risk agent.

"I believe that our ethylene oxide emissions do not pose a significant health risk to the community. I also believe that our emissions pose a much less serious problem than our hazardous waste problem, which is daily becoming more serious because the repositories in our state are filled and none are being built."

e. Comparisons with other specific causes of the same disease, illness, or injury.

"One way to look at the cancer risk from emissions of ethylene oxide in our community is to compare the risk with the cancer risk from the X-rays you get during a health checkup. One chest X-ray per year presents a risk of developing cancer that is twice that of developing cancer from our plant's emissions of ethylene oxide."

FIFTH-RANK COMPARISONS (last choice—rarely acceptable—use with extreme caution!)

The comparisons provided below are placed in the bottom rank because they disregard distinctions that the public considers important in judging the acceptability of a risk. Unless there is already a high level of trust between you and your audience, this sort of comparison is likely not only to fail but to provoke outrage.

There is seldom if ever a compelling reason to present fifth-rank risk comparisons. But if you think that you must use one, precede the comparison with an acknowledgement of its limitations. For example, you might want to say: "A final way to get some perspective on the risk of ethylene oxide emissions is by comparing it to some of the risks that we all face in our daily lives, such as being struck by lightning and driving. My purpose in making such a comparison is only to put the size of the risk in context. I recognize that such comparisons are like comparing apples and oranges. Still, I think the comparison can help us all understand and gain some perspective on the size of the risk we are talking about...."

If you find this too laborious an introduction, your best strategy may be to find a less irrelevant or more legitimate comparison.

a. Comparisons of unrelated risks. (Warning: Using these comparisons may severely damage your credibility.)

"To help gain some perspective on this risk for ethylene oxide, it may be useful to compare it to other risks that we are exposed to as a result of contaminants in our food supply. For example, the risk of death by salmonella poisoning from poultry bought at the local supermarket is at least five times greater than the risk of cancer from the highest exposure to ethylene oxide in this community."

"You may be wondering, 'But what does that mean to me as a resident of this community? What's the risk to me and my family?' First let me tell you that I am convinced that there is no threat to the health or safety of any member of our community at these extremely low exposure levels. However, I recognize that the data still may be troubling. So it would probably be helpful to put these levels of risk from exposure to ethylene oxide into the context of other risks that you're exposed to in your daily lives. For example, the risk of death from lightning is at least 140 times greater than the risk of cancer from the highest exposure to ethylene oxide. Hurricanes and tornadoes also pose a risk about 140 times greater. Insect bites pose a risk about 70 times greater. The additional 0.007 risk is about the same as the additional risk you would incur spending four hours in Denver rather than at sea level because of Denver's high altitude and higher radiation level."

Again, the general rule of thumb in using risk comparisons is: *Select from the highest-ranking risk comparisons whenever possible. When you have no choice but to use a low-ranking risk comparison, do so cautiously, being aware that it could well backfire.*

V ANTICIPATING OBJECTIONS TO EXPLANATIONS OF CHEMICAL RISKS

Various objections can be anticipated in response to explanations of risk-related information, including risk comparisons. Some of these objections have already been discussed. However, other objections can be anticipated that are related to (1) data uncertainties, (2) information disclosure, and (3) demands for zero risk.

Data Uncertainties

Since risk data are often highly uncertain, some people are likely to object that the data are too uncertain to trust. In addressing this issue, several guidelines can be helpful. (For more details, see Hance, Chess and Sandman, 1987.)

(a) Acknowledge—do not hide—uncertainty. Sounding more certain than the data can justify is a sure path to losing trust and credibility. Sources of uncertainty—for example, uncertainties due to generalizing from animal data to humans, gaps in the data, and differences of interpretation—should all be acknowledged up front, not "admitted" belatedly when an opposing interest group points them out. But acknowledging uncertainty is not the same thing as asserting total randomness or declaring ignorance.

Degree of certainty can be represented along a scale or continuum, from "total confidence" in the data to "guesswork" (in science there is *never* complete certainty, since new evidence can always overturn previous beliefs). When you have total confidence in the data, do not hesitate to say so. Most of the data produced by risk assessments, however, are somewhere in the middle of the scale. Such data are characterized by uncomfortably large margins of error; often they are based on disputable assumptions, models, and extrapolations, such as those from animals to people, from high doses to low doses. Nonetheless, such data are a much better basis for decision and action than guesswork. In these cases, assert frankly that the information is helpful but far from certain. Then explain that risk assessments deal with this uncomfortable level of uncertainty by making assumptions in the direction of overestimating the risk.

Somewhere near the "guesswork" end of the scale are risk assessments based on very inadequate data. When that is the case, say so. State as much as is known and explain (a) what you propose to do to get better risk data, and (b) what you propose to do in the meantime to reduce or protect people against the risk. Projecting this attitude is crucial. Under Title III, communities may begin asking about many possible health and environmental consequences for thousands of different chemicals. In many cases little or no data are available to answer these questions. When you have no evidence one way or the other, such as in the case of data on the relationship between air toxic *X* and miscarriages, never respond with "There is no evidence to show that air toxic *X* causes miscarriages." The statement is technically correct—but profoundly misleading. If similar compounds have been tested and found not to cause miscarriages, say that. If there are theoretical reasons for doubting that air toxic *X* could interfere with pregnancies, say that. If you have carefully kept track of and monitored female plant employees and found no miscarriage problems, say that. And if the possible connection is still untested and deserves to be studied, say that.

(b) In some cases, risk estimates are very uncertain because the risk is very low and measurement is very difficult, such as in cases of the chronic effects of chemicals with extremely low toxicity.

In these cases you are best off explaining that the data are uncertain because it is so hard to measure such improbable effects.

(c) In acknowledging and explaining data uncertainties, talk about how the risk estimate was obtained, and by whom. Demystifying the risk assessment process is a public benefit in its own right and will help your audience understand why you are simultaneously claiming (a) that your risk estimate is uncertain and (b) that your estimate is based on the best available scientific data. Explaining this process will also enable you to make points that are important for the audience to understand. Two points of special relevance and importance for the chemical industry are as follows.

First, the presence of a toxic chemical in the environment, such as an emission from a manufacturing plant, does not necessarily signify a significant health or environmental risk. This point is often extremely difficult to communicate, especially to those worried about long-term, low-dose effects. Even if hundreds or thousands of tons of air toxics are emitted into the air each year, there may be no significant health or environmental risk to people. For a toxic chemical to pose a risk, *an exposure must occur.* There must be a way for the air toxic to get from where it is (the manufacturing plant) to where people or the things they value are. Routes of exposure are as important in risk assessment as toxicity measurements are.

Second, when a route of exposure exists, the next important question is the concentration of the chemical that may reach people. This concentration amount, typically far lower than the concentration at the source, will often become even lower with the passage of time as the substance breaks down. Risk assessors consider not only *whether* a toxic substance is in the air or groundwater but also *how much* is in the air or groundwater.

This distinction becomes more important as measurement equipment becomes better. By means of their ability to measure parts per trillion and parts per quadrillion, scientists are now able to detect "low but measurable" chemical concentrations that were unknown before. Thus the proper question is not "How risky is a toxic substance?" but rather "How risky is the concentration of the toxic substance to which people are being exposed?"

(d) Regardless of how you explain uncertainty in risk estimates, some people will still be dissatisfied. The demand for certainty is a natural human trait, especially in stressful situations when we feel helpless, angry, or at the mercy of other people. Often community members will suggest ways of improving the quality of risk assessment data. These suggestions are worth taking seriously, not only for their technical information, such as information on exposure routes that may have been overlooked, but as a means for reassuring the community that you are listening, that you care about their concerns, and that you are willing to be responsive. Although absolute certainty can never be achieved, community proposals for striving for that goal deserve respectful attention. But remember: Never promise you will do something if you cannot do it.

Information Disclosure

In some cases, risk data are quite preliminary. The company may want to delay releasing the information until further testing has been done. In addressing this issue, two general guidelines can be helpful to you. (For more detail see Hance, Chess and Sandman, 1987.)

(a) Uncertainty is seldom if ever an acceptable excuse for waiting to communicate risk information. Especially if the information is alarming, it should be released promptly (with appropriate reservations about its reliability). This disclosure may be a legal obligation in some situations, and an ethical obligation in nearly all situations.

(b) Almost without exception, it is better to announce a possible problem right away than to be accused later of having covered one up. Of course common sense is the rule. Often the preliminary data are highly unreliable and emergency action would not be warranted. In such cases, you may prefer to wait a week or two for retesting and quality control, rather than start a furor over nothing. But no plant manager with unsettling risk data is likely to be tempted to announce the data prematurely. Rather, your temptation—a very dangerous one—will be to wait too long. The worst of all possible worlds is to have an investigative reporter, an environmental activist, a disaffected employee, or a regulatory agency discover and announce the problem. Do not wait for that to happen (it will). And do not wait until the problem is solved or until all the scientific data are in. As soon as you reasonably can, announce what you know and what you propose to do about it.

Demands for Zero Risk

One of the predictable things that will happen when you explain a risk number is that someone in the audience will point out that it is not zero, following up with the assertion that it should be. Explain that zero risk does not exist. Explain that we all habitually—if ignorantly—tolerate quite substantial and avoidable risks, including smoking and driving without seatbelts fastened. Explain that it is an impossible demand to expect zero risk from a chemical company.

How you specifically respond to the demand for zero risk will depend on your assessment of its source. Consider five possibilities:

(a) The demand for zero risk may be reasonable. The plant may be able to (in effect) eliminate virtually all the risk in question through some change in procedure. If so, consider the costs and benefits of doing so. If the situation warrants, you should agree to take action.

(b) The demand for zero risk may be an exaggerated way of making the point that the risk is too high. In these cases, the demand is in effect a negotiating position. Your response to this demand may be complicated by the fact that although further risk reduction is entirely feasible, the remaining risk is insignificant and such action simply makes no economic sense. However, for several reasons, you should *not* point out the economic benefits that compensate for risks that will not be eliminated. First, given the high value people attach to good health, the public will generally reject the argument that the reduced risk to the community does not justify the added costs to the company. Second, if you contend that the benefits compensate for the risks, you expose the company to accusations of bribery and blackmail. Finally, since economic benefits are typically distributed differently from health and environmental risks, such arguments often raise serious problems of fairness and equity.

(c) The demand for zero risk may be sincere but ill-informed. The people making it may simply not understand why something that is known to be risky can be allowed to continue. If so, respond *gently* with some fundamental risk education. Explain (as above) that zero risk is non-existent. Point out that all of life's activities carry some risk, which we usually ignore if the risk is small enough and if the activity is beneficial enough. Be sure to agree that the risk *should* be made as low as possible, and discuss what you are doing to achieve the lowest possible level.

(d) The demand for zero risk may be politically motivated. The demand may be designed to win followers, influence politicians, or attract the interest of journalists. Such political activity is perfectly legitimate in a democracy. Groups opposed to the chemical industry—whether they are staffed by volunteers or paid organizers—are often highly dedicated and committed to their cause. Just as the chemical industry—as an industry—is entitled to build its political case, opponents of the chemical industry are also entitled to build their political câse. With occasional exceptions, the strategies used by opponents are legitimate political strategies. For example, an opposing group may appeal to the community's health concerns, just as the chemical industry may appeal to the community's economic concerns. An opposing group may recruit and mobilize experts to support its view, just as the chemical industry may recruit and mobilize experts to support its view. Given that such activities are entirely legitimate in a democracy, you will find it unwise to attack the sincerity or legitimacy of opposing groups. A plant manager—or the chemical industry as a whole—has a legitimate right to disagree with the view of an opposing group. Disagreeing, however, is not the same as questioning the integrity of an opposing group or the right of the opposing group to use legitimate political strategies to promote its views.

If the demand for zero risk is politically motivated, you are unlikely to make much headway in meetings held in public settings. One of your main options is to try to arrange a private or semi-private meeting, where frank discussion and negotiation might be possible. In public settings, your best strategy is to clarify your position as best you can, following the advice offered in this manual.

(e) Finally, the demand for zero risk may be a reflection of emotional distress stemming from outrage, anger, and distrust. Some people in the community may have decided that you are the enemy; that the company is uncaring, arrogant, and dishonest; or that chemical manufacturing is an industry that does society little benefit at great cost. Risk, then, may not be the central issue. If a small number of community residents adopt a hostile view, you can probably do little to change their minds. But if the outrage, anger, and distrust are widespread, consider those reactions as symptoms of serious problems in your overall communication effort or in your overall health and environmental protection effort. You must address yourself to the underlying antagonism and begin the slow, hard work of building bridges. In short, talking about risk to an audience that *wants* to believe that the risk is high is a pointless undertaking. Figure out why the audience feels as it does, and pay more attention to those issues than to the battle over zero risk.

CONCLUSION

As stated in the beginning of this manual, there are no easy prescriptions for effective risk communication. There are also limits on what one chemical plant manager—no matter how skilled, committed, and sincere—can do. However, the rules, guidelines, advice, and specific examples offered in this manual can help. Over the next few years, effective risk communication will become increasingly important for the chemical industry. The industry as a whole, and plant managers in particular, will continually be challenged and asked to provide information about chemical risks to employees, customers, and the general public. As a plant manager, your response to this challenge will have an effect on public response to the chemical industry for years to come.

APPENDIX A: CONCENTRATION AND QUANTITY COMPARISONS

TABLE A.1: CONCENTRATION COMPARISONS ORGANIZED BY UNIT CATEGORIES

TABLE A.2: MISCELLANEOUS CONCENTRATION COMPARISONS

FIGURE A.1: AIR EMISSIONS FROM CHEMICAL PRODUCTION: TONS PER YEAR PROJECTED THROUGH 1988 FOR THE DOW CHEMICAL COMPANY, MIDLAND DIVISION

WARNING NOTES ON TABLES:

1. The data in the tables are designed to stress how *small* small really is. By minimizing magnitude, the comparisons tend to minimize risk.

2. When the data in the tables are used by those with an obvious interest in minimizing risk, they often lack credibility. They are also likely to provoke the same sort of backlash provoked by self-serving risk comparisons.

3. The data often lack relevance and meaning unless coupled with data on the toxic potency of a particular chemical.

4. Efforts to minimize small quantities through the comparisons given in the tables may backfire by making the quantity easier to visualize. While an image such as "a drop of vermouth in 500 barrels of gin" may be intended to convey smallness, for some in the audience it serves as an easily visualized and memorable metaphor.

TABLE A.1. CONCENTRATION COMPARISONS ORGANIZED BY UNIT CATEGORIES

Unit	1 Part per million	1 Part per billion	1 Part per trillion
Length	1 in./16 mi.	1 in./16,000 mi.	1 in./16,000,000 mi. (a 6-in. leap on a journey to the sun)
Time	1 min./2 years	1 sec./32 years	1 sec./320 centuries (or 0.06 sec. since the birth of Jesus Christ)
Money	1 cent/$10,000	1 cent/$10,000,000	1 cent /$10,000,000,000
Weight	1 oz./31 tons	1 pinch salt/10 tons of potato chips	1 pinch salt/10,000 tons of potato chips
Volume	1 drop vermouth/80 "fifths" of gin	1 drop vermouth/ 500 barrels of gin	1 drop of vermouth in a pool of gin covering the area of a football field 43 ft. deep
Area	1 square ft./23 acres	1 in./160-acre farm	1 square ft./the state of Indiana; or 1 large grain of sand on the surface of Daytona Beach
Action	1 lob/1,200 tennis matches	1 lob/1,200,000 tennis matches	1 lob/1,200,000,000 tennis matches
Quality	1 bad apple/2,000 barrels	1 bad apple/2,000,000 barrels	1 bad apple/2,000,000,000 barrels

Source: Adapted from Warren B. Crumett, Dow Chemical Company (as reproduced in Rowe, W.D. et al., 1984, *Evaluation Methods for Environmental Standards*. CRC Press Inc., Boca Raton, Florida.

WARNING! USE OF DATA IN THIS TABLE FOR RISK COMPARISON PURPOSES CAN DAMAGE YOUR CREDIBILITY (SEE TEXT).

TABLE A.2: MISCELLANEOUS CONCENTRATION COMPARISONS

Parts per million:	• One automobile in bumper-to-bumper traffic from Cleveland to San Francisco • One drop of gasoline in a full-size car's tankful of gas • One facial tissue in a stack taller than the Empire State Building • One pancake in a stack four miles high
Parts per billion:	• One silver dollar in a roll of silver dollars stretching from Detroit to Salt Lake City • One kernel of corn in enough corn to fill a 45-foot silo, 16 feet in diameter • One sheet in a roll of toilet paper stretching from New York to London
Parts per trillion:	• One square foot of floor tile on a kitchen floor the size of Indiana • One drop of detergent in enough dish-water to fill a train of railroad tank cars ten miles long • One mile on a two-month journey at the speed of light
Parts per quadrillion:	• One postage stamp on a letter the size of California and Oregon combined • The palm of one's hand resting on a table the size of the United States • One human hair out of all the hair on all the heads of all the people in the world • One mile on a journey of 170 light years

Source: Adapted from data supplied by Jim Callaghan, Hill and Knowlton, Inc., as reproduced in P. Sandman, D. Sachsman, and M. Greenberg, 1987, *Risk Communication for Environmental News Sources*. Industry/University Cooperative Center for Research in Hazardous and Toxic Substances: New Brunswick, New Jersey.

WARNING! USE OF DATA IN THIS TABLE FOR RISK COMPARISON PURPOSES CAN DAMAGE YOUR CREDIBILITY (SEE TEXT).

FIGURE A.1: AIR EMISSIONS FROM CHEMICAL PRODUCTION: TONS PER YEAR PROJECTED THROUGH 1988 FOR THE DOW CHEMICAL COMPANY, MIDLAND DIVISION

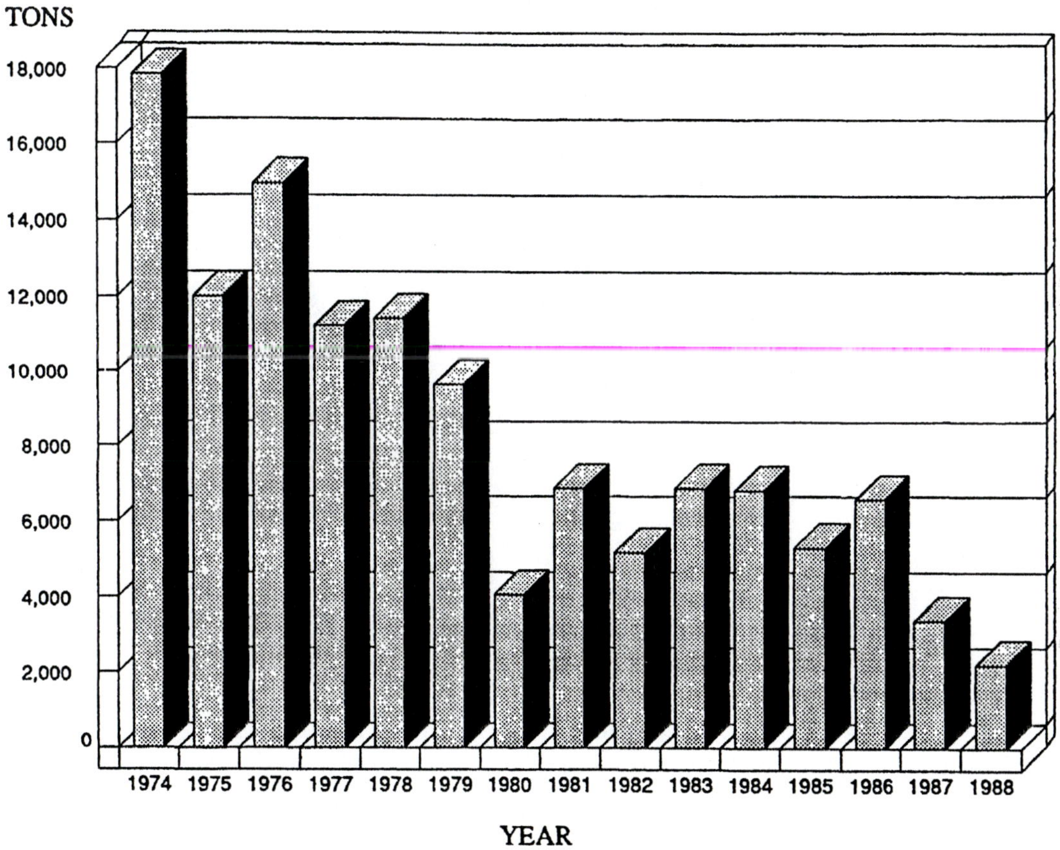

Source: Adapted from Midland Daily News, June 5, 1987.

APPENDIX B: RISK COMPARISON TABLES AND FIGURES

TABLES

FIGURES

WARNING NOTES:

1. Since the data in these tables and figures have been calculated or assembled by others, their technical accuracy cannot be guaranteed. CMA makes no representations or warranties concerning their accuracy.

2. Some of the data are old and need to be updated. For some risks, this can make a significant difference, either because the risk itself has changed significantly or because its measurement has improved. In general, rates (e.g., number of deaths per million population) tend to change less over time than fatalities (counts).

3. It is not always clear what is included in the specific risk entries. For example, do deaths from smoking include cardiovascular disease and emphysema or just lung cancers? What is included in the categories "falling objects" or "toxic gas?" When in doubt, do not use the statistic.

4. Most tables of risk comparisons in the literature contain a hodgepodge of risks characterized by different levels of uncertainty. For risks such as driving, where fatalities can be counted, the number is likely to be reliable. But for risks such as radiation or food additives—based not on counting and actuarial statistics but on theoretical modeling and extrapolation—the number is likely to be highly uncertain. In general, data based on theoretical models and extrapolation are more likely to be a target for debate and criticism than data based on counts and actuarial statistics.

5. Most risk comparison tables offer only single number risk estimates, with no range or error term.

6. Most tables of risk comparisons in the literature have been developed to make a particular point. No matter how often the table has been reprinted, it is important to be sensitive to biases in the calculation of risks.

7. A careful risk comparison requires a good deal of background information about data sources, assumptions, and other qualifiers. Just because a risk statistic is published does not mean it is reliable. Published data often take on a life of their own. The original publication may discuss a number of qualifying uncertainties but these may be left out by the next person who reproduces the statistic. This may make the data look more certain, but in fact it makes them far less reliable. Keep in mind, however, that even if a risk estimate in a table is slightly off, it still could prove useful for comparisons in which risks differ by factors of 10, 100 or more.

8. The tables are often neither clear nor consistent about the population used to calculate the risk. Within the same table, some risk estimates are based on the entire population (e.g., the United States), while others are based only on the population that is exposed (e.g., only people who hunt or live in tornado-prone regions). Every risk looks more risky if only the most exposed population is considered, less risky if lots of unexposed people are considered.

9. Even if the risk comparison data are carefully and accurately reported, they can be misleading. For example, the risk calculation for driving includes many different driving situations. Yet speeding home from a party just before dawn is two orders of magnitude more dangerous than driving to the supermarket. Similarly, the risk of being hit by lightning for people who remain on a golf course during a thunderstorm is much higher than the risk for the U.S. population provided in these tables.

10. Risk comparisons raise all the same framing issues as risk quantification generally. That is, there are many different ways to express risk comparison data. Each of these expressions is likely to have a somewhat different impact on the audience.

11. The primary intent of these cautionary statements is to warn against casual acceptance of data in comparison tables, to emphasize the importance of acting fairly and responsibly in constructing comparisons, and to indicate the advisability of having someone carefully cross-check the comparison data. Whenever possible, avoid the use of secondary data sources. Track down the original source of the statistic and, if it seems accurate and appropriate, use that number.

12. Remember that a useful risk comparison must be accurate *and* appropriate. Comparing chemical plant risks to voluntary lifestyle choices such as smoking or driving without a seatbelt is seldom appropriate or successful, even if the comparison is technically accurate.

TABLE B.1. Annual Risk of Death in the United States

Cause	Risk Per Million Persons
Motor vehicle accidents (total)	240.0
Home accidents	110.0
Falls	62.0
Motor vehicle pedestrian collisions	42.0
Drowning	36.0
Fires	28.0
Inhalation and ingestion of objects	15.0
Firearms	10.0
Accidental poisoning	
Gases and vapors	7.7
Solids and liquids (Not drugs or medicaments)	6.0
Electrocution	5.3
Tornadoes	.6
Floods	.6
Lightning	.5
Tropical cyclones and hurricanes	.3
Bites and stings by venomous animals and insects	.2

SOURCE: Adapted from Wilson, R. and Crouch, E., *Risk/Benefit Analysis*. Cambridge: Ballinger, 1982.

WARNING! USE OF DATA IN THIS TABLE FOR RISK COMPARISON PURPOSES CAN DAMAGE YOUR CREDIBILITY (SEE TEXT).

Illustrative Verbal Interpretation

Every year approximately 60 persons per million die from falls in the United States. In a city of 100,000 persons, we could expect approximately 6 persons to die from falls annually. In the United States as a whole, we could expect approximately 15,000 deaths from falls per year.

TABLE B.2: Annual Risk of Death in the United States

Hazard	Total Number of Deaths	Risk Per Million Persons
All causes	1,973,003	9000.0
Heart Disease	757,075	3400.0
Cancer	351,055	1600.0
Motor vehicle accidents	46,200	210.0
Work Accidents	13,400	150.0
Homicides	20,465	93.0
Falls	16,300	74.0
Drowning	8,100	37.0
Fires, burns	6,500	30.0
Poisoning by solids or liquids	3,800	17.0
Suffocation, ingested objects	2,900	13.0
Firearms, sporting	2,400	11.0
Railroads	1,989	.9
Civil aviation	1,757	.8
Water transport	1,725	.7
Poisoning by gases	1,700	.7
Pleasure boating	1,446	.6
Lightning	124	.5
Hurricanes	93	.4
Tornadoes	91	.4
Bites and Stings	48	.2

Source: Adapted from Atallah, S., "Assessing and Managing Industrial Risk," *Chemical Engineering*, September 8, 1980: 99-103.

WARNING! USE OF DATA IN THIS TABLE FOR RISK COMPARISON PURPOSES CAN SEVERELY DAMAGE YOUR CREDIBILITY (SEE TEXT).

Illustrative Verbal Interpretation.

Every year approximately 1,500 persons die in pleasure boating accidents in the United States. This represents .6 deaths per million persons. Of course, since everyone in the United States is not exposed to this risk, the rate per million boaters would be higher.

TABLE B.3. Risk Comparisons (Involuntary Risks Only)

Risk	Risk of Death/ Person/Year
Influenza	1 in 5000
Leukemia	1 in 12,500
Struck by an automobile (United Kingdom)	1 in 16,600
Struck by an automobile (United States)	1 in 20,000
Floods (United States)	1 in 455,000
Tornadoes (Midwest United States)	1 in 455,000
Earthquakes (California)	1 in 588,000
Bites of venomous creatures (United Kingdom)	1 in 5 million
Lightning (United Kingdom)	1 in 10 million
Falling aircraft (United States)	1 in 10 million
Release from nuclear power plant	
At site boundary (United States)	1 in 10 million
At one kilometer (United Kingdom)	1 in 10 million
Flooding of dike (the Netherlands)	1 in 10 million
Explosion, pressure vehicle (United States)	1 in 20 million
Falling aircraft (United Kingdom)	1 in 50 million
Meteorite	1in 100 billion

Adapted from Dinman, B.D., "The Reality and Acceptance of Risk," *Journal of the American Medical Association*, Vol. 244 (11) : 1126-1128, 1980.

WARNING! USE OF DATA IN THIS TABLE FOR RISK COMPARISON PURPOSES CAN SEVERELY DAMAGE YOUR CREDIBILITY (SEE TEXT).

Illustrative Verbal Interpretation.

The risk of tornadoes in the tornado-prone midwestern United States is 1 death per 455,000 persons per year, or about 2.2 deaths per million persons. This is much greater than the risk across the U.S. as a whole (.4 deaths per million persons per year—See Table B.2).

TABLE B.4: Estimated Loss of Life Expectancy Due to Various Causes

Cause	Days	Cause	Days
Cigarette smoking (male)	2250	Job with radiation exposure	40
Heart disease	2100	Falls	39
Being 30% overweight	1300	Accidents to Pedestrians	37
Being a coal miner	1100	Safest job (accidents)	30
Cancer	980	Fire (burns)	27
Being 20% Overweight	900	Generation of energy	24
Cigarette smoking (female)	800	Illicit drugs (U.S. average)	18
Stroke	520	Poison (solid, liquid)	17
Living in unfavorable state	500	Suffocation	13
Cigar smoking	330	Firearms accidents	11
Dangerous job (accidents)	300	Natural radiation	8
Pipe smoking	220	Medical X rays	6
Increasing food intake		Poisonous gases	7
100 calories/day	210	Coffee	6
Motor vehicle accidents	207	Oral contraceptives	5
Pneumonia (influenza)	141	Accidents to bicycles	5
Alcohol (U.S. average)	130	All catastrophes combined	3.5
Accidents in home	95	Diet drinks	2
Suicide	95	Reactor accidents (UCS)	2 *
Diabetes	95	Reactor accidents (NRC)	0.02*
Being murdered (homicide)	90	PAP test	-4
Legal drug misuse	90	Smoke alarm in home	-10
Average job (accidents)	74	Air bags in car	-50
Drowning	41	Mobile coronary care units	-125

Source: Adapted from Cohen, B. and Lee, I. "A Catalog of Risks." *Health Physics*, 36, June, 1979, 707-722.

Notes: (*) These items assume that all U.S. power is nuclear. UCS stands for the Union of Concerned Scientists, a leading critic of nuclear power. NRC stands for the U.S. Nuclear Regulatory Commission.

WARNING! USE OF DATA IN THIS TABLE FOR RISK COMPARISON PURPOSES CAN SEVERELY DAMAGE YOUR CREDIBILITY (SEE TEXT).

Illustrative Verbal Interpretation

The average coal miner in the United States lives three years less than the national average. Although not indicated in the table, this is presumably due to the increased risk of accidents and disease (e.g., black and brown lung disease). However, other characteristics of coal miners, such as their smoking habits, diet, and access to medical care, may also affect this statistic.

TABLE B.5: Risks Estimated to Increase the Probability of Death in Any Year by One Chance in a Million

ACTIVITY	CAUSE OF DEATH
Smoking 1.4 cigarettes	cancer, heart disease
Drinking .5 liter of wine	cirrhosis of the liver
Spending 1 hour in a coalmine	black lung disease
Spending 3 hours in a coalmine	accident
Living 2 days in New York or Boston	air pollution
Traveling 6 minutes by canoe	accident
Traveling 10 miles by bicycle	accident
Traveling 300 miles by car	accident
Flying 1000 miles by jet	accident
Flying 6000 miles by jet	cancer caused by cosmic radiation
Living 2 months in Denver	cancer caused by cosmic radiation
Living 2 months in average stone or brick building	cancer caused by natural radio-activity
One chest X ray taken in a good hospital	cancer caused by radiation
Living 2 months with a cigarette smoker	cancer, heart disease
Eating 40 tablespoons of peanut butter	liver cancer caused by aflatoxin B
Drinking Miami drinking water for 1 year	cancer caused by chloroform
Drinking 30 12 oz cans of diet soda	cancer caused by saccharin
Living 5 years at site boundary of a typical nuclear power plant	cancer caused by radiation
Drinking 1000 24-oz soft drinks from plastic bottles	cancer from acrylonitrile monomer
Living 20 years near a polyvinyl chloride plant	cancer caused by vinyl chloride (1976 standard)
Living 150 years within 20 miles of of a nuclear power plant	cancer caused by radiation
Living 50 years within 5 miles of a nuclear power plant	cancer caused by radiation
Eating 100 charcoal-broiled steaks	cancer from benzopyrene

Source: Adapted from Wilson, R., "Analyzing the Daily Risks of Life." *Technology Review*, 81, 1979, pp. 40-46.

Note: These data are based on simple extrapolations from population averages. Some data are based on actuarial statistics (e.g., coal mine accidents) and others are based on theoretical models (e.g., cancers from chlorinated water).

WARNING! USE OF DATA IN THIS TABLE FOR RISK COMPARISON PURPOSES CAN SEVERELY DAMAGE YOUR CREDIBILITY (SEE TEXT).

TABLE B.6: Average Risk of Death to an Individual from Various Natural and Human-caused Accidents

ACCIDENT TYPE	TOTAL NUMBER	INDIVIDUAL CHANCE PER YEAR
Motor Vehicle	55,791	1 in 4,000
Falls	17,827	1 in 10,000
Fires and Hot Substances	7,451	1 in 25,000
Drowning	6,181	1 in 30,000
Firearms	2,309	1 in 100,000
Air Travel	1,778	1 in 100,000
Falling Objects	1,271	1 in 160,000
Electrocution	1,148	1 in 160,000
Lightning	160	1 in 2,000,000
Tornadoes	91	1 in 2,500,000
Hurricanes	93	1 in 2,500,000
All Accidents	111,992	1 in 1,600

SOURCE: Nuclear Regulatory Commission, *Reactor Safety Study.* WASH-1400 (NUREG/74/104), Washington, D.C., 1975.

WARNING! USE OF DATA IN THIS TABLE FOR RISK COMPARISON PURPOSES CAN SEVERELY DAMAGE YOUR CREDIBILITY (SEE TEXT).

TABLE B.7: Average Risk of Death from Various Human-caused and Natural Accidents

TYPE OF EVENT	PROBABILITY OF 100 OR MORE FATALITIES	PROBABILITY OF 1,000 OR MORE FATALITIES
HUMAN-CAUSED		
Airplane Crash	1 in 2 yrs.	1 in 2,000 yrs.
Fire	1 in 7 yrs.	1 in 200 yrs.
Explosion	1 in 16 yrs.	1 in 120 yrs.
Toxic Gas	1 in 100 yrs.	1 in 1,000 yrs.
NATURAL		
Tornado	1 in 5 yrs.	very small
Hurricane	1 in 5 yrs.	1 in 25 yrs.
Earthquake	1 in 20 yrs.	1 in 50 yrs.
Meteorite Impact	1 in 100,000 yrs.	1 in 1 million yrs.

SOURCE: Nuclear Regulatory Commission, *Reactor Safety Study*. WASH-1400 (NUREG/74/104), Washington, D.C., 1975.

WARNING! USE OF DATA IN THIS TABLE FOR RISK COMPARISON PURPOSES CAN SEVERELY DAMAGE YOUR CREDIBILITY (SEE TEXT).

TABLE B.8. Ranking of Possible Cancer Risks from Common Substances

RANKING	RISK SOURCE
0.2	PCBs (daily dietary intake): exposure through industrial residues
0.3	DDE/DDT (daily dietary intake): exposure through pesiticide residues; DDE is a by-product of DDT
1	Tap water (1 liter a day): contains chloroform, a by-product of chlorination
3	Cooked bacon (100 g/about 15 slices a day): contains dimethyl-nitrosamine, a preservative by-product
4	Contaminated well water (1 liter a day): from worst well in Silicon Valley; contains trichloroethylene
4	EDB (daily dietary intake): exposure through pesticide and other residues in grains and grain products
8	Swimming pool (1 hour a day for a child): exposure to chloroform by swallowing chlorinated water
30	Peanut butter (32 g/2 tablespoons a day): contains aflatoxin, a natural mold
30	Comfrey herb tea (1 cup a day): contains symphytine, a natural pesticide
60	Diet cola (12 ounces a day): contains saccharin
100	Raw mushroom (1 a day): contains hydrazines, natural pesticides
100	Dried basil (1 g of dried leaf): contains estragole, a natural pesticide
300	Phenacetin pill (average dose): ingredient in pain reliever

RANKING	RISK SOURCE
600	Indoor air (homes) (14 hours a day): formaldehyde emitted from furniture, carpets, and wall coverings
2,800	Beer (12 ounces a day): contains ethyl alcohol
4,700	Wine (250ml/8 ounces a day): contains ethyl alchohol
5,800	Formaldehyde (6.1 mg/workers' average daily intake): exposure through the inhalation
16,000	Phenobarbitol (1 pill a day): a sleeping pill
140,000	EDB (150 mg/workers' daily intake at high exposure): exposure through inhalation; workers' maximum legal exposure

Source: Adapted from Ames, B. N., Magaw, R., and Gold, L. S., "Ranking Possible Carcinogenic Hazards," *Science*, 1987, Vol. 236, (17 April 1987), 271-285; and J. Tierney (1988), "Not to Worry...," *Hippocrates*, January/February 1988, pp. 29-38.

WARNING! USE OF DATA IN THIS TABLE FOR RISK COMPARISON PURPOSES CAN SEVERELY DAMAGE YOUR CREDIBILITY (SEE TEXT).

Illustrative Verbal Interpretation.

The risk from industrial formaldehyde is 5800 times greater than the risk from tap water.

FIGURE B.1: Health Risk Ladder

ANNUAL NUMBER OF DEATHS PER MILLION PEOPLE

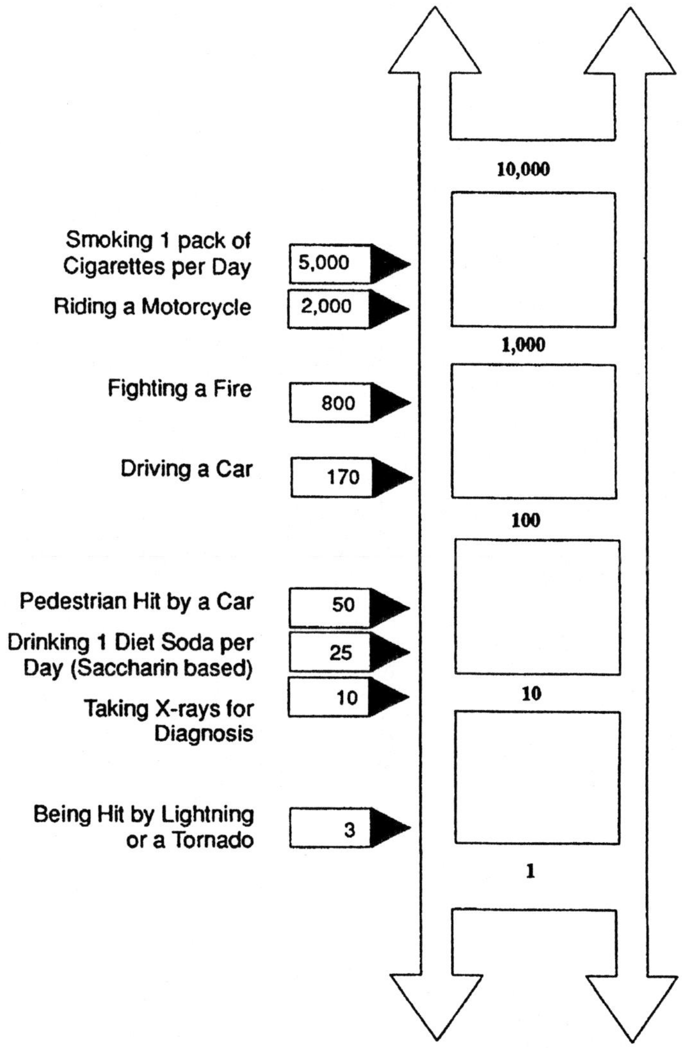

Source: Adapted from Schultz, W., G. McClelland, B. Hurd, and J. Smith (1986), *Improving Accuracy and Reducing Costs of Environmental Benefits Assessment.* Vol. IV. Boulder: University of Colorado, Center for Economic Analysis.

WARNING! USE OF DATA IN THIS FIGURE FOR RISK COMPARISON PURPOSES CAN SEVERELY DAMAGE YOUR CREDIBILITY (SEE TEXT).

FIGURE B.2: Upper Bound Estimates of Deaths for Different Energy Systems

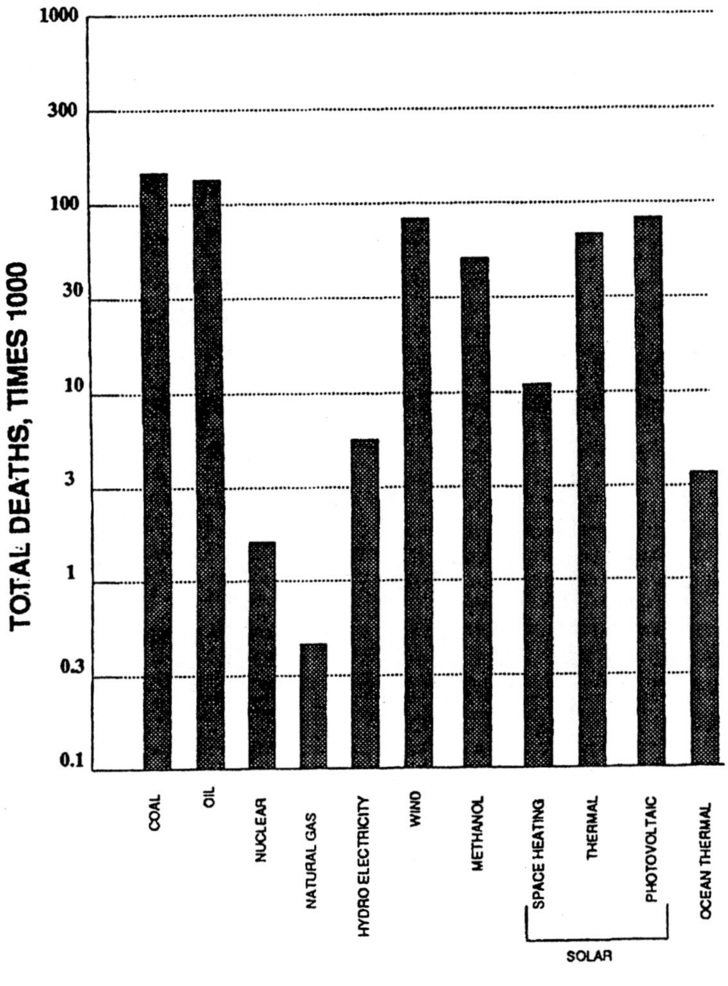

Source: Adapted from Inhaber, H. (1979), "Risks with energy from conventional and non-conventional Sources." *Science* 203, 1979, 718-723. Also Inhaber, H., *Risk of Energy Production.* Report No. AECB 119/rev. 3, 4th edition. Ottawa: Atomic Energy Control Board, 1979.

WARNING! USE OF DATA IN THIS FIGURE FOR RISK COMPARISON PURPOSES CAN SEVERELY DAMAGE YOUR CREDIBILITY (SEE TEXT).

FIGURE B.3: Comparisons of Different Sources of Radiation Exposure

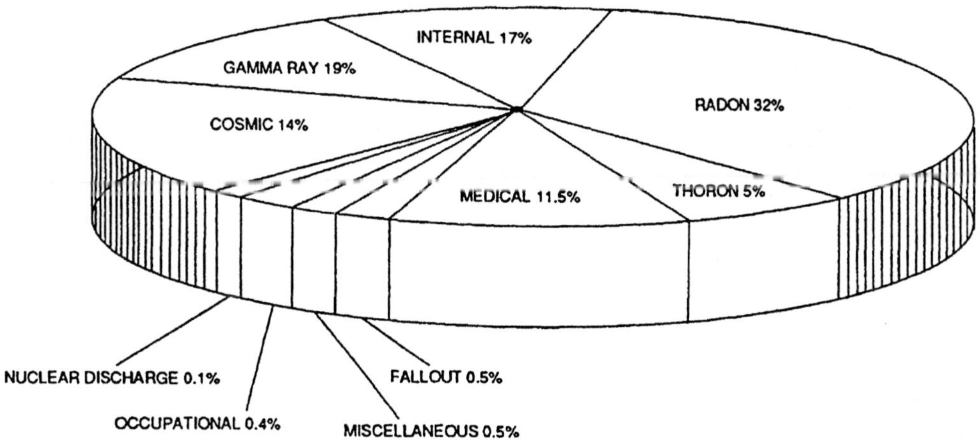

Source: Adapted from the National Radiological Protection Board (1986), *Living with Radiation*, London: HMSO.

WARNING! USE OF DATA IN THIS FIGURE FOR RISK COMPARISON PURPOSES CAN SEVERELY DAMAGE YOUR CREDIBILITY (SEE TEXT).

FIGURE B.4 The Causes of Cancer: Quantitative Estimates of the Avoidable Risk of Cancer in the U.S.

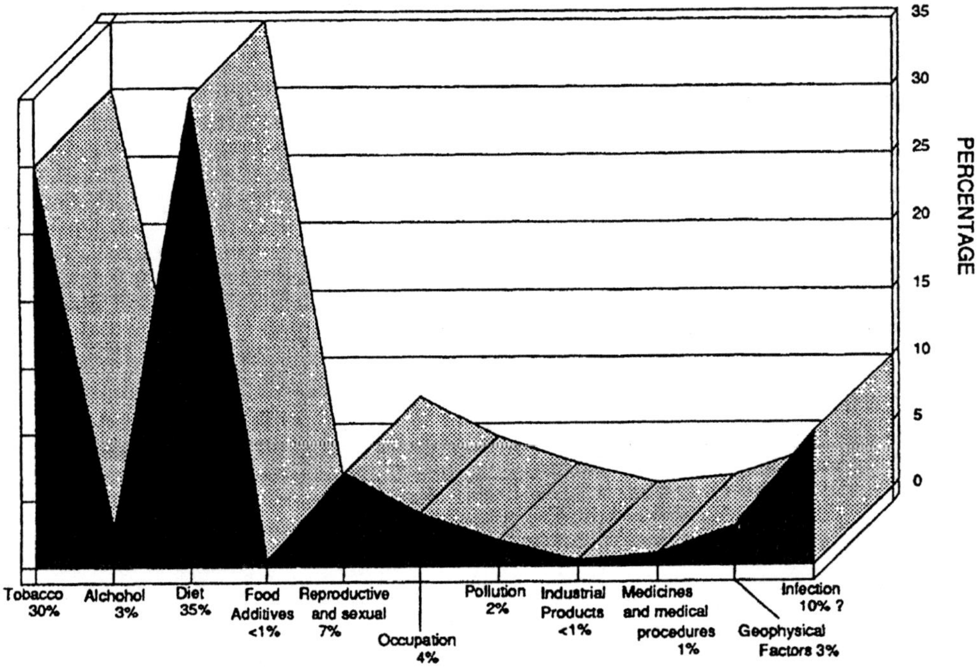

Note:

Due to rounding error, percentage figures do not add up to one hundred percent.

Source: Adapted from Doll, R. and Peto, R. (1981), "The Causes of Cancer: Quantitative Estimates of the Avoidable Risk of Cancer in the U.S. Today." *Journal of the National Cancer Institute*, 1981, Vol. 66, 1191-1308.

WARNING! USE OF DATA IN THIS FIGURE FOR RISK COMPARISON PURPOSES CAN SEVERELY DAMAGE YOUR CREDIBILITY (SEE TEXT).

FIGURE B.5: Radon Risk Charts

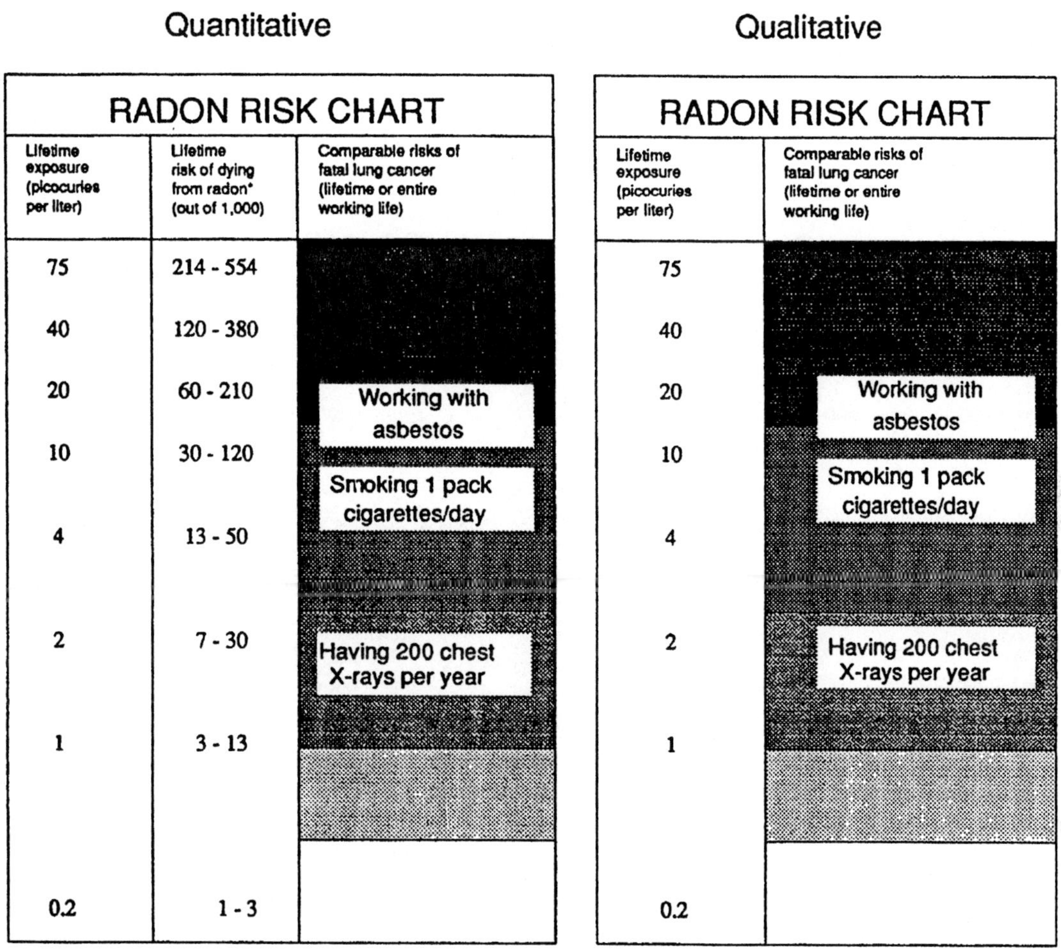

U.S. Environmental Protection Agency lifetime risk estimates. The National Council on Radiation Protection has estimated lower risk, but it still considers radon a serious health concern. (original chart in color)

Source: Adapted from Smith, V.K., W.D. Desvousges, and A. Fisher (1987), *Communicating Radon Risk Effectively: A Mid-Course Evaluation*, Report No. CR-811075. Washington, D.C.: U.S. Environmental Protection Agency, Office of Policy Analysis.

WARNING! USE OF DATA IN THIS FIGURE FOR RISK COMPARISON PURPOSES CAN SEVERELY DAMAGE YOUR CREDIBILITY (SEE TEXT).

APPENDIX C: RISK PERCEPTION FACTORS

TABLE C.1: FACTORS IMPORTANT IN RISK PERCEPTION AND EVALUATION

Factor	Conditions Associated With Increased Public Concern	Conditions Associated With Decreased Public Concern
Catastrophic Potential	Fatalities and Injuries Grouped in Time and Space	Fatalities and Injuries Scattered and Random
Familiarity	Unfamiliar	Familiar
Understanding	Mechanisms or Process Not Understood	Mechanisms or Process Understood
Uncertainty	Risks Scientifically Unknown or Uncertain	Risks Known to Science
Controllability (Personal)	Uncontrollable	Controllable
Voluntariness of Exposure	Involuntary	Voluntary
Effects on Children	Children Specifically at Risk	Children Not Specifically at Risk
Effects Manifestation	Delayed Effects	Immediate Effects
Effects on Future Generations	Risk to Future Generations	No Risk to Future Generations
Victim Identity	Identifiable Victims	Statistical Victims
Dread	Effects Dreaded	Effects Not Dreaded
Trust in Institutions	Lack of Trust in Responsible Institutions	Trust in Responsible Institutions
Media Attention	Much Media Attention	Little Media Attention
Accident History	Major and Sometimes Minor Accidents	No Major or Minor Accidents
Equity	Inequitable Distribution of Risks and Benefits	Equitable Distribution of Risks and Benefits
Benefits	Unclear Benefits	Clear Benefits
Reversibility	Effects Irreversible	Effects Reversible
Origin	Caused by Human Actions or Failures	Caused by Acts of Nature or God

Note: In selecting risks to be compared, it is helpful to keep these distinctions in mind. Risk comparisons that ignore these distinctions are likely to backfire (e.g. comparing voluntary to involuntary risks) unless appropriate qualifications are made (see text).

SELECTED BIBLIOGRAPHY ON RISK COMMUNICATION

Bean, M. (1987), "Tools for Environmental Professionals Involved in Risk Communication at Hazardous Waste Facilities Undergoing Siting, Permitting, or Remediation." Report No. 8730.8. Reston, Virginia: Air Pollution Control Association.

Covello, V. T. (1983), "The Perception of Technological Risks: A Literature Review." *Technological Forecasting and Social Change*, 23, 1983, 285-297.

Covello, V.T. (1988), "Informing the Public About Health and Environmental Risks: Problems and Opportunities for Effective Risk Communication," in N. Lind (ed.), *Risk Communication: A Symposium*, Waterloo: University of Waterloo

Covello, V. and F. Allen (1988), *Seven Cardinal Rules of Risk Communication*, Washington, D.C.: U.S. Environmental Protection Agency, Office of Policy Analysis.

Covello, V., D. von Winterfeldt, and P. Slovic (1987), "Communicating Risk Information to the Public," in J.C. Davies, V. Covello, and F. Allen, eds., *Risk Communication*: Washington, D.C.: The Conservation Foundation.

Covello, V., D. McCallum, and M. Pavlova, eds. (1988), *Effective Risk Communication: The Role and Responsibility of Government*. New York: Plenum.

Davies, J.C., V.T. Covello, and F.W. Allen, eds. (1987), *Risk Communication*. Washington, D.C.: The Conservation Foundation.

Fessenden-Raden, J., J. Fitchen, and J. Heath (1987), "Risk Communication at the Local Level: A Complex Interactive Process," *Science, Technology and Human Values*, December, 1987.

Fischhoff, B. (1985), "Protocols for Environmental Reporting: What to Ask the Experts. *The Journalist*, Winter, 1985, pp.11-15.

Fischhoff, B., S. Lichtenstein, P. Slovic, S.L. Derby and R.L. Keeney, (1981), *Acceptable Risk*. Cambridge University Press: New York.

Fischhoff, B. (1985), "Managing Risk Perception." *Issues in Science and Technology*, 2, 1985, 83-96.

Fischhoff, B., P. Slovic, and S. Lichtenstein, (1979), "Weighing the Risks," *Environment, 21*, 1979.

Hance, B., C. Chess, and P. Sandman (1987), *Improving Dialogue with Communities: A Risk Communication Manual for Government*. Trenton, New Jersey, Office of Science and Research, New Jersey Department of Environmental Protection, December, 1987.

Johnson, B. and V. Covello, eds. (1987), *The Social and Cultural Construction of Risk: Essays on Risk Selection and Perception*. Boston: Reidel.

Kahneman, D., P. Slovic, and A. Tversky eds. (1982), *Judgment Under Uncertainty: Heuristics and Biases*. New York: Cambridge University Press.

Kasperson, R. (1986), "Six Propositions on Public Participation and Their Relevance to Risk Communication." *Risk Analysis*, 1986, 6, 275-282.

Kasperson, R. and J. Kasperson (1983), "Determining the Acceptability of Risk: Ethical and Policy Issues," in J. Rogers and D. Bates, (eds.), *Risk: A Symposium*, Ottawa: The Royal Society of Canada, 1983.

Klaidman, S. (1985), "Health Risk Reporting," Washington, D.C.: Institute for Health Policy Analysis, Georgetown University.

Mazur, A. (1981), "Media Coverage and Public Opinion on Scientific Controversies," *Journal of Communication*, pp. 106-115.

Nelkin, D. (1984), *Science in the Streets*. New York: Twentieth Century Fund.

President's Commission on the Accident at Three Mile Island (1979), *Report of the Public's Right to Information Task Force*. Washington, D.C.: U.S. Government Printing Office.

Ruckelshaus, W.D. (1983), "Science, Risk, and Public Policy," *Science*, 221: 1026-1028.

Ruckelshaus, W.D. (1984), "Risk in a Free Society," *Risk Analysis*, September 1984, pp. 157-163.

Ruckelshaus, W. D. (1987), "Communicating About Risk," pp. 3-9 in J.C. Davies, V.T. Covello, and F.W. Allen (eds.). *Risk Communication*. Washington, D.C.: The Conservation Foundation, 1987.

Press, F. (1987), "Science and Risk Communication," pp. 11-17 in J.C. Davies, V.T. Covello, and F.W. Allen (eds.). *Risk Communication*. Washington, D.C.: The Conservation Foundation, 1987.

Sandman, P.M. (1986), "Getting to Maybe: Some Communications Aspects of Hazardous Waste Facility Siting," *Seton Hall Legislative Journal*, Spring 1986.

Sandman, P.M. (1986), *Explaining Environmental Risk*. Washington, D.C.: U.S. Environmental Protection Agency, Office of Toxic Substances.

Sandman, P., D. Sachsman, M. Greenberg, and M. Gotchfeld, (1987), *Environmental Risk and the Press*, New Brunswick: Transaction Books.

Sandman, P., D. Sachsman, and M. Greenberg (1987), *Risk Communication for Environmental News Sources*. Industry/University Cooperative Center for Research in Hazardous and Toxic Substances: New Brunswick, New Jersey.

Sharlin, H. (1987), "EDB: A Case Study in the Communication of Health Risk," in B. Johnson and V. Covello, (eds.), *The Social and Cultural Construction of Risk: Essays on Risk Selection and Perception*, Boston: Reidel.

Slovic, P. (1987), "Perception of Risk," *Science* 236: 280-285.

Slovic, P. (1986),"Informing and Educating the Public About Risk." *Risk Analysis*, vol. 4: 403-415.

Slovic, P., B. Fischhoff, and S. Lichtenstein (1982), "Facts Versus Fears: Understanding Perceived Risk," in D. Kahneman, P. Slovic, A. Tversky, (eds.), *Judgment Under Uncertainty: Heuristics and Biases.* Cambridge University Press: Cambridge, 1982.

Slovic, P., and B. Fischhoff (1982), "How Safe is Safe Enough? Determinants of Perceived and Acceptable Risk." In L. Gould and C. Walker (eds.), *Too Hot to Handle,* Yale University Press, New Haven, 1982.

Thomas, L. M. (1987), "Why We Must Talk About Risk," pp. 19-25 in J.C. Davies, V.T. Covello, and F.W. Allen (eds.). *Risk Communication.* Washington, D.C.: The Conservation Foundation, 1987.

Wilson, R. and E. Crouch (1987), "Risk Assessment and Comparisons: An Introduction." *Science,* Vol. 236 (17 April 1987): 267-270.

Note: The views expressed in this manual are solely those of the authors and do not necessarily represent the views of their organizations.

D

Encouraging Effective Risk Communication in Government: Suggestions for Agency Management

Caron Chess

Government agencies are frequently frustrated by communities that seem alarmed by relatively minimal environmental health risks, yet are unresponsive to serious ones. Communities are equally frustrated by what they see as government inattention to their concerns. Although agencies may understandably long for the "right" combination of words to transform community response, their process for dealing with communities typically has more impact than their explanations of risk.

While risk communication cannot (and should not) replace effective risk management, it can help agencies to:

- Understand public perception and more easily anticipate community response to agency actions;
- Increase the effectiveness of risk management decisions by involving concerned publics;
- Reduce unwarranted tension between communities and agencies;
- Explain risks more effectively; and
- Alert communities to risk in productive ways.

Although effective risk communication hinges largely on how agency staff interact with the public day to day, consistent support is needed from management for risk communication principles to become consistent agency practice. This report recommends ways in which management can promote effective risk communication throughout the agency.

Caron Chess • Environmental Communication Research Program, New Jersey Agricultural Experiment Station, Cook College, Rutgers University, New Brunswick, New Jersey 08903.

Although the suggestions in this report vary in specificity and in the ease with which they can be implemented, all are grounded in an appreciation of agencies' limited time and resources. The recommendations also assume that risk communication should complement, not replace, agencies' primary commitment to sound science and meaningful policy.

A. ORGANIZATIONAL CLIMATE

An agency's organizational climate will determine in part whether effective risk communication can thrive. Put simply, if the internal agency climate is cold and closed, interaction with the public is less likely to be warm and open. On the other hand, if an agency's internal environment encourages dialogue, informal interaction, and creative problem solving, staff are more likely to interact similarly with communities.

A1. Promote effective risk communication by agency management. Agency managers act as role models for the rest of the agency. For example, when agency leadership enters into dialogue with communities, this action sets a tone for the department and provides a model for staff to emulate.

A2. Open communication within the agency. Internal decisionmaking processes that involve staff and encourage expression of diverse viewpoints are likely to foster similar openness to differing opinions outside the agency.

B. DECISIONMAKING

One of the keys to successful interaction with the public is involving communities early and often in the decisionmaking process. Communities are far more likely to respect decisions that involve rather than exclude them. Consequently, battles are less likely to erupt over issues of agency control.

B1. Develop internal policies requiring public participation. Public participation can be made literally the rule rather than the exception through internal guidelines that stress the need for ongoing community input at all levels in the agency. (Ideally, representatives of environmental groups would have input into developing the guidelines, so that the process is consistent with the content.)

Management can also (1) routinely raise questions about the adequacy of public participation during internal discussions of plans and policies; (2) consider withholding approval of agency actions, programs, regulations, and policies that have been developed without input from those affected; and (3) take care to consult with the public before promoting their own policies.

B2. Institutionalize early release of information. Because communities prefer to be involved early in the decisionmaking process rather than after risk management decisions have been reached, meaningful participation is closely linked to early release of information. Unnecessary delay can erode public trust.

Management can encourage early communication by (1) serving as models for early release of information; (2) advocating this approach in discussions of forthcoming agency actions and development of agency policies; (3) supporting agency personnel who develop communication strategies and risk management plans that involve early release of information; (4) requiring more justification from staff for delaying release of information than for promoting release; and (5) developing agency guidelines that establish a mandate for early release of information to the public yet allow for flexibility.

B3. Develop alternative models for public input. Agency staff turn to public hearings, in part, because this forum is institutionalized. However, if agencies rely on public hearings and formal meetings for community input, citizen concerns will usually be heard too late in the agency's decisionmaking process to be meaningful. In addition, such forums may encourage posturing rather than problem-solving dialogue.

Management can promote alternative approaches to soliciting input from the public, including informal meetings, hotlines, community-based task forces, and "out-of-office hours" when staff are available in the local community for questions and concerns. In addition, agencies can consider development of "environmental town meetings" for the public to transmit ideas, suggestions, and concerns to the agency when there aren't pressing controversies. Such forums might allow agencies to respond routinely to community interests and to build trust that might transfer to controversial issues.

B4. Hold routine, informal meetings with representatives of community and environmental groups. Top management can hold bi-monthly or quarterly meetings with representatives of community and environmental groups to listen to their concerns *outside of crisis situations*. This allows policy-makers to develop ongoing relationships with environmental leaders and address their concerns on a regular basis. It also provides a model for similar interactions on the program level.

B5. Use innovative means to resolve disputes. Agencies can develop mechanisms to deal with community dissatisfaction so that citizens have alternatives to taking to the courts or to the streets. For example, agencies can explore development of internal ombudsman positions or consider means to offer negotiation or mediation involving neutral outsiders.

C. ORGANIZATIONAL STRUCTURE

If an agency is structured such that there are a variety of ways for the public to gain access and provide input, meaningful interaction is more likely. Just as important, the agency's organizational chart can reflect the priority it places on public input. Communicating with the public can be respected as a function that requires a great deal of expertise, rather than dismissed as a task that anyone could do but no one should want to do.

C1. Create communication positions at all levels of the agency to promote interaction with communities. Agencies can bring the same expertise to explaining risk assessments as they bring to developing them. Hiring sufficient communication staff can reduce the drain of agency resources by agency proposals mired in public opinion.

Care should be taken to hire communication staff who can promote dialogue with communities, not merely explain agency policy. Staff with two-way communication experience are at least as essential as writers and media specialists.

C2. Use communication staff to amplify community concerns within the agency. Too often communication staff become buffers between the community and other agency staff. Instead, community relations people can act as amplifiers, bringing community needs and concerns back to others in the agency *before* communities feel the need to shout.

To place more of a priority on listening, the agency can also allocate some positions specifically to alerting the agency to community concerns. For "community input specialists" to be effective, managers need to listen to their observations and recommendations as attentively as the specialists listen to community concerns.

C3. Use communication staff to assist technical and policy staff to interact effectively with communities. Because communities usually prefer to talk directly with people making technical and policy decisions, much direct communication with communities should be handled by staff and policy-makers with the expertise and authority to address community concerns. Communication staff can advise agencies about process, act as liaisons with communities, and identify community concerns, rather than attempt to fulfill all the communication functions of the agency.

C4. Consider communication abilities and experience when developing job descriptions and hiring. Because technical, policy, and secretarial staff play a vital role in communicating with the public, communication experience can play a useful role in hiring decisions. An agency's ability to communicate effectively with the public improves significantly when there are more agency staff with good communication skills and fewer who are "communication averse."

C5. Coordinate communication functions within the agency. Communication functions need to be coordinated sufficiently in order to be efficient and consistent. Yet programs must also interact with communities routinely and easily. One model to balance these competing needs is a communication office that serves as a resource to communication staff throughout the agency, facilitating consistency, reducing duplication, and handling a limited number of projects that are outside program boundaries.

The following suggestions may help strike the appropriate balance: (1) the agency staffs communication positions at all levels; (2) the communication office assists program staff rather than speaking for them or dictating to them; (3) interaction between the communication office and communication staff throughout the agency is two-way; and (4) communication staff, while coordinating with each other, work most closely with the technical staff of their particular program.

C6. Involve communication staff in developing policy. Agencies sometimes use communication specialists to transmit policy rather than to help formulate it. This approach sells short the agency (which may develop policies without the benefit of understanding community concerns), the public (which may feel disenfranchised), and the communicators (who may become messengers for policies they feel have inherent problems). Instead, staff who are most likely to understand community concerns can be intimately involved in developing policy. Communication specialists can also help policy-makers determine when and how to involve the public directly in decisionmaking.

C7. Develop mechanisms to make the agency "user-friendly" to those outside the government. Government agencies are often regarded as mazes that only the initiated can navigate with any ease. The agency can place a priority on developing ways to address routine inquiries from the public, such as: (1) an easy-access directory for the public that explains agency structure and lists frequently asked questions with appropriate phone numbers for responses; (2) central numbers for citizen inquiries with staff responsible for facilitating responses, not merely bouncing calls; (3) staff within divisions whose responsibilities explicitly include responding to citizen inquiries by referring them within the division or responding directly; (4) training of secretarial and professional staff that stresses the importance of responding to citizen inquiries as well as the ways to handle them; and (5) answering machines to ensure that calls are answered after hours or other times when clerical and professional staff are unavailable.

D. STAFF SUPPORT

Dealing with the public is acknowledged by agency staff to be one of the toughest tasks they face; it is generally regarded as more difficult to deliver test results to an anxious family than to conduct the sampling. Yet risk communication functions often seem to be poorly supported by agencies. In fact, the great majority of both the agency staff within New Jersey who served on the advisory committee to a related project and the government personnel from out of state who were interviewed for a manual on government risk communication disagreed or strongly disagreed with the statement: "People in my position are given adequate training and support for their risk communication activities."

D1. Provide information about risk communication in orientation for new staff. If the agency wishes to place a priority on effective risk communication, that message needs to begin during the hiring process and soon after hiring. All staff can be made aware that communicating with the public is considered an important function of the agency. This message is important for secretarial staff, who are often the public's first contact with the agency, as well as for top staff who will be spokespersons. An orientation program can include some or all of the following components: a brief risk communication guide similar to the one developed for this project; a workshop or videotape to introduce people to the subject; and checklists for staff to monitor their own attitudes and performance.

D2. Provide training for agency staff. Consideration can be given to conducting both introductory risk communication workshops and more in-depth workshops on specific subjects of concern, such as handling public meetings, dealing with the media, developing communication plans, etc. Development of training programs can be preceded by a formal or informal needs assessment of the agency to ensure that the program meets staff needs. Such training programs, whether developed in-house or by outside contractors, can also involve agency staff in providing feedback on the training design. Finally, staff can be encouraged to attend courses, workshops, and conferences about risk communication outside the agency.

D3. Disseminate information about risk communication successes through an internal "good-news letter" and working groups. Most agencies have had positive experiences conducting dialogues of mutual respect and consideration with communities. Sharing information about such interactions—from a full case study to a few minutes in a public hearing when effective communication makes a difference—can provide ideas and guidance to staff throughout the agency. One method for disseminating such information is a monthly or quarterly internal report on agency communication successes, based on staff descriptions of positive interactions. Such an internal "good-news letter" would not only help staff dealing with risk communication problems, but would also, by recognizing staff efforts, show that risk communication is valued within the agency. Consideration can also be given to development of "risk communication work groups" to bring together on a regular basis both communication staff and those technical staff who routinely interact with the public.

D4. Reward staff communication efforts. Agency staff may feel that communication with the public is a no-win proposition. Staff may receive little recognition when they do well. But when communication problems receive adverse attention, regardless of whether staff are at fault, they may feel vulnerable to blame. To provide incentive for staff to develop and use their communication skills, agencies can recognize and reward staff who make communication a priority in their work and improve their skills. When communication efforts misfire, agencies can reassure affected staff that it is better to have communicated and "lost" than never to have communicated at all.

E. PLANNING AND EVALUATION

Agencies are more likely to attend to the middle of the communication process—transmitting and receiving information—than to the equally critical ends—planning and evaluation.

Planning is as essential to communication as development of sampling plans is to monitoring. As with environmental monitoring, communication efforts that are carefully planned tend to be more useful and ultimately less resource-intensive. Yet agency staff may start in the middle of a communication process, developing newsletters or brochures, before assessing whether these are the best ways to meet communication goals. As a result, agencies may "fight fires" instead of developing comprehensive approaches to prevent communication flare-ups.

Communication efforts, like technical ones, can also improve with feedback. Evaluation that goes beyond merely noting unqualified disasters and stunning successes may help agencies avoid mistakes and duplicate successes.

E1. Conduct an agencywide assessment of communication needs. A formal or informal assessment of communication problems and concerns can help an agency develop priorities for communication-related changes. Just as important, a properly designed needs assessment can give staff at all levels opportunities to articulate priorities so that changes are ultimately workable and realistic.

E2. Incorporate communication planning in planning efforts. When staff feel they don't have time to involve the public, it may be in part because they think of public participation very late in project development. Involving the public is apt to be easier and less labor-intensive if public participation is planned from the outset as an ongoing part of project, regulatory, or policy development. This type of planning is more likely to occur if planning documents are required to consider public participation.

E3. Encourage evaluation of communication efforts. Although agencies cannot easily afford resource-intensive evaluations, they need feedback to increase effectiveness. At minimum, agencies can (1) document their communication efforts so they have a record from which to build; (2) debrief efforts with staff involved and develop recommendations for future efforts based on such sessions; and (3) solicit feedback and suggestions from those outside the agency involved in the dialogue.

F. RESOURCE ALLOCATION

Funding technical efforts generously while scrimping on communication budgets is false economy. As pointed out previously, if agencies fail to communicate with the public, their technical efforts are less likely to be understood. While agencies may never have the budgets to fund communication efforts at ideal levels, they can make communication a greater funding priority than is often the case.

F1. Require funding for communication efforts in project budgets. Program budgets can include input from communication staff in order to reflect communication planning and allocate reasonable funds for communication programs. Agencies can also routinely include funding for public participation programs in funding packages submitted to legislatures. The more controversial a program, the greater the funds that should be allocated to communication. Similarly, programs to alert communities to risks for which people must take individual action (such as naturally occurring radon) will require greater communication funding.

F2. Maximize existing resources. Agencies usually have many technical staff with good communication skills. With training, encouragement, and clear mandates, agency technical staff can make significant communication contributions during the course of their routine activities.

G. INTERAGENCY COOPERATION

Competition for funds and credit can take their toll on agencies' efforts to coordinate effectively. But it is painfully obvious that both communities and agencies ultimately lose when agencies fail to cooperate.

G1. Inform all agencies potentially affected by your agency's actions. Notification might occur more routinely if those agencies that are alerted "reward" the communication by striving to cooperate at least as much as they criticize. This response is more likely if agencies are notified and involved early in the process. Notification and involvement should also include affected local and county agencies, which often resent policies being imposed without their input.

G2. Communicate routinely. Often agencies must coordinate efforts in the middle of a crisis. Crisis communication improves when working relationships are developed through routine communication at all levels.

A FINAL NOTE

Agencies do not expect to resolve thorny environmental problems quickly or easily. Neither can they expect speedy resolution of difficult communication problems with communities. In many cases distrust has grown over a long period of time, and trust may need an equally long time to build. Similarly, agencies may want "freeze-dried risk communication" programs that are prepackaged and need few resources to become ready to use. However, only monologues can be prepackaged. The dialogue with communities that is key to successful risk communication requires commitment from agency management as well as implementation by agency staff.

Index

Printed in the United States
55908LVS00005B/41-54

9 780306 484971